Radiographic Pathology
for
Technologists

Radiographic Pathology for Technologists

Fourth Edition

James D. Mace, MBA, RT(R)
PACS Specialist
Medical IT
Philips Medical Systems
Powell, Ohio

Nina Kowalczyk, MS, RT(R)(QM)
Lecturer/Clinical Instructor
The Ohio State University
Columbus, Ohio

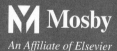
Mosby
An Affiliate of Elsevier

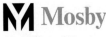

An Affiliate of Elsevier

11830 Westline Industrial Drive
St. Louis, Missouri 63146

NOTICE

Radiography is an ever-changing field. Standard safety precautions must be followed, but as new research and clinical experience broaden our knowledge, changes in treatment and drug therapy may become necessary or appropriate. Readers are advised to check the most current product information provided by the manufacturer of each drug to be administered to verify the recommended dose, the method and duration of administration, and contraindications. It is the responsibility of the licensed prescriber, relying on experience and knowledge of the patient, to determine dosages and the best treatment for each individual patient. Neither the publisher nor the author assumes any liability for any injury and/or damage to persons or property arising from this publication.

Previous editions copyrighted 1988, 1994, 1998

Library of Congress Cataloging-in-Publication Data

Mace, James D.
    Radiographic pathology for technologists / James D. Mace, Nina Kowalczyk.--4th ed.
        p. ; cm.
    Includes bibliographical references and index.
    ISBN 0-323-01893-9
        1. Diagnosis, Radioscopic. 2. Diagnostic imaging. 3. Pathology. 4. Radiologic technologists. I. Kowalczyk, Nina. II. Title.
        [DNLM: 1. Pathology--methods. 2. Radiology--methods. QZ 4 M141r 2004]
    RC78.M185 2004
    616.07'57--dc22

2003065104

Publishing Director: Andrew Allen
Executive Editor: Jeanne Wilke
Senior Developmental Editor: Linda Woodard
Publishing Services Manager: Melissa Lastarria
Project Manager: Joy Moore
Design Manager: Bill Drone

Printed in United States of America

Last digit is the print number: 9 8 7 6 5 4 3

Contributors

Kevin D. Evans, MS, MA, RT(R)(M), RDMS, FSDMS

Chapters 4, 5, 6, 7, 8 & 10
Manager of Radiology and Cardiovascular
  Ultrasound
The Ohio State University Hospitals East
The Ohio State University
Columbus, Ohio

Beth McCarthy, BSRT (R) (CV)

Chapters 2, 3, 4 & 5
Research Assistant
The Ohio State University Medical Center
Columbus, Ohio

Bryan Pfeiffer, BA, RT(R)

Chapters 2, 4, 5, 6, 7, 8 & 10
Assistant Manager of Radiology
Grant Medical Center
Columbus, Ohio

Reviewers

Mark A. Hagy, MS, RT(R)
Clinical Coordinator/Assistant Professor
East Tennessee State University
Johnson City, Tennessee

Paul Howard Littlefield, EdS, RT(R)(ARRT)
Program Director
Baptist Medical Center South School of Radiologic
  Technology
Montgomery, Alabama

Lauren B. Noble, EdD, RT(R)
Instructor, Radiography
Vance-Granville Community College
Henderson, North Carolina

Linda Rarey, MA, AART, CNMT
PET Technologist
Molecular Imaging Corp.
San Diego, California

Carol Southern, EdD, RT(R)(CT)
Radiography Program Director
Southern Union State Community College
Opelika, Alabama

Homer Terry, BUS, RT(R)(M)(QM)
Radiography Program Director/Associate Professor
Hazard Community College/Southeast Community
  College
Hazard, Kentucky

Preface

Radiography is a front-line diagnostic tool for a wide variety of pathologies. Familiarity with the radiographic appearance and origins of a disease or injury, as well as a likely prognosis, helps the technologist produce optimal quality radiographs, so physicians have the information they need to make accurate diagnoses. *Radiographic Pathology for Technologists* is a well-illustrated textbook that concisely presents the pathologic processes most likely to be diagnosed using medical imaging.

CONTENT AND ORGANIZATION

Radiographic Pathology for Technologists is a practical and easy-to-use reference for both students and practicing radiographers. The chapters are organized by body system; each starts with an explanation of anatomy and physiology, then moves on to imaging considerations. When imaging modalities other than plain-film radiography are used to diagnose a particular disease, images from those modalities are included along with discussions of why the particular modalities are used. Each disease is categorized by type, with a description of its radiographic appearance, signs and symptoms, and treatment.

Key terms, chapter outlines, and objectives at the beginning of each chapter orient students to the material. Multiple-choice and discussion questions are included at the end of each chapter to aid in assessing comprehension and to provide the instructor with questions for classroom discussion. Summary tables of the pathology discussed in each chapter provide a quick and easy reference for students and practitioners.

NEW CONTENT AND FEATURES

This edition features the most current information on new imaging techniques, such as MRI, CT, ultrasound, and PET scanning, as appropriate for diagnosis of a particular disease, injury, or abnormality. Over 200 new images, including images from alternative modalities, have been added to update existing content, to illustrate new discussions, and to more comprehensively represent the pathologies discussed.

New or expanded information has been added for the following pathologies: myocardial infarction, cor pulmonale, hydronephrosis, esophageal atresia, Meckel's diverticulum, gastroesophageal reflux (GERD), cholecystitis, ascites, current types of hepatitis, and brain abscesses. New pathology and imaging modality summary tables provide a quick and easy reference for students and practitioners.

ELECTRONIC ANCILLARIES
Electronic Image Collection

An electronic image collection on CD-ROM that includes the images from this book is available for those teaching a course with the text, providing an easy-to-use and cost-effective alternative to traditional pathology slide sets.

Evolve—Online Course Management

Evolve is an interactive learning environment designed to work in coordination with

Radiographic Pathology for Technologists. Instructors may use *Evolve* to provide an Internet-based course component that reinforces and expands on the concepts delivered in class. *Evolve* may be used to publish the class syllabus, outlines, and lecture notes; set up "virtual office hours" and e-mail communication; share important dates and information through the online class calendar; and encourage student participation through chat rooms and discussion boards. *Evolve* allows instructors to post exams and manage their grade book online. For more information, visit **http://www.evolve.elsevier.com** or contact an Elsevier sales representative.

ACKNOWLEDGMENTS

As with the previous three editions, I certainly could not have completed the revisions to this book without a great team of people who wanted this text to be successful and accomplish its primary mission. First and foremost, I thank my husband, Doug, and son, Nick, for going on without me at the most inopportune moments as a deadline from my publisher was coming. Their support is, in large part, why I succeeded. I also want to thank Mosby for their unending patience, and particularly Linda Woodard, who helped to keep me to a timeline.

As with the last edition, the images come from a variety of fine organizations that are to be thanked for graciously allowing us to use their material. They include the American College of Radiology, as well as The Ohio State University Medical Center, Riverside Methodist Hospitals, Grant Medical Center, and Children's Hospital—all located in Columbus, Ohio. Also, thanks to the technologists, sonographers, and others who provided support and encouragement. You made our job so much easier.

Nina Kowalczyk
J.D. Mace

Contents

Introduction to Pathology

UPON COMPLETION OF CHAPTER 1, THE READER SHOULD BE ABLE TO:

- Define common terminology associated with the study of disease.
- Differentiate between signs and symptoms.
- Distinguish between a disease diagnosis and its prognosis.
- Describe the different types of disease classifications.
- Cite characteristics that distinguish benign from malignant neoplasms.
- Describe the system used to stage malignant tumors.
- Identify the difference in origin for carcinoma and sarcoma.

1

Pathology is the study of disease. Many types of disease exist, and, in general, many conditions can be readily demonstrated radiographically. The radiography student who wants to better understand specific pathologic conditions must first have a working knowledge of common pathologic terms. It is also important to understand the role of the Centers for Disease Control and Prevention (CDC) in terms of tracking, monitoring, and reporting trends in health and aging. This information is captured and reported by the National Center for Health Statistics (NCHS). This chapter serves as a brief introduction to terms associated with pathology and recent health trends.

PATHOLOGIC TERMS

Any abnormal disturbance of the function or structure of the human body as a result of some type of injury is called a **disease**. After injury, **pathogenesis** occurs. This refers to the sequence of events producing cellular changes that ultimately lead to observable changes known as manifestations. These manifestations can display in a variety of fashions. A **symptom** refers to the patient's perception of the disease. Symptoms are subjective, and only the patient can identify these manifestations. For example,

a headache is considered a symptom. A **sign** is an objective manifestation that can be detected by the physician during examination. Fever, swelling, and skin rash are all considered signs. A group of signs and symptoms that characterizes a specific abnormal disturbance is a **syndrome**. However, some disease processes, especially in the early stages, do not produce symptoms and are termed **asymptomatic**.

Etiology is the study of the cause of a disease. In addition to the normal agents that can cause disease (e.g., viruses, bacteria, trauma, heat), a number of other causes are known. Proper infection control practices are important in a health care environment to prevent **nosocomial** disease. Staphyloccocal infection following hip replacement surgery is an example of a nosocomial disease, that is, one acquired from the environment. The cause of the disease in this case could be poor infection-control practices. **Iatrogenic** reactions are those adverse responses that occur from medical treatment itself (e.g., a collapsed lung that occurs in response to a complication that arises during arterial line placement). If no causative factor can be identified, the disease is termed **idiopathic**.

The length of time over which the disease is displayed may vary. **Acute** diseases usually have a quick onset and last a short period of time, whereas a **chronic** disease may present more slowly and last a very long time. An example of an acute disease is pneumonia, whereas multiple sclerosis is considered a chronic condition.

Two additional terms refer to the identification and outcome of a disease. A **diagnosis** is the name of a disease an individual is believed to have, and the prediction of the course and outcome of the disease is called a **prognosis**. Pathologic conditions can alter the normal body tissue in a variety of ways. Sometimes the disease process is destructive, decreasing the normal tissue density. This occurs when the tissue composition is altered by decreasing its atomic number, the compactness of the cells, or changes in the tissue thickness, such as atrophy from limited use. Such disease processes are radiographically classified as subtractive, lytic, or destructive disease processes and require a decrease in the exposure technique. Conversely, some pathologic conditions cause an increase in normal tissue density, resulting in a higher atomic number or increased compactness of the cells. These are classified as additive or sclerotic disease processes and require an increase in the exposure technique. It is important for the radiographer to know common pathologic conditions that require an alteration of the exposure technique so that quality radiographs can be obtained to assist in the diagnosis and treatment of the disease.

Government agencies compile statistics annually regarding the incidence, or rate of occurrence, of disease. **Epidemiology** is the investigation of disease in large groups. The prevalence of a given disease refers to the number of cases found in a given population. The incidence of disease refers to the number of new cases found in a given time period. Diseases of high prevalence in an area where a given causative organism is commonly found are said to be endemic to that area. For example, histoplasmosis is a fungal disease of the respiratory system endemic to the Ohio and Mississippi River valleys. It is not uncommon to see a relatively high prevalence of it in these areas. Its appearance in great numbers in the western United States, however, could represent an epidemic.

Monitoring Disease Trends

Over the past century, life expectancy in the United States has continued to increase. The majority of children born at the beginning of the twenty-first century are expected to live well into their eighth decade. The principal causes of death have shifted from acute infections to chronic diseases over the past 100 years. These changes have occurred as a result of biomedical and pharmaceutical advances, public health initiatives, and social changes over the past century (Fig. 1-1). But experts disagree if life expectancy can continue advancing into the twenty-first century. Some believe that increased knowledge of disease etiology and continued development of medical technology in combination with screening, early intervention, and treatment of disease could have positive results. However, many experts express concern about the quality of life of the elderly. In other words, there is a concern that the added years may be spent in declining health and lingering illness instead of as active, productive years.

The **mortality rate** is the number of deaths caused by a particular disease averaged over a population. Death certificates are collected by each state, forwarded to NCHS, and subsequently processed and published as information on mortality statistics and trends. One common mortality rate monitored by the NCHS is the infant mortality rate. In 2000, the infant mortality rate was at an all-time low of 6.9 deaths per 1000 live births. In addition, the NCHS and the U.S. Department of Health and Human Services monitors and reports mortality rates in terms of leading causes of death, according to sex, race, age, and specific causes of death such as heart disease or breast cancer (see Chapter 11, Table 11-1). Trends in these mortality patterns are identified and tracked to help identify

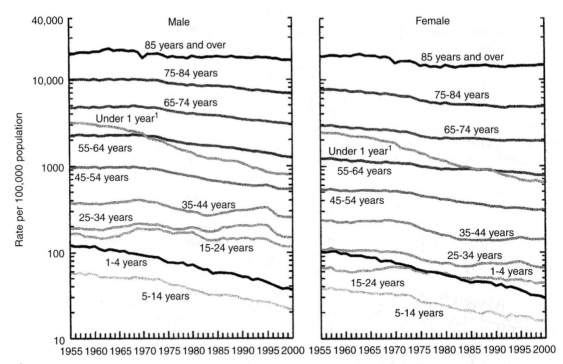

^{1}Death rates for "Under 1 year" (based on population estimates) differ from infant mortality rates (based on live births).

FIG. 1-1 Death rates by age and sex: United States, 1955–2000.

necessary interventions. For instance, the age-adjusted death rate for diseases of the heart has demonstrated a downward trend since the 1970s, declining 30% to 40% for both women and men over the past 20 years. This decline has resulted, in part, from health education and changes in lifestyle behaviors. Because mortality information is gathered from death certificates, changes in the descriptions and coding of "cause of death" and the amount of information forwarded to the NCHS, can alter these statistics. For instance, changes in the way deaths were recorded and ranked in terms of the leading causes of death most recently occurred between 1998 and 1999. As of 1999, mortality data and cause-of-death statistics are gathered and classified according to the *Tenth Revision, International Classification of Diseases (ICD-10).*

Chronic diseases continue to be the leading causes of death in the United States. Diseases of the heart and malignant neoplasms were the top two causes of deaths in 2000, responsible for over 50% of all deaths. Emphasis has been placed on reducing the deaths associated with these chronic diseases, and decline was noted through 2000 (Table 1-1). The decrease in heart disease deaths may clearly be attributed to advances in prevention and treatment of cardiac disease. An increased understanding of the genetics of cancer (the goal of the Cancer Genome Anatomy Project) is certainly responsible for better screening and treatment of many types of cancer. Advances in diagnostic

TABLE 1-1 DEATH RATES BY AGE AND AGE-ADJUSTED DEATH RATES FOR THE 15 LEADING CAUSES OF DEATH IN 2000: UNITED STATES, 1999-2000[1]

Cause of death (based on the Tenth Revision, International Classification of Diseases, 1992) and year	All ages[2]	Under 1 year[3]	Age											Age-adjusted rate
			1-4 years	5-14 years	15-24 years	25-34 years	35-44 years	45-54 years	55-64 years	65-74 years	75-84 years	85 years and over	
All causes													
2000	873.1	728.7	32.9	18.7	81.6	108.1	200.0	431.6	1,004.6	2,428.6	5,688.4	15,321.5	872.0
1999	877.0	731.4	34.7	19.2	81.2	108.3	199.2	427.3	1,021.8	2,484.3	5,751.3	15,476.1	881.9
Diseases of heart (I00-I09,I11,I13,I20-I51)													
2000	258.2	12.8	1.2	0.7	2.7	7.9	29.4	95.5	264.5	673.8	1,787.1	5,848.7	257.9
1999	265.9	13.7	1.2	0.7	2.8	8.1	30.3	97.7	274.3	709.5	1,861.8	6,032.5	267.8
Malignant neoplasms (C00-C97)													
2000	200.9	2.4	2.8	2.6	4.5	10.5	36.8	129.3	371.3	826.4	1,340.8	1,795.6	201.0
1999	201.6	1.8	2.8	2.6	4.6	10.6	37.3	130.4	380.8	836.2	1,340.0	1,796.7	202.7
Cerebrovascular diseases (I60-I69)													
2000	60.9	3.2	0.3	0.2	0.5	1.6	5.8	16.2	41.5	130.2	463.1	1,568.4	60.8
1999	61.4	2.7	0.3	0.2	0.5	1.5	5.7	15.5	41.3	132.2	472.8	1,606.7	61.8
Chronic lower respiratory diseases (J40-J47)													
2000	44.3	0.9	0.3	0.4	0.5	0.8	2.1	8.8	44.8	171.5	387.6	640.1	44.3
1999	45.5	0.9	0.4	0.4	0.6	0.9	2.0	8.7	48.3	179.2	400.4	642.7	45.8

*Figure does not meet standards of reliability or precision.
... Category not applicable.
[1]Rates on an annual basis per 100,000 population in specified group; age-adjusted rates per 100,000 U.S. standard population based on year 2000 standard. Populations used for computing death rates are postcensal estimates based on the 1990 census, estimated as of July 1.
[2]Figures for age not stated included in "All ages" but not distributed among age groups.
[3]Death rates for "Under 1 year" (based on population estimates) differ from infant mortality rates (based on live births).

TABLE 1-1 DEATH RATES BY AGE AND AGE-ADJUSTED DEATH RATES FOR THE 15 LEADING CAUSES OF DEATH IN 2000: UNITED STATES, 1999-2000—cont'd

Cause of death (based on the Tenth Revision, International Classification of Diseases, 1992) and year	All ages	Age												Age-adjusted rate
		Under 1 year	1-4 years	5-14 years	15-24 years	25-34 years	35-44 years	45-54 years	55-64 years	65-74 years	75-84 years	85 years and over	
Accidents (unintentional injuries) [V01-X59, Y85-Y86]													
2000	35.6	22.9	12.1	7.5	36.8	31.4	34.3	33.0	31.3	42.4	95.5	269.9	35.5
1999	35.9	22.1	12.6	7.8	36.2	31.3	34.0	32.5	31.1	45.1	101.1	280.9	35.9
Diabetes mellitus (E10-E14)													
2000	25.2	*	*	0.1	0.4	1.7	4.3	13.3	38.3	91.8	180.2	315.6	25.2
1999	25.1	*	*	0.1	0.4	1.5	4.3	13.2	38.9	92.8	179.1	315.6	25.2
Influenza and pneumonia (J10-J18)													
2000	23.7	7.5	0.7	0.2	0.5	1.0	2.4	4.8	12.0	39.6	161.0	734.4	23.7
1999	23.4	8.4	0.9	0.2	0.5	0.9	2.4	4.7	11.2	37.7	158.0	748.0	23.6
Alzheimer's disease (G30)													
2000	18.0	*	*	*	*	*	*	0.2	2.0	18.9	140.1	659.0	18.0
1999	16.3	*	*	*	*	*	*	0.2	1.9	17.6	130.4	598.3	16.5
Nephritis, nephrotic syndrome, and nephrosis (N00-N07, N17-N19, N25-N27)													
2000	13.5	4.2	*	0.1	0.2	0.7	1.6	4.4	12.9	38.5	101.2	274.2	13.5
1999	13.0	4.3	*	0.1	0.2	0.7	1.6	4.1	12.2	37.6	98.2	267.5	13.1
Septicemia (A40-A41)													
2000	11.3	7.1	0.7	0.2	0.3	0.7	2.0	5.0	12.1	31.4	80.7	212.9	11.4
1999	11.3	7.4	0.6	0.2	0.3	0.7	1.8	4.7	11.6	31.6	79.9	219.5	11.3

Cause of death (based on the Tenth Revision, International Classification of Diseases, 1992) and year	All ages	Under 1 year	1-4 years	5-14 years	15-24 years	25-34 years	35-44 years	45-54 years	55-64 years	65-74 years	75-84 years	85 years and over	Age-adjusted rate
Intentional self-harm (suicide) (X60-X84,Y87.0)													
2000	10.7	...	...	0.8	10.4	12.8	14.6	14.6	12.3	12.6	17.7	19.4	10.6
1999	10.7	...	...	0.6	10.3	13.5	14.4	14.2	12.4	13.6	18.3	19.2	10.7
Chronic liver disease and cirrhosis (K70,K73-K74)													
2000	9.6	*	*	*	0.1	1.1	7.5	17.9	24.1	30.2	31.1	22.8	9.6
1999	9.6	*	*	*	0.1	1.1	7.4	17.8	24.1	31.0	32.1	23.1	9.7
Essential (primary) hypertension and hypertensive renal disease (I10,I12)													
2000	6.6	*	*	*	*	0.2	0.8	2.4	6.0	15.3	45.7	160.8	6.6
1999	6.2	*	*	*	*	0.2	0.7	2.2	5.6	15.4	43.8	151.3	6.3
Assault (homicide) (X85-Y09,Y87.1)													
2000	6.1	9.1	2.3	0.9	12.9	11.1	7.2	4.7	3.1	2.4	2.4	2.3	6.1
1999	6.2	8.7	2.5	1.1	13.2	11.2	7.2	4.7	3.1	2.6	2.5	2.4	6.2
Pneumonitis due to solids and liquids (J69)													
2000	6.0	*	*	*	0.1	0.2	0.4	1.0	2.5	10.5	44.7	185.2	6.0
1999	5.6	*	*	*	0.1	0.2	0.4	0.8	2.5	9.6	41.4	174.7	5.6

body is entered by puncture or incision.

and therapeutic radiologic procedures have also played a role in helping to reduce deaths associated with these chronic diseases.

As the mortality rate for heart disease, cancer, and human immunodeficiency virus (HIV) infection have declined over the past 5 years, increases have been noted in both acute infections such as septicemia and chronic diseases such as hypertension, chronic lower respiratory diseases, and diabetes. In addition, several chronic renal diseases and Alzheimer's disease have increased as causes of death among the elderly, with Alzheimer's disease ranked eighth among the leading causes of death in 2000. Among children and young adults, injury remains the leading cause of death.

Mortality rates from any specific cause may fluctuate from year to year, so trends are monitored over a 3-year time period. These data are used to evaluate the health status of U.S. citizens and identify segments of the population at greatest risk from specific diseases and injuries. Current data are available on the NCHS Web page and may be accessed at *www.cdc.gov/nchs/about/major/dvs/mortdata.htm.*

The incidence of sickness sufficient to interfere with an individual's normal daily routine is referred to as the **morbidity rate**. The Centers for Disease Control and Prevention (CDC) is also responsible for trending morbidity rates in the United States. States must submit death certificates to the NCHS, making it fairly easy to obtain accurate data concerning the mortality rate of a specific population. It is more difficult to obtain accurate data about the morbidity rate. This information comes primarily from physicians and other health care workers reporting morbidity statistics and information to the various governmental and private agencies.

Health Care Resources

Since the early 1990s, there have been major changes in the delivery of health care with an increase in the use of ambulatory care centers, especially among the elderly. Increases in ambulatory surgery in combination with less invasive and improved surgical techniques developed over the past 20 years, as well as improvements in cardiovascular/interventional radiologic procedures have greatly contributed to this shift from inpatient to outpatient services. Ambulatory care centers range from hospital outpatient and emergency departments to physicians' offices. In response to this shift, emphasis has been placed on increasing the numbers of physician generalists including family practitioners, internal medicine physicians, and pediatricians. Inpatient services and hospital length of stay have continued to decline, averaging less than 5.0 days in 1999, down from 7.3 days in 1980. Heart disease is still the most frequent cause of hospitalization.

Although the rate of growth in U.S. health expenditures slowed during the 1990s, the cost associated with health care in the United States is staggering. In 1998, U.S. health spending accounted for 13.0% of gross domestic product, a larger share than in any other major industrialized country. In 1999, U.S. health care expenditures totaled $1.2 trillion. The major sources of funding for health care include Medicare, funded by the Federal government for elderly and disabled individuals; Medicaid, funded by Federal and State governments for the poor; and privately funded health care plans. In 1999, approximately 70% of the U.S. population had private insurance; however, approximately 17% of the U.S. population under the age of 65 had no health care coverage. Emphasis on wellness and disease prevention must continue to help reduce these costs. Studies have shown that it is much more cost-effective to provide preventive care than to wait until a disease has progressed. One good example of this trend is the emphasis placed on mammography in the management of breast disease. The percentage of women 50 years of age or older having routine mammograms has more than doubled in the last decade, again in part because of aggressive health education programs.

DISEASE CLASSIFICATIONS

Diseases can be grouped into several broad categories. Those in the same category may not necessarily be closely related, but groupings such as those discussed in the following tend to produce lesions that are similar in morphology, that is, their form and structure. Pathologies discussed in this text are generally grouped into classifications of

1. Congenital and hereditary
2. Inflammatory
3. Degenerative
4. Metabolic
5. Traumatic
6. Neoplastic

Congenital and Hereditary Disease

Diseases that are present at birth and result from genetic or environmental factors are termed **congenital**. It is estimated that 2% to 3% of all live births show one or more congenital abnormalities, although some of these may not be visible until a year or so after birth. A major category of congenital diseases is caused by abnormalities in the number and distribution of chromosomes. In somatic cells (those other than germ cells), chromosomes exist in the nucleus of each cell in pairs, with one member from the male parent and the other from the female parent. In humans, chromosomes are normally composed of 22 pairs of autosomes (those other than the sex chromosomes) and one pair of sex chromosomes. Down syndrome is a congenital condition caused by an autosomal mitosis error leading to an extra twenty-first chromosome so that the affected individual has 47 chromosomes rather than the normal 46.

Hereditary diseases are caused by developmental disorders genetically transmitted from either parent to child through abnormalities of individual genes in chromosomes and are derived from ancestors. For example, hemophilia is a well-known hereditary disease in which proper blood clotting is absent. A genetic abnormality present on the sex chromosome is a sex-linked inheritance; those on one of the other 22 chromosomes are an autosomal inheritance. The inherited disease may be dominant (transmitted by a single gene from either parent) or recessive (transmitted by both parents to an offspring). Amniocentesis, typically guided by ultrasound, is a standard procedure used prenatally to assess the presence of certain hereditary disorders.

A congenital defect is not necessarily hereditary because it may have been acquired in utero. Intrauterine injury during a critical point in development can occur from maternal infections, radiation, or drugs. Abnormalities of this type occur sporadically and cannot generally be recognized before birth. However, their likelihood is greatly lessened by following proper precautions against infection, avoiding radiation (particularly during the early term of pregnancy), and avoiding drugs or agents not specifically recognized by a physician as safe.

Inflammatory Disease

An **inflammatory** disease results from the body's reaction to a localized injurious agent. Types of inflammatory diseases include infective diseases, which result from invasion by microorganisms such as viruses, bacteria, or fungi; toxic diseases, which result from poisoning by biologic substances; and allergic diseases, which are an overreaction of the body's own defenses. Pneumonia is a type of inflammatory disease.

Some diseases in this classification are considered autoimmune disorders. Under normal conditions, antibodies are formed in response to foreign antigens. In certain diseases, however, they form against and injure the patient's own tissues. These are known as **autoantibodies,** and diseases associated with them are **autoimmune disorders**. Rheumatoid arthritis is an example of an autoimmune disorder.

An inflammatory reaction (i.e., inflammation) is a generalized pathologic process that is nonspecific to the agent causing the injury. The body's purpose in creating an inflammatory reaction is to localize the injurious agent and prepare for subsequent repair and healing of the injured tissues. Substances released from the damaged tissues can cause both local and systemic effects (Fig. 1-2). Those effects seen local to the injury include capillary dilatation to allow fluids and leukocytes, specifically, to infiltrate into the area of damage. Cellular necrosis (death) is common to acute inflammation, and the leukocytes serve to remove the dead material through phagocytosis. The characteristics of such acute inflammation include heat, redness of skin, swelling, pain, and some loss of function as the body tends to protect the injured part. If the inflammatory process is significant, systemic effects such as an elevation of body temperature become evident.

Chronic inflammation differs from that of the acute stage in that damage caused by an injurious agent may not necessarily result in tissue death. In fact, necrosis is relatively uncommon in cases of chronic inflammation. It differs also in the duration of the inflammation, with chronic conditions lasting for long periods.

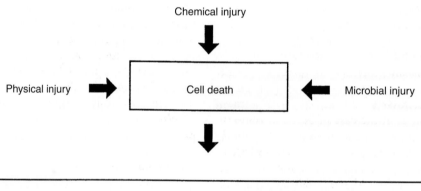

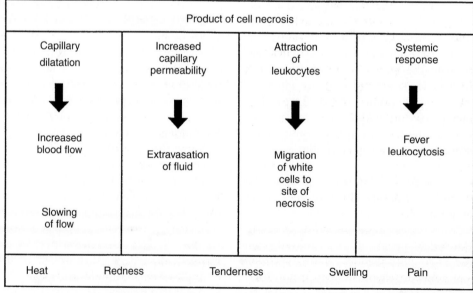

FIG. 1-2 Local and systemic effects of cell necrosis induced by various agents.

Certain conditions discussed in this text evidence chronic inflammation (e.g., pulmonary emphysema, as described in Chapter 3).

The repair of tissues damaged from an inflammatory process attempts to return the body to normal. Tissue regeneration is the process in which damaged tissues are replaced by new tissues that are essentially identical to those replaced. Although this is the most desirable type of repair, tissues vary in their ability to replace themselves. Damaged nerve cells, for example, are not likely to readily regenerate. Fibrous connective tissue repair is the alternative to regeneration, but it is less desirable because it leads to scarring and fibrosis. Damaged tissues are replaced by a scar and lack the structure and function of the original tissue.

Debridement (removal of dead cells and materials) is an essential component of the healing process. It may be accomplished at both the cellular level and through human intervention, as in the case of burns or removal of foreign objects such as glass. The repair process begins with the migration of adjacent cells into the injured area and replication of the cells via mitosis to fill the void in the tissue. This new growth includes capillaries, fibroblasts, collagen, and elastic fibers. Remodeling of the new tissue, the last phase in the healing process, occurs in response to normal use of the tissue. For instance, remodeling of the bone following a skeletal fracture may take months, but the results often return the injured bone to its original contour.

Infection refers to an inflammatory process caused by a disease-causing organism. Under favorable conditions, the invading pathogenic agent multiplies and causes injurious effects. Generally, localized infection is usually accompanied by inflammation, but inflammation can occur without infection. Virulence refers to the ease with which an organism can overcome body defenses. An organism with high virulence is likely to produce progressive disease in susceptible persons; one of low virulence can produce disease only in highly susceptible persons under favorable conditions.

Degenerative Disease

Degenerative diseases are caused by a deterioration of the body. Although they are usually associated with the aging process, some degenerative conditions may exist in younger patients. For instance, an individual may develop a degenerative disease following a traumatic injury, regardless of age.

The process of aging results from the gradual maturation of physiologic processes that reach a peak, then gradually fade (i.e., degenerate) to a point where the body can no longer survive. Heredity, diet, and environmental factors are known to affect the rate of aging. Over time, the functional abilities of tissues decrease because either their cell numbers are reduced or the function of each individual cell declines, with both typically participating in pathologies resulting from aging. Atherosclerosis, osteoporosis, and osteoarthritis are three diseases commonly associated with the aging process. Each is discussed later in this text.

Metabolic Disease

Metabolism is the sum of all physical and chemical processes in the body. Diseases caused by a disturbance of the normal physiologic function of the body are classified as metabolic diseases. These include endocrine disorders (e.g., diabetes and hyperparathyroidism) and disturbances of fluid and electrolyte balance.

Endocrine glands secrete their product (hormones) into the bloodstream to regulate various metabolic functions. The major endocrine glands include the pituitary, thyroid, parathyroids, adrenal glands, pancreatic islets, ovaries, and testes. An endocrine disorder may consist of hypersecretion, causing an overactivity of the target organ, or insufficient secretion, resulting in underactivity. The clinical effects of an endocrine disturbance depend on the degree of dysfunction and the age and sex of the individual.

Dehydration is the most common disturbance of fluid balance. It is caused by insufficient intake of water or excessive loss of it. Electrolytes are mineral salts (most commonly sodium and potassium) dissolved in the body's water. Depletion of them may occur because of vomiting, diarrhea, or use of diuretics (substances that promote the excretion of salt and water). Disturbance of either the fluid or electrolyte balance upsets homeostasis, the body's normal internal resting state.

Traumatic Disease

Another general classification of diseases is **traumatic**. These diseases may result from mechanical forces such as crushing or twisting of a body part or from the effects of ionizing radiation on the human body. In addition, disorders resulting from extreme hot or cold temperatures, such as burns and frostbite, are also classified as traumatic.

Trauma may injure a bone, resulting in fractures, which are covered extensively in Chapter 11. It may also injure soft tissues. A wound is an injury of soft parts associated with rupture of the skin. Traumatic injuries may injure soft tissues even if the skin is not broken. Bleeding into the tissue spaces as a result of capillary rupture is known as a bruise or contusion.

Neoplastic Disease

Neoplastic disease results in new, abnormal tissue growth. Normally, growing and maturing cells are subject to mechanisms that control their growth rate. When this control mechanism goes awry, an overgrowth of cells develops, resulting in a neoplasm. Lesion is a term used to describe the many types of cellular change that can occur in response to disease. Some lesions may be visible immediately; others may be detectable initially only through diagnostic means such as laboratory testing.

An abnormal growth of cells leads to the formation of either a benign or malignant tumor, or neoplasm. A **benign neoplasm** remains localized and is generally noninvasive, as opposed to a **malignant neoplasm**, which continues to grow, spread, and invade other tissues. Cancer is a general term often used to denote various types of malignant neoplasms. Sometimes it is difficult to classify abnormal cells as either benign or malignant because they may exhibit characteristics of both types. Often the abnormal growth is graded depending on the composition of the particular cells. Cells are classified as either differentiated or undifferentiated depending on the resemblance of the new cells to the original cells in the host organ or site. If the differences are small, the growth is termed differentiated and has a low probability for malignancy. If the cells within the neoplasm exhibit atypical characteristics, they are termed poorly differentiated or undifferentiated and have a higher probability of malignancy.

The spread of malignant cancer cells is termed metastasis. **Metastatic spread** can occur in a variety of ways. If the cancerous cells invade the circulatory system, they may be spread via blood vessels, termed **hematogenous spread**; or via the lymphatic system, termed **lymphatic spread**. If the cancerous cells spread into surrounding tissue by virtue of the close proximity of the areas, it is termed **invasion**. However, if the cancerous cells travel to a distant site or distant organ system, it is termed **seeding**. Certain types of cancer appear more often as metastases from other areas rather than originating in a given organ.

Note that the terms cancer and carcinoma are not synonymous. A **carcinoma** is one type of cancer and is derived from epithelial tissue. Other cancers include **sarcoma**, which arises from connective tissue, and **leukemias** and **lymphomas**, which arise from blood cells and lymphatic cells, respectively. Both benign and malignant tumors are also named according to the tissue type of origin (Table 1-2). In the case of a benign neoplasm, the word root is added to "oma," for instance, *adenoma*. Malignant neoplasms are named by adding the word root to the name of the tissue type, for instance, *adenocarcinoma*. Radiography plays a major

TABLE 1-2 TUMOR WORD ROOTS BASED ON TISSUE TYPE

Common Word Root	Cells of Origin
Adeno-	Gland
Angio-	Vascular
Chondro-	Cartilage
Fibro-	Fibrous tissue
Hemangio-	Blood vessels
Lipo-	Adipose
Myo-	Muscle
Neuro-	Nerve
Osteo-	Bone

role in the diagnosis and staging of a variety of neoplastic diseases.

The treatment of cancer consumes enormous financial, emotional, and other resources in health care. Although the state of the art is continually advancing, the primary treatment modalities are surgery, chemotherapy, and radiation therapy. The choice of which modality or combination of modalities depends on many factors, including the type of cancer, its location and stage, and the treating oncologist. The goal of treatment may be curative, allowing the patient to remain free of disease for 5 years or more, or palliative, which is designed to relieve pain when curing is not possible.

The Staging of Cancer

Decisions regarding the appropriate treatment of malignant tumors and in determining prognosis and end results are guided by classifications that "stage" the disease. Although several clinical classifications of cancer exist, the TNM system emerged in the 1950s and is now considered a recognized standard, as endorsed by the American Joint Committee on Cancer (AJCC). The AJCC is cosponsored by several prominent health organizations, including the American Cancer Society and the American College of Radiology.

The TNM system is based on the premise that cancers of similar histology or origin are similar in their patterns of growth or extension. The *T* refers to the size of the untreated primary cancer or tumor. As the size increases, lymph node involvement *(N)* occurs, eventually leading to distant metastases *(M)*. The addition of numbers to these three letters indicates the extent of malignancy and the progressive increase in size or involvement of the tumor. For example, T0 indicates that no evidence of a primary tumor exists, whereas T1, T2, T3, and T4 indicate an increasing size or extension. Lack of regional lymph node metastasis is indicated by N0, and N1, N2, and N3 indicate increasing involvement of regional lymph nodes. Finally, M0 indicates no distant metastasis, and M1 indicates the presence of distant metastasis.

In addition, other descriptors are used to categorize a given tumor further according to its primary site, histopathologic type and grade, lymphatic or venous invasion, and residual tumor classification. Neoplastic cells are examined histologically, and these growths are categorized or "graded" according to their degree of differentiation. The degree of differentiation or grading is used to distinguish among degrees of malignancy, with grade 1 categorized as least malignant and grade 4 as most malignant. The combination of all of these allows the TNM system to serve as a shorthand notation for description of the clinical extent of a given malignant tumor. It facilitates treatment planning, provides an indication of prognosis, assists in evaluating treatment results, facilitates information exchange between treatment centers, and allows unambiguous categorization of malignancies to aid in the continuing investigation of cancer.

CONCLUSION

There is no doubt that technological advances in the field of radiology have done much to relieve human suffering, but medical imaging alone cannot provide a definitive diagnosis. Medical imaging must be used in conjunction with other diagnostic and therapeutic modalities to provide the best treatment for each specific disease process. The following chapters provide the student radiographer with a better understanding of the disease processes of the various physiologic systems. This information should help students to analyze and critique each radiograph to ensure that it provides optimal information to assist physicians in their diagnosis.

QUESTIONS

1. The prediction of the course and end of a disease and an outlook based on that prediction best define its:
   - a. diagnosis
   - b. etiology
   - c. prognosis
   - d. syndrome

2. A compression fracture of the lumbar spine that results from steroid treatments for pain reduction of arthritis would be an example of _____ disease.
   - a. degenerative
   - b. iatrogenic
   - c. idiopathic
   - d. traumatic

3. A disease such as Tay-Sachs syndrome that is transmitted genetically is termed:
   - a. congenital
   - b. hereditary
   - c. metabolic
   - d. neoplastic

4. Sickness sufficient to interfere with normal daily routines is termed:
   - a. etiology
   - b. morbidity
   - c. mortality
   - d. pathogenesis

5. Which of the following would be considered a symptom of a disease process?
   - a. bloody stool
   - b. nausea
   - c. skin rash
   - d. swelling

6. A disease that presents slowly and lasts over a long period of time is said to be:
   - a. acute
   - b. asymptomatic
   - c. chronic
   - d. congenital

7. Which of the following types of disease classifications is usually associated with the normal aging process?
   - a. congenital
   - b. degenerative
   - c. inflammatory
   - d. metabolic

8. If 4000 cases of a given disease are found in the inhabitants of a given population, its _____ is defined.
   - a. incidence
   - b. morphology
   - c. metabolism
   - d. prevalence

9. The relative ease with which an organism can overcome normal bodily defenses against the organism refers to its:
   - a. infection
   - b. necrosis
   - c. pestilence
   - d. virulence

10. A neoplastic growth is evaluated to determine its degree of histologic differentiation. This is termed:
    - a. grading
    - b. metastasis
    - c. morphology
    - d. staging

11. Specify two pathologies that are iatrogenic in origin and explain the probable cause of each pathology. Are any specific to the use of ionizing radiation?

12. What is the difference between mortality and morbidity rates? How is each important to the practice of medicine and to public health agencies?

13. Differentiate between an acute illness and a chronic illness. Give two examples of each type of disease.

14. Explain the concept of neoplastic disease. Are all neoplasms cancer?

15. Describe the TNM classification system and specify how it may be used by physicians in a health care setting.

The Skeletal System

UPON COMPLETION OF CHAPTER 2, THE READER SHOULD BE ABLE TO:

- Describe the anatomic components of the skeletal system on a macroscopic and basic microscopic level.
- Identify and explain the criteria for assessing technical adequacy of skeletal radiographs.
- Characterize a given condition as congenital, inflammatory, arthritic, metabolic, traumatic, or neoplastic.
- Specify the pathogenesis, signs and symptoms, and prognosis of the skeletal pathologies cited in this chapter.
- Explain the role of various imaging modalities in the diagnosis and treatment of skeletal pathologies.

KEY TERMS

Achondroplasia	Gouty arthritis	Osteoporosis
Acromegaly	Hyperostosis frontalis interna	Paget's disease
Albers-Schönberg disease	Hyperparathyroidism	Polydactyly
Anencephaly	Involucrum	Pott's disease
Ankylosing spondylitis	Juvenile rheumatoid arthritis	Pyogenic arthritis
Arthritis	Medullary canal	Rheumatoid arthritis
Bursitis	Metaphysis	Rickets
Cancellous bone	Osteoarthritis	Scoliosis
Chondrosarcoma	Osteoblasts	Sequestrum
Clubfoot	Osteoblastoma	Simple bone cyst
Compact bone	Osteochondroma	Spina bifida
Congenital hip dislocation	Osteoclasts	Spondylolisthesis
Craniosynostoses	Osteoclastoma	Spondylolysis
Craniotubular dysplasias	Osteogenesis imperfecta	Staphylococcus aureus
Diaphysis	Osteoid osteoma	Syndactyly
Diploë	Osteoma	Tenosynovitis
E. coli	Osteomalacia	Trabeculae
Endochondroma	Osteomyelitis	Trabecular pattern
Ewing's sarcoma	Osteosarcoma	Transitional vertebra
Exostosis	Osteopenia	Tuberculosis
Ganglion	Osteopetrosis	Whiplash
Giant cell tumor (GCT)	Osteophytes	

ANATOMY AND PHYSIOLOGY

The skeletal system is comprised of 206 separate bones and is responsible for body support, protection, movement, and blood cell production. It contains more than 98% of the body's total calcium and up to 75% of its total phosphorus. The system is commonly divided into the axial skeleton (Fig. 2-1), which contains 80 bones, and the appendicular skeleton (Fig. 2-2), which contains 126 bones. Bone is a type of connective tissue, but it differs from other connective tissue because of its matrix of calcium phosphate. The construction of this matrix further classifies bone tissue as either compact (dense) or cancellous (spongy) (Fig. 2-3).

The outer portion of bone is composed of **compact bone**, and the inner portion, termed the **medullary canal**, is made up of cancellous bone. Bone marrow is located within the medullary canal and is interspersed between the *complex* **trabeculae**. This intricate, web-like bony structure is visible on a properly exposed radiograph of the skeletal system and is often referred to as the **trabecular pattern**. The term **diploë** is specific to the cancellous bone located within the skull. The red bone marrow is responsible for the production of bone erythrocytes and leukocytes. Red bone marrow is found, in a normal adult, primarily in the bones of the trunk. At the approximate age of 20 years, the majority of the red bone marrow is replaced by yellow bone marrow composed mainly of fat.

Osteoblasts are the bone-forming cells that line the medullary canal and are interspersed throughout the periosteum. They are responsible for bone growth and thickening, ossification, and regeneration. **Osteoclasts** are specialized cells that break down bone to enlarge the medullary canal and allow for bone growth. This production and breakdown of

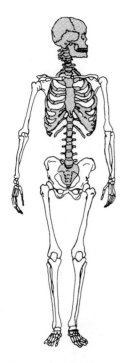

FIG. 2-1 Axial skeleton.

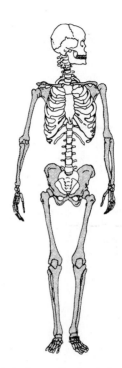

FIG. 2-2 Appendicular skeleton.

bone play an important role in serum calcium and phosphorus equilibrium. Certain metabolic disease processes may alter the percentage of calcium, resulting in either hypocalcemia or hypercalcemia.

The bones of the skeletal system may also be classified according to their shape to include long, short, flat, and irregular bones. The **diaphysis** of a long bone refers to the shaft portion, whereas the epiphysis refers to the expanded end portion (Fig. 2-4). The **metaphysis** refers to the growth zone between the epiphysis and diaphysis. It is the area of greatest metabolic activity in a bone. A cartilaginous growth plate is located between the metaphysis and the epiphysis in the bone of a growing child. Radiographically, these growth areas appear radiolucent. As the body matures, this cartilage calcifies and is no longer radiographically visible in the adult.

The periosteum is a fibrous membrane that encloses all of the bone except the joint surfaces

and is crucial to supplying blood to the underlying bone. Osteoblasts located within the periosteum increase bone thickness relative to individual activities. The more physical stress a bone is under, the thicker the compact portion develops; therefore, it is common medical practice to allow patients with healing fractures of the hip or femur to bear weight on the injured bone, thus helping to reduce the healing period. Disuse atrophy occurs when a bone is not allowed to bear weight and results in significant decalcification and thinning of the bone.

The 206 bones of the body are connected to each other by one of three types of joints. Fibrous (synarthrodial) joints form firm, immovable joints such as the sutures of the skull. Cartilaginous (amphiarthrodial) joints, such as those found between the vertebral bodies, are slightly movable. Synovial (diarthrodial) joints, such as the knee, are freely movable. The ends of the bones composing a synovial joint are

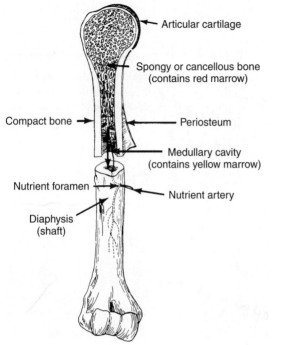

FIG. 2-3 Bone composition.

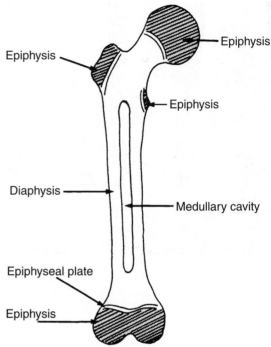

FIG. 2-4 Endochondral ossification.

lined with articular cartilage and are held together by ligaments. The joint capsules are lined by a synovial membrane responsible for the secretion of synovia, a lubricating fluid containing mucin, albumin, fat, and mineral salts.

IMAGING CONSIDERATIONS

Radiography

In examining a skeletal radiograph, it is important to begin by properly orienting the film and recognizing the radiographic projection. When film/screen technology is used, the radiographic exposure technique selected can be very important in achieving a proper diagnosis. Proper technique is achieved when the soft tissues and bony structures of interest are both visible. Any motion of the part in question impairs the visibility of the detail present.

Soft tissue areas often hold clues to the diagnosis and are examined by the interpreting physician. Any signs of muscle wasting, soft tissue swelling, calcifications, opaque foreign bodies, or the presence of gas may indicate disease. Analysis of the configuration of the bone and its relationship to other bones serves to detect or exclude fractures, dislocations, congenital anomalies, or acquired deformities.

The interface between cortical (compact) bone and soft tissue is also important. Any periosteal new bone formation seen may be a response to trauma, tumors, or infection. Juxta-articular erosions are often seen in cases of arthritis. Cortical reabsorption can be demonstrated as smudgy, irregular loss of the cortical margin. In addition, the internal bone structure is important and should be examined for abnormally altered texture, alterations in the amount of mineralization, or foci of destruction. Careful consideration of all areas mentioned assists the physician in achieving the correct diagnosis.

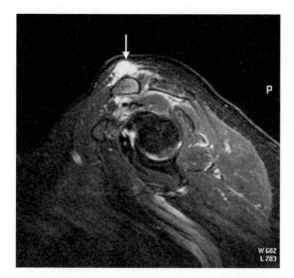

FIG. 2-5 MRI (Short-tau inversion recovery sequences) showing a subcutaneous cyst on the scapula.

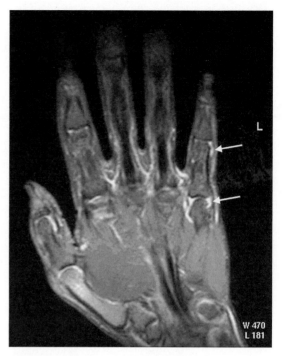

FIG. 2-6 MRI (Short-tau inversion recovery sequences) showing synovitis of the metacarpophalangeal and interphalangeal joints.

Magnetic Resonance Imaging

Magnetic resonance imaging (MRI) is an important modality utilized in imaging of skeletal pathology, particularly in providing soft tissue detail, because of its superior contrast resolution. It is considered the modality of choice for detection and staging of soft tissue tumors involving the extremities. It is also extremely useful in evaluation of joints, particularly the knee and shoulder (Fig. 2-5). Newer imaging techniques, faster scan times, and high-speed computers allow MR to detect a greater number of musculoskeletal subtleties with higher-resolution imaging (Fig. 2-6). Sometimes these subtleties mimic bone pain but involve soft tissues instead—an important distinction. Bone marrow imaging done with MR is superior to the older nuclear medicine bone scan, particularly for subtle abnormalities (e.g., edema). Also, MR may play a larger role in trauma medicine, particularly with the refinement of open-bore and short-bore technologies.

Computed Tomography

Computed tomography (CT) is an important tool in skeletal imaging because with newer technology the examination can be performed quickly and noninvasively, even in cases of trauma. CT has the ability to define the presence and extent of fractures or dislocations, to assess joint abnormalities and associated soft tissues, and to help diagnose spinal disorders (Fig. 2-7). Cortical bone gives no signal in MRI, but CT provides ready visualization of bony detail and is often used as a follow-up for improved detail to plain film imaging. Bone tumors, in particular, are now usually imaged with spiral or helical CT because of its excellent ability to display bony margins and trabecular patterns and to assess both bony and soft tissue involvement of tumors. Although CT possesses greater contrast resolution than radiography,

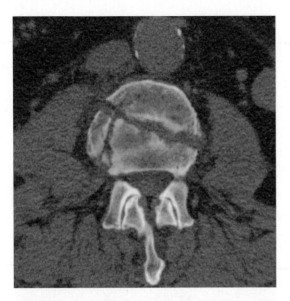

FIG. 2-7 CT demonstrating a burst fracture of the third lumbar vertebra.

much of the role for imaging other related soft tissues has been usurped by MRI. Quantitative computed tomography (QCT) is also used in evaluating bone mass loss, especially within the vertebral bodies of the spine.

Nuclear Medicine Procedures

Nuclear medicine retains an advantage not offered by either MRI or CT in skeletal imaging: the ability to look at the entire body at one time in a convenient fashion (Fig. 2-8). It allows ready decision making as to whether any pathology shown is an old injury or a new problem, with activity indicating that the bone involved is affected by some new process. Additionally, the bone scan is still the standard of care for examination of metastatic processes because it demonstrates metabolic reaction of the bone to the disease process and is more sensitive than comparative radiographic studies. This is also true in many other traumatic or inflammatory diseases of the skeletal system.

Bone Mineral Densitometry

Double-energy x-ray absorbtiometry (DEXA) or bone mineral densitometry is also important in evaluation of osteoporosis. DEXA units readily show bone density by evaluating the bone mass of the distal radius, femoral neck, and lumbar spine. The results of bone densitometry are used in combination with routine laboratory tests of blood and urine to determine when loss of bone mass is evident. Bone mineral densitometry reports indicate the amount of bone mass present and compare the density of a particular individual to norms used in evaluation. A "T-score" is used to reflect standard deviations above or below the 30-year-old national reference population because it is assumed that this is the age of peak bone mass. Based on criteria established by the World Health Organization, a T-score greater than −1.0 is normal. T-scores less than −1.0 but greater than −2.49 are classified as osteopenia, and T-scores less than −2.5 reflect osteoporosis. The "Z-score" reports standard deviation above or below a population matched for age, sex, weight, and ethnicity. Z-scores less than −2 suggest bone disease.

CONGENITAL AND HEREDITARY DISEASES

Osteogenesis Imperfecta

Osteogenesis imperfecta (OI), sometimes called brittle bone disease, is a quite serious and rather rare heritable or congenital disease affecting the skeletal system. It is caused by mutations in the two structural genes that encode the α_1 and α_2 peptides of type I collagen, the main collagen of bone, tendon, and skin. Thus, deficient and imperfect formation of osseous tissue, skin, sclera, inner ear, and teeth are noted in individuals presenting with this disease. There are two main clinical groups of OI, depending on the age of onset and the severity of the disease. Osteogenesis imperfecta congenita is present at birth. Infants afflicted with this disease usually have multiple fractures

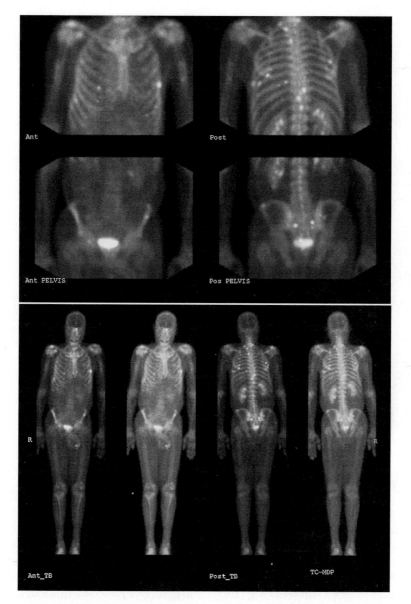

FIG. 2-8 Bone scan demonstrating metastatic disease throughout the ribs, thoracic vertebrae, and pelvis due to carcinoid disease.

at birth that heal only to give way to new fractures (Fig. 2-9). This results in limb deformities, dwarfism, and may lead to death. In osteogenesis imperfecta tarda, fractures might not appear for some years after birth and then generally stop once adulthood is reached. In some cases, however, a hearing disorder persists because of otosclerosis, abnormal connective tissue around the auditory ossicles. Radiographic evaluation will demonstrate multiple fractures

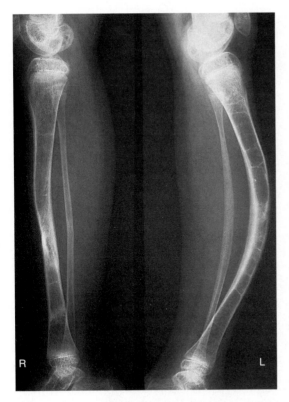

FIG. 2-9 Tibia-fibula radiograph demonstrating bowed lower extremities resulting from osteogenesis imperfecta tarda. This condition was recognized shortly after the child began to walk.

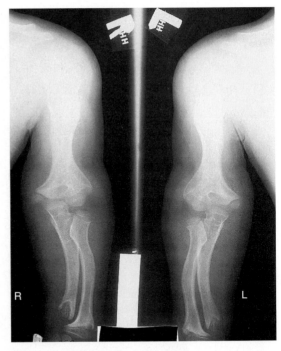

FIG. 2-10 Radiographs of shortened upper extremities caused by a defect in the endochondral bone formation associated with achondroplasia.

in various stages of healing and a general decrease in bone mass. The bone cortex is thin and porous, and the trabeculae are thin, delicate, and widely separated.

Achondroplasia

The most common inherited disorder affecting the skeletal system is **achondroplasia**, which results in bone deformity and dwarfism. Because of a disturbance in endochondral bone formation, the cartilage located in the epiphyses of the long bones does not convert to bone in the normal manner, impairing the longitudinal growth of the bones. Thus, patients with this type of osteochondrodysplasia present with a normal trunk size and shortened extremities

(Fig. 2-10). An adult with achondroplasia is usually no more than 4 feet in height, with lower extremities usually less than half the normal length. Additional clinical manifestations of this disorder include extreme lumbar spine lordosis, bow legs, and a bulky forehead. Occasionally, orthopedic surgery may be necessary in management of complications associated with achondroplasia. In addition, these patients may receive genetic and social counseling.

Osteopetrosis

Osteopetrosis and marble bone are terms used to characterize a variety of disorders involving an increase in bone density and defective bone contour, often referred to as skeletal modeling. With osteopetrosis, bones are abnormally heavy and compact but nevertheless brittle. The disorders characterizing osteopetrosis include

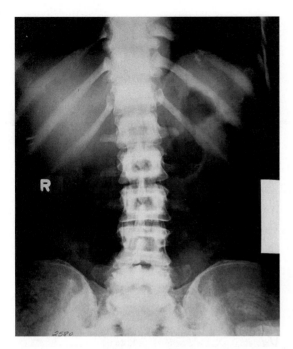

FIG. 2-11 AP lumbar spine radiograph demonstrating uniform sclerosis of the bone associated with osteopetrosis.

osteoscleroses, craniotubular (affecting the cranium and tubular long bones) dysplasias, and craniotubular hyperostoses. It is important for the technologist to be aware that both the osteosclerotic and craniotubular hyperostotic disorders require an increase in exposure factors to adequately penetrate the bony anatomy because of abnormal bone density (Fig. 2-11). In some cases, adequate radiographic density may never be achieved. All bones are affected, but the most significant changes occur in the long bones of the extremities, vertebrae, pelvis, and base of the skull. Radiographs demonstrate an increase in the density and thickness of the bony cortex as well as an increase in the number and size of trabeculae with a marked reduction of the marrow space.

Albers-Schönberg disease is a fairly common form of osteosclerotic osteopetrosis. This benign skeletal anomaly involves increased bone density in conjunction with fairly normal bone contour. If fact, many patients afflicted with Albers-Schönberg disease are asymptomatic, and it is often discovered after radiographing the patient for an unrelated problem. Although this is a hereditary disorder, the bone sclerosis is not radiographically visible at birth. As the individual ages, radiographic manifestations of the osteopetrosis become visible, especially in the region of the cranium and spine; however, general health is unimpaired.

Craniotubular dysplasias are a group of hereditary diseases mainly resulting in abnormal or defective bone contour of the cranium and long bones. Radiographs are useful in demonstrating this alteration in contour, scleroses, and changes within the cortical bone. Craniotubular hyperostoses include a variety of fairly rare hereditary diseases, causing both an increase in bone density and abnormal bone modeling. Both of these craniotubular anomalies present in childhood. Although these disorders do not normally impair the individual's general health, bony overgrowth may entrap cranial nerves, resulting in some dysfunction such as facial palsy or deafness.

Hand and Foot Malformations

A variety of abnormalities of the fingers and toes may occur during fetal development but can be surgically corrected at birth. Failure of the fingers or toes to separate is called **syndactyly** and gives the physical appearance of webbed digits. **Polydactyly** (Fig. 2-12) refers to the presence of extra digits.

Clubfoot (talipes) is a congenital malformation of the foot that prevents normal weight bearing. The foot is most commonly turned inward at the ankle. This congenital malformation is more common in males than in females and may occur bilaterally. It is generally corrected by casting or splinting the foot in correct anatomic position.

Congenital Dislocation of the Hip

A malformation of the acetabulum often results in **congenital hip dislocations.** Because the

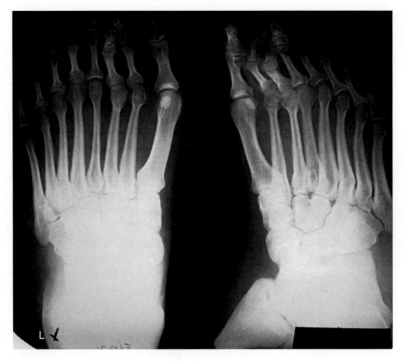

FIG. 2-12 Foot radiograph demonstrating additional digits associated with familial polydactyly.

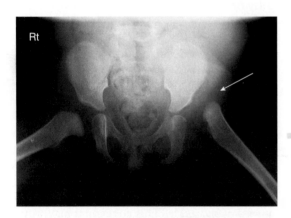

FIG. 2-13 Frog leg lateral projection of the pelvis on an infant demonstrating congenital dislocation of the left hip.

acetabulum does not completely form, the head of the femur is displaced superiorly and posteriorly (Fig. 2-13). Many times, the ligaments and tendons responsible for proper placement of the femoral head are also affected. Congenital dislocations of the hip occur more frequently in females than in males. This anomaly is most commonly treated with immobilization through casting or splinting the affected hip.

Vertebral Anomalies

Scoliosis refers to an abnormal lateral curvature of the spine (Fig. 2-14). The lateral curves are usually convex to the right in the thoracic region and to the left in the lumbar region of the spine. Up to 80% of all scolioses are idiopathic, although factors such as connective tissue disease and diet have been implicated. Scoliosis does not generally become visually apparent until adolescence. It tends to affect girls more frequently than boys and can generate numerous complications, including cardiopulmonary complications, degenerative spinal arthritis, and fatigue and joint dysfunction syndromes.

Radiography is important in the diagnosis and treatment of scoliosis. Initial evaluation

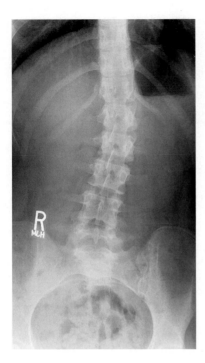

FIG. 2-14 AP lumbar spine radiograph demonstrating congenital scoliosis.

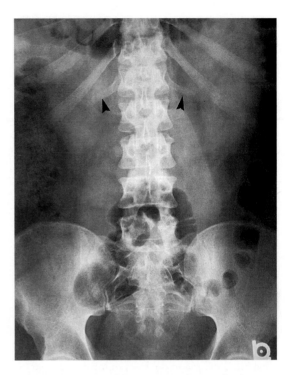

FIG. 2-15 AP lumbar spine radiograph demonstrating bilateral lumbar ribs.

requires initial anteroposterior (AP) or posteroanterior (PA) and lateral standing radiographs with follow-up radiographs on a fairly routine basis. Radiologists use one of several methods to measure the spine's curvature, so consistent quality from one examination to another is important. Good radiation protection techniques are vital because of the large size of the exposure field, the young age of the patient, and the frequency of the examinations. Special attention is necessary in shielding the breasts of young, female patients during radiographic examination throughout the treatment process. Scoliosis may be corrected surgically or by placing the individual in a brace or body cast. Treatment depends on the site of the deformity and the severity of the curvature.

A **transitional vertebra** is one that takes on the characteristics of both vertebrae on each side of a major division of the spine. Most frequently, such vertebrae occur at the junction between the thoracic and lumbar spine or at the junction between the lumbar spine and the sacrum. The first lumbar vertebra may have rudimentary ribs articulating with the transverse processes (Fig. 2-15), as may the seventh cervical vertebra. A cervical rib most commonly occurs at C7 and may exert pressure on the brachial nerve plexus or the subclavian artery, requiring surgical removal of the rib.

Spina bifida is an incomplete closure of the vertebral canal that is particularly common in the lumbosacral area (Fig. 2-16). Frequently, such patients have no visible abnormality or neurologic deficit, but failure of bony fusion of the two laminae is visible radiographically (spina bifida occulta). In more severe cases, the spinal cord or nerve root may be involved, which results in varying degrees of paralysis. Treatment of spina bifida is determined based on the extent of the anomaly and requires the services of a variety of physicians.

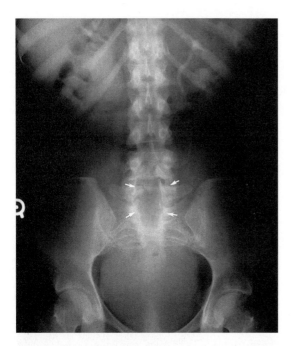

FIG. 2-16 Abdominal radiograph of a patient with spina bifida occulta of the lower lumbar vertebrae.

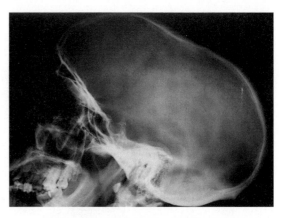

FIG. 2-17 Lateral skull radiograph demonstrating premature closure of the sagittal suture. This results in dolichocephaly and prominent convolutional markings caused by the increased intracranial pressure.

Cranial Anomalies

The premature or early closure of any of the cranial sutures is called **craniosynostoses**. This congenital anomaly causes an overgrowth of the unfused sutures to accommodate brain growth, thus altering the shape of the head (Fig. 2-17). Although this defect may be corrected with surgery, brain damage may occur.

Anencephaly is a congenital abnormality in which the brain and cranial vault do not form (Fig. 2-18). In most cases, only the facial bones are formed. This abnormality results in death shortly after birth and may be diagnosed before birth by sonography.

INFLAMMATORY DISEASE

Osteomyelitis

Osteomyelitis is an infection of the bone and bone marrow caused by a pathogenic micro-

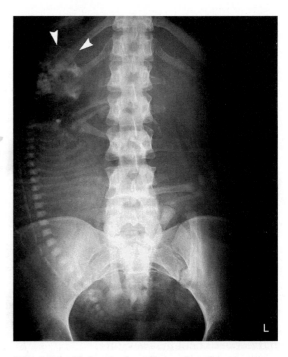

FIG. 2-18 Abdominal radiograph of a pregnant woman carrying a fetus with anencephaly. Notice the lack of the cerebral cranial bones.

organism spread via the bloodstream (hematogenous), from an infection within a contiguous site, or through direct introduction of the microorganism. Generally, hematogenous osteomyelitis develops at the ends of the long bones such as the distal femur, proximal tibia and humerus, and radius in children and in the vertebrae in adults. Infants and children are more commonly affected by acute hematogenous osteomyelitis because of increased vascularity and rapid growth of their long bones. In addition, children often have a lowered resistance to the pathogenic organism, most commonly *Staphylococcus aureus.* Infection may be spread to the marrow space via the nutrient artery from an infection of the skin, ear, or pharynx. In infants, hematogenous osteomyelitis may also be caused by group B streptococci and *E. coli*. In adults, hematogenous osteomyelitis is commonly secondary to bacteremia caused by genitourinary tract, soft tissue, or respiratory infections. As in children, *S. aureus* and streptococci are the pathogenic microorganisms primarily responsible for the infections.

Osteomyelitis resulting from contiguous infections is often associated with burns, sinus disease, periodontal infection, soft tissue infection, or skin ulcers resulting from peripheral vascular disease. Pathogenic microorganisms may also be directly introduced to the bone by penetrating wounds, open fractures, fractures treated with internal fixation devices, or prosthetic replacements.

No specific bone changes may be demonstrated radiographically in the very early stage of infection. But the infection spreads rapidly, with the acute stage of osteomyelitis characterized by the formation of an abscess, leading to an inflammatory reaction within the bone that causes a rise in internal bone pressure. Because of the constriction of periosteum, blood vessels compress and thrombose, leading to bone necrosis within 24 to 48 hours. Unfortunately, not until about 10 to 14 days later is new periosteal bone repair evident

radiographically to indicate the presence of the disease. Therefore, it is imperative that the condition be recognized clinically and treated with antibiotics and local drainage.

Initially, radiographs may demonstrate soft tissue swelling in the area around the affected bone. Follow-up radiographs may be performed 10 to 14 days after medical treatment to aid in the diagnosis.

With the effective use of antibiotics, osteomyelitis seldom passes the acute stage. When it does, antibiotics in combination with surgical drainage of pus from under the periosteum often result in a complete cure of the bone lesion in a majority of cases. Chronic osteomyelitis, however, is characterized by extensive bone destruction with irregular, sclerotic reaction throughout the bone (Fig. 2-19). A **sequestrum** is the essentially dead, devascularized bone that appears very dense. An **involucrum** is a shell of new supporting bone laid down by the periosteum around the sequestrum. An accurate diagnosis is extremely important to distinguish osteomyelitis from a neoplastic bone disease.

Radiography is not a very sensitive means of diagnosing the condition because a 30% to 50% loss of bone calcium is required before the destructive changes of osteomyelitis are visible radiographically. Nuclear medicine bone scan studies and MR images are much more sensitive in detecting ostemyelitis.

Tuberculosis

Tuberculosis of the bone is a chronic inflammatory disease, usually more advanced, often long untreated as compared to pulmonary tuberculosis. Its incidence has sharply declined in the last few decades as the incidence of pulmonary tuberculosis has declined. It most commonly affects the hip, knee, and spine. Radiographically, the ends of the long bones display a "worm-eaten" appearance, with the disease slowly destroying the epiphyses, spreading to the articular cartilage, and in some cases infecting the joint space (Fig. 2-20).

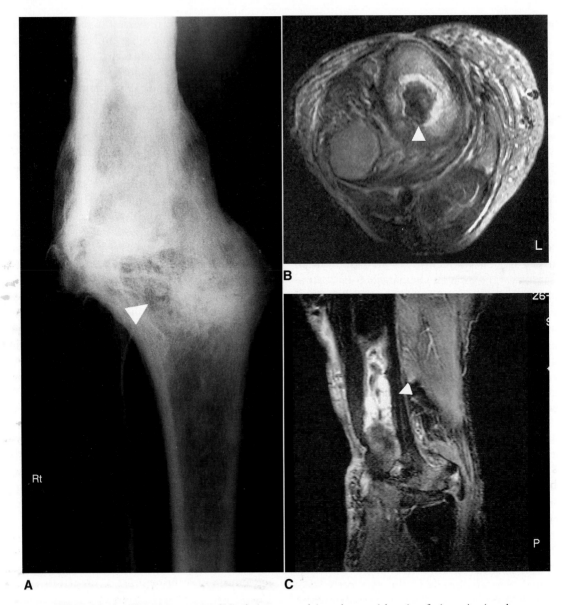

FIG. 2-19 A, Chronic osteomyelitis demonstrated in a knee with prior fusion. An involucrum surrounded by fluid densities is seen in the middle of a large intramedullary cavity approximately 3 cm above the fusion site. **B,** The involucrum demonstrated on a sagittal MRI on the same patient. **C,** The sequestrum demonstrated on an axial MRI of the same patient, appearing as very dense bone as a result of devascularization.

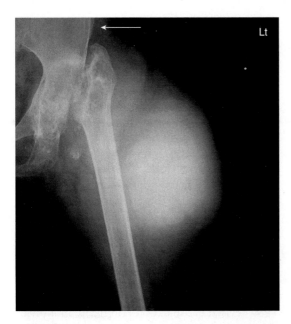

FIG. 2-20 Hip radiograph of a 47-year-old man with extensive destruction of the femoral head and neck caused by tuberculosis of the hip with a cold abscess.

Tuberculosis of the spine is also called **Pott's disease**. Recognized in ancient times, it has been described in Egyptian mummies dating back to 3000 BC. It destroys the spine, causing softening and eventual collapse of the vertebrae, which results in paravertebral abscess formation and exerts abnormal pressure on the spinal cord.

Arthritis

Joint inflammation is known as **arthritis** and may be caused by a variety of etiologic factors. It can generally be divided into two main types: (1) degenerative, in which pathologic changes begin in the articular cartilage of joints, and (2) inflammatory, in which pathologic changes begin in the synovial membrane of joints. An accurate clinical history is of extreme importance because different types of arthritis are characterized by specific features. For example, it is important to identify the number of joints involved, the location of the joints involved,

and the presence of any other disease process. Some types of arthritis involve several joints, but others involve only one joint. In addition, certain types of arthritis have a predilection for specific joints while sparing others. Finally, some types of arthritis are associated with specific disease processes caused by a host of factors, such as bacteria or autoimmune response. Arthritis may be further classified as acute or chronic; the most common forms are chronic and disabling.

Acute Arthritis

Acute arthritis is commonly called **pyogenic arthritis**, and it is caused by a variety of factors including staphylococci, streptococci, and gonococci. Common clinical symptoms of acute arthritis are pain, redness, and swelling of the affected joint, often accompanied by a fever. Generally, the pyogenic or pus-forming organisms enter the body via a wound, as in the case of an open fracture, or the organisms may spread to the joint from a bone infected with osteomyelitis. Pyogenic arthritis usually responds rapidly to antibiotic therapy. The early radiographic changes demonstrate an increase in joint space, bony destruction, and joint dislocation. Radiographs obtained during the healing stage demonstrate recalcification and sclerosis, often resulting in joint ankylosis.

Rheumatoid Arthritis

Rheumatoid arthritis (RA) is a chronic autoimmune disease that may fluctuate in severity. It is triggered by exposure of an immunogenetically susceptible host to an arthritogenic antigen and is characterized by chronic inflammation and overgrowth of the synovial tissues, most often in the extremities. RA develops slowly, and as the synovial tissues proliferate, they progressively destroy the cartilage, bone, and supporting structures. Genetic factors also are believed to predispose an individual to RA: analysis of blood chemistry identifies the presence of an autoantibody against γ-globulin, also known as the serologic rheumatoid factor (RF).

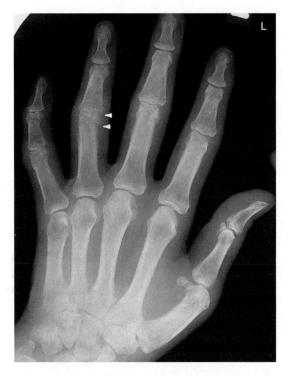

FIG. 2-21 Hand radiograph demonstrating soft tissue joint swelling associated with early rheumatoid arthritis.

It usually occurs between the ages of 30 and 40 years and is three times more common in women than in men. In the United States, approximately 2.5 million adults are affected by RA. The juvenile form of RA also affects nearly 100,000 American children. Symptoms include pain, swelling, and stiffness of the affected joint with periods of activity or exacerbations and remissions of the disease process.

Although any joint may be involved, RA typically begins in the peripheral joints, particularly in the small bones of the hands and feet and in the knee. The radiographic changes seen early in this disease are soft tissue swelling and osteoporosis of the affected bones (Fig. 2-21). As the disease progresses, cortical erosion with joint space narrowing occurs because of the overgrowth of synovial tissue into the articular spaces. This severe damage makes the joint unstable and leads to deformity caused by the displacement of the bones. The late changes of this condition can be quite severe, resulting in bone and cartilage destruction and subluxation or dislocation of the involved joint (Fig. 2-22). Eventually, the joints become ankylosed (fused), which requires surgical intervention. Surgical procedures such as synovium excision, dislocation corrections, joint reconstructions, and prosthetic joint replacements may be performed to improve joint function (Fig. 2-23). Overall, life expectancy is reduced by 3 to 7 years with RA, with deaths usually resulting from complications such as gastrointestinal (GI) bleeding related to long-term use of aspirin. Diagnosis of RA in adults is based on the American College of Radiology (ACR)'s 1987 revised classification criteria. If an individual meets four of the seven criteria listed, a positive diagnosis of RA is indicated. The seven criteria indicating the presence of RA are (1) morning stiffness in and around the joints, (2) simultaneous soft tissue swelling or fluid of at least three joint areas, lasting for at least 6 weeks and observed by a physician, (3) arthritis of the hand joints—at least one area swollen in a proximal interphalangeal joint (PIP), metacarpophalangeal joint (MCP), or wrist joint for at least 6 weeks, (4) symmetric arthritis—simultaneous involvement of the same joint areas on both sides of the body for at least 6 weeks, (5) rheumatoid nodules or lumps of tissue, (6) abnormal amounts of serum RF, and (7) radiographic changes demonstrating bone erosion or decalcification.

Juvenile rheumatoid arthritis affects children under 16 years of age and is similar to the adult form of RA. There are differences, however, in the pattern of involvement and prognosis. Generally, there is less fibrosis and proliferation than in the adult form. Prognosis is generally good, with fewer than 20% having progressive destructive disease. The majority have long periods of remission without signifi-

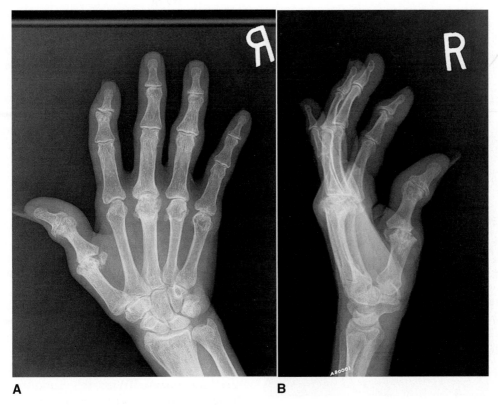

A   **B**

FIG. 2-22 PA (**A**) and lateral (**B**) hand images demonstrating advanced rheumatoid arthritis with subluxation of the first metacarpophalangeal joint.

cant joint damage. The ACR criterion for diagnosis of juvenile RA differs from the adult. Juvenile RA is indicated if (1) the child is younger than 16 years at the onset of the disease, (2) symptoms of arthritis (swelling or effusion) are present in one or more joints for at least 6 weeks, and (3) the onset can be assigned to one of three JRA onset types: pauciarticular, polyarticular, and systemic.

Ankylosing Spondylitis

Ankylosing spondylitis (Marie-Strümpell disease) is a progressive form of arthritis, mainly involving the spine, in which joints and articulations become ankylosed, especially the sacroiliac joints. It tends to affect men between the ages of 20 and 40 years and is believed to have a genetic predisposition because it is 20 times more common in the first-degree relatives of individuals known to have this disorder. Most commonly, an individual will present with low back pain varying in intensity, often nocturnal in nature and associated with morning stiffness. Other early symptoms include a low-grade fever, fatigue, weight loss, and anemia. Early radiographic changes demonstrate bilateral narrowing and fuzziness of the sacroiliac joints. Eventually, the sacroiliac joints become obliterated, and the condition progresses up the spine. Later radiographic changes show calcification of the bones of the spine with ossification of the vertebral ligaments. The articular cartilage is

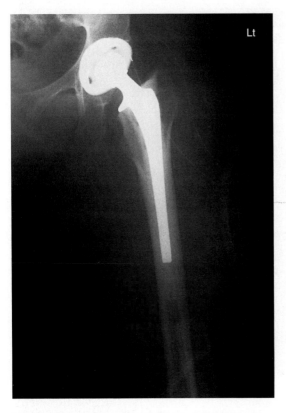

FIG. 2-23 Portable radiograph of a left hip demonstrating proper placement of a prosthetic hip replacement.

destroyed, and fibrous adhesions develop. These adhesions lead to bone fusion and calcification of the annulus fibrosis of the intervertebral disks and the anterior and lateral spinal ligaments. The spine becomes a rigid block of bone, giving the condition its characteristic nickname of "bamboo spine" (Fig. 2-24). In addition to radiographic indications, blood serum analysis is utilized in the diagnosis of ankylosing spondylitis. It is treated by the use of nonsteroidal antiinflammatory drugs, COX-2 inhibitors, therapeutic exercise, and postural training.

Osteoarthritis

The most common type of arthritis is **osteoarthritis**, also known as degenerative joint disease. It affects men and women equally, although patients are usually asymptomatic until they are in their fifties. Osteoarthritis is a disease of cartilage and is classified as primary or secondary. Primary osteoarthritis may be inflammatory or erosive and destructive, resulting from a noninflammatory deterioration of the joint cartilage that occurs with the normal wear and tear of aging. In some cases, individuals may have a genetic predisposition for developing osteoarthritis. Secondary osteoarthritis occurs as a result of bone stress associated with trauma, congenital anomalies, or other diseases that alter the hyaline cartilage and surrounding tissue. Osteoarthritis generally affects the large, weight-bearing joints of the body such as the hip, where it is particularly disabling, or the knees and ankles (Fig. 2-25), because they serve as the primary weight-bearing joints of the body. Osteoarthritis can also affect the interphalangeal joints of the fingers. Osteoarthritis of the fingers is thought to be hereditary and affects women more often than men, especially after menopause. With this condition, the fingers become enlarged and often develop bony knobs termed Heberden's nodes and Bouchard's nodes. Osteoarthritis of the fingers is most often managed with the use of medications, splints, and heat treatments.

In joints afflicted with this disease, the articular cartilage degenerates and is gradually worn away, exposing the underlying bone. Radiographically, this loss of articular cartilage appears as a narrowing of the joint space. An overgrowth of articular cartilage occurs on the peripheral surfaces of the joint and often calcifies, which results in **osteophytes** or bone spurs that are visible radiographically (Fig. 2-26). In terms of radiographic diagnosis, the formation of osteophytes is indicative of osteoarthritis, helping to distinguish it from other types of arthritis.

Clinically, an individual with osteoarthritis presents with pain and progressive stiffening of the affected joint. Methods of halting its gradual progression are few; it is second only to cardiovascular disease in causing long-term dis-

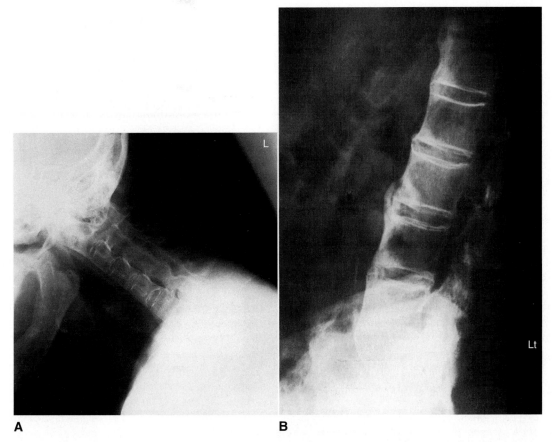

A   B

FIG. 2-24 A, Lateral cervical spine radiograph depicting ankylosing spondylitis with granulation tissue beneath the anterior longitudinal ligament destroying the corners of the contiguous vertebra. **B,** Lateral lumbar spine radiograph on a 64-year-old man with ankylosing spondylitis. Notice the fusion of the vertebrae into a solid block of bone.

ability. Treatment consists of the use of medications such as nonsteroidal antiinflammatory drugs, COX-2 inhibitors, and acetaminophen. Exercise is one of the best treatments to decrease pain, increase flexibility, and help with weight control. The use of walking aids, rest, and heat treatment may also be incorporated in the treatment regimen. Surgery may also be utilized to resurface or reposition bones, remove loose pieces of bone or cartilage, and, in cases of severe pain, for surgical prosthetic joint replacement, which greatly relieves the pain and allows a return of joint mobility.

Inflammation of Associated Joint Structures

The specialized connective tissues that attach muscle to bone are called tendons. They are enclosed in a sheath that is susceptible to inflammation, a condition known as **tenosynovitis** (Fig. 2-27). Tenosynovitis may spread to the associated tendon, resulting in tendinitis. Chronic tendinitis may also cause the formation of calcium deposits in either the affected tendon or an associated sheath. These calcium deposits that form in the shoulder joint as a result of chronic trauma often cause rotator cuff tears, which can be detected on shoulder

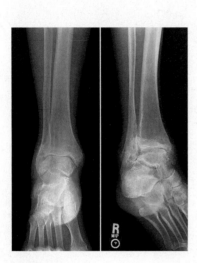

FIG. 2-25 AP and oblique ankle radiographs demonstrating osteoarthritis.

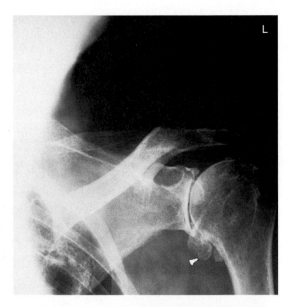

FIG. 2-26 Shoulder radiograph demonstrating the formation of an osteophyte at the inferior lip of the glenoid labrum caused by primary osteoarthritis.

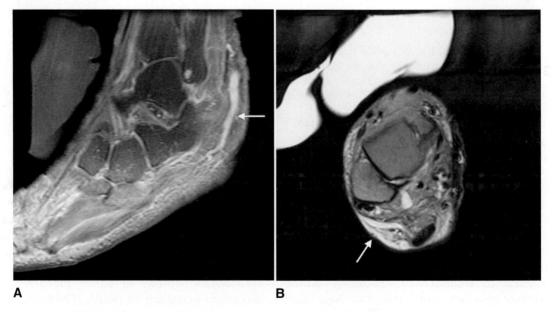

A   B

FIG. 2-27 MR images (**A,** sagittal; **B,** axial) of right ankle demonstrate tenosynovitis involving the posterior tibialis muscle following a strain injury.

arthrogram and magnetic resonance examinations of the shoulder. Bursae are sacs lined with a synovial membrane, and they are found in locations where tendons pass over bony prominences. If the bursa becomes inflamed, it is called **bursitis**. Inflammation of these associated structures may be caused by acute or chronic trauma (e.g., housemaid's knee), acute or chronic infection, inflammatory arthritis, gout, and, rarely, pyogenic or tuberculous organisms. These inflammatory conditions are characterized by pain, localized tenderness, and limited motion of the involved joint. In cases of chronic bursitis, the walls of the bursa become thickened, and calcium deposits may be visible radiographically within the bursa (Fig. 2-28).

Common medical treatment of bursitis and tendinitis include nonsteroidal antiinflammatory agents in combination with analgesics. In severe cases, corticosteroid injections may be used. In cases in which the tendons or bursae ossify, surgical intervention is necessary, especially in conjunction with rotator cuff tears. A **ganglion** is a cystic swelling that develops in connection with a tendon sheath (Fig. 2-29). These commonly occur on the back of the wrist, but they can occur in any joint space.

Gouty Arthritis

Gouty arthritis is an inherited metabolic disorder in which excess amounts of uric acid are produced and deposited in the joint and adjacent bone. The condition occurs more frequently in men and most commonly affects the metatarsophalangeal joint of the great toe. It is characterized by acute attacks with intervals of remission. This disease may occur in patients placed on long-term diuretics, as in the case of congestive heart failure.

The crystallization of uric acid within the joint causes an acute inflammatory reaction. Large masses of these sodium urate crystalline deposits in joints and other sites are called tophi. Bony changes include erosion (Fig. 2-30) with overhanging edges. One long-term

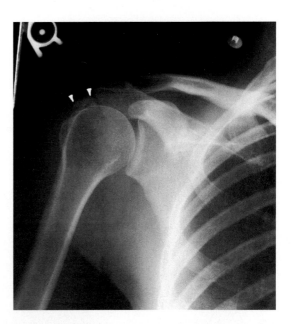

FIG. 2-28 Shoulder radiograph demonstrating radiopaque calcium deposits within the bursa caused by chronic bursitis.

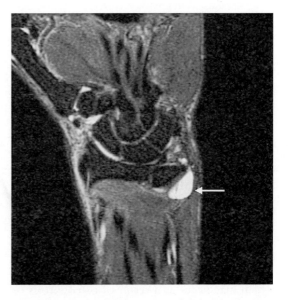

FIG. 2-29 Coronal MR image of the wrist demonstrating a cystic lesion on the volar aspect of the wrist along the ulnar side.

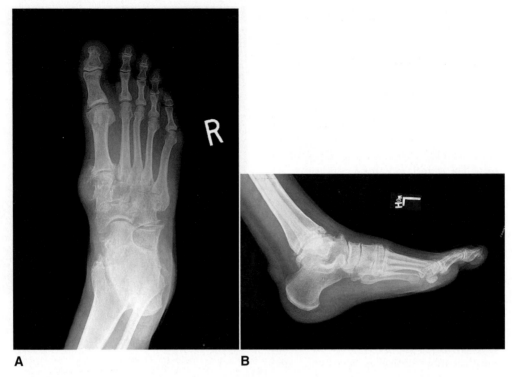

FIG. 2-30 PA (**A**) and lateral (**B**) foot radiographs demonstrating bony erosion of the tarsal bones from gout.

complication of gout is the formation of radiolucent kidney stones caused by increased excretion of uric acid by the kidneys. Treatment of gout consists of medications either to promote excretion of uric acid by the kidneys or to inhibit the production of uric acid within the body.

METABOLIC DISEASE

Osteoporosis

A prime determinant of radiographic film density is the amount of calcium present in the bone structure. A radiographically visible decrease in bone density is termed **osteopenia**, which may occur as a result of osteoporosis or osteomalacia. **Osteoporosis** is a commonly known metabolic bone disorder that may be classified by age groups as postmenopausal, senile, idiopathic, and juvenile. Postmenopausal osteoporosis is the most common form of the disease. Estimates are that more than half of the women in North America over age 60 have osteoporosis, and it is a major cause of fractures of the hip, spine, and wrist in women over the age of 45 years. The disease is characterized by an abnormal decrease in bone density. Although the formation of bone is normal, the bone reabsorption rate is abnormally high in individuals with osteoporosis. Thus, osteoporosis results in a thinning of the cortical bone and an enlargement of the medullary canal without a change in the actual diameter of the bone. The normal equilibrium associated with osteoid production and withdrawal is quite complicated and depends on a combination of dietary intake and absorption, hormonal interplay, and normal stress or muscular activity. In postmenopausal women, for example, the lack of the hormone estrogen creates a weakened bony matrix, contributing to the development of "porous" bones. As this condition becomes more severe, these bones are subject to compression fractures, and they can literally cave in from the weakness. As the vertebral bodies of the thoracic and lumbar spine are weakened, they collapse anteriorly, causing a kyphotic deformity of the spine often termed a "dowager's hump."

These bony changes are well demonstrated in radiographs of the spine (Fig. 2-31), where decreased bone density stands out clearly against the bony cortex. Osteoporosis is a subtractive or destructive pathologic condition and requires a decrease in exposure technique. However, conventional radiographs can only identify a loss of bone mass when it is advanced or the bone has lost approximately 30% to 50% of its original mass. Therefore, conventional

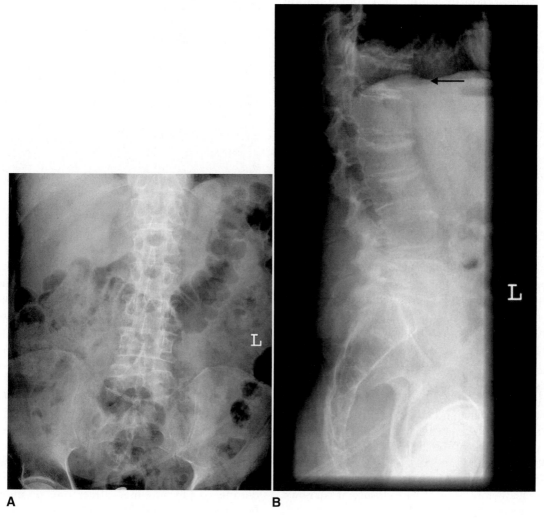

FIG. 2-31 AP (**A**) and lateral (**B**) lumbar spine radiographs demonstrating osteopenia secondary to long-term steroid use.

radiography is of little value in diagnosing early stages of osteopenia. The best method for evaluating early stages of osteoporosis is bone mineral densitometry of the hip and lumbar spine using either double-energy x-ray absorptiometry (DEXA) or QCT.

Osteopenia may be caused by other diseases such as pathologies of the endocrine system, neoplastic disease, malnutrition, chronic renal failure, or hereditary diseases of the skeletal system or be a result of drug therapy. However, osteoporosis is by far the most common form of metabolic bone disease and can be differentiated from other causes by examining serum enzyme levels, especially alkaline phosphatase. For example, patients with osteoporosis have normal or elevated serum alkaline levels, whereas patients with osteomalacia present with a decrease in these serum levels. Elevated alkaline phosphatase is an indication of increased bone activity because it is found on the outside of osteoclast cell. Treatment of osteoporosis generally includes an increase in dietary intake of calcium and vitamin D in combination with hormone replacement therapy.

Osteomalacia

Osteomalacia is a condition caused by a lack of calcium in the tissues and a failure of bone tissue to calcify. This normally results from inadequate intake or absorption of calcium, phosphorus, or vitamin D, most commonly as a consequence of intestinal malabsorption of fats. Osteomalacia may be associated with hepatic disease, chronic pancreatitis, regional ileitis, and resections of the GI system because these conditions may inhibit the body from absorbing fat-soluble vitamin D. It is often also present in individuals with chronic renal failure secondary to the loss of renal parenchyma and the kidneys' inability to convert vitamin D into a form useful to the human body. If osteomalacia occurs before growth plate closure, it is known as **rickets** (Fig. 2-32).

With this condition, the bones are spongelike and demonstrate osteopenia on radiographic

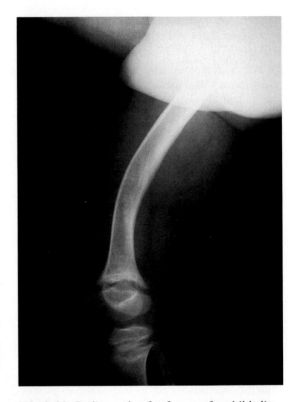

FIG. 2-32 Radiograph of a femur of a child diagnosed with vitamin D–resistant rickets. Notice the bowing of the extremity.

evaluation. Radiographically, osteomalacia appears similar to osteoporosis except for the presence of bands of radiolucency within the bone, termed pseudofractures or "Looser's zones." Laboratory analysis and other testing are necessary to differentiate the diagnosis, and bone biopsy remains the definitive method of determining the presence of osteomalacia.

Paget's Disease (Osteitis Deformans)

Paget's disease is a metabolic disorder of unknown etiology that is fairly common in the elderly population, affecting men twice as frequently as women. It usually begins in the fifth decade of life and may affect one or more bones, most commonly the pelvis, spine, skull (Fig. 2-33), and the long bones (Fig. 2-34). Paget's disease is characterized by two stages in

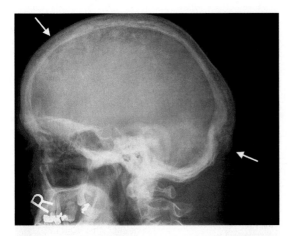

FIG. 2-33 Lateral skull radiograph depicting an advanced proliferative phase of Paget's disease. Notice the changes within the inner and outer tables of the skull.

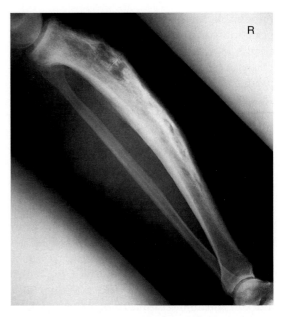

FIG. 2-34 Radiograph of the tibia of the patient in Fig. 2-33 demonstrating the effect of advanced proliferative Paget's disease on the tibia.

which the bone undergoes continuous destruction, called the osteolytic stage, and simultaneous replacement by abnormally soft and poorly mineralized material, called the osteoblastic stage. The osteoid material that replaces the normal bone tissue is very bulky and porous, with exceptional vascularity. Although this osteoid matrix is thicker than the normal bone, its softness often leads to weight-bearing, stress-induced deformities and fractures. As the skull enlarges, additional complications may occur because of impingement on the cranial nerves. These complications include hearing and vision disturbances. In addition, individuals with Paget's disease have an increased risk of developing osteogenic sarcoma, a malignant neoplastic disease of the skeletal system. Radionuclide bone scans readily detect Paget's disease, even in its very early stages. Radiographically, the affected bones typically demonstrate cortical thickening with a coarse, thickened trabecular pattern. Mixed areas of radiolucent osteolysis and radiopaque osteosclerosis may be seen. Blood chemistry results indicate very high alkaline phosphatase levels with normal serum calcium and phosphorus. There is no known

cure for this disease. Most cases are mild and asymptomatic; no treatment is necessary. In symptomatic cases, medications are administered to decrease bone resorption.

Hyperparathyroidism

Hyperparathyroidism is a fairly common disease of the endocrine system, but it is discussed in this chapter because of its effect on the skeletal system. This disease is often very mild and may go undetected for a long time. Like all metabolic bone diseases, the entire skeleton is affected in hyperparathyroidism, with some sites more affected than others.

Remember that the skeletal system is involved in the balance of serum calcium and phosphorus levels and that the body strives to keep this ratio constant. Hyperparathyroidism applies to any disorder that disrupts the calcium–phosphate ratio and results in an elevated level of parathyroid hormone (PTH). Excess PTH secretion overstimulates the osteoclasts that are responsible for bone removal, thus leading to bone destruction. This osteoclastic activity results in a decreased bone density, so a decrease in radiographic exposure is necessary to produce a high-quality radiographic image.

There are basically three types of hyperparathyroidism: primary hyperparathyroidism, secondary hyperparathyroidism, and a third type caused by ectopic production of a parathyroid-like hormone. Treatment varies with each specific cause of hyperparathyroidism and is very complex.

Primary hyperparathyroidism most frequently affects adults in their 30s or 50s and arises from an adenoma, carcinoma, or hyperplasia of the parathyroid gland. The excess production of PTH causes bone destruction, an increased absorption of calcium by the intestines and kidneys, and an increase in urine calcium, which predisposes the individual to renal stones. The net effect of these reactions to the high level of PTH is an increase in serum calcium with a decrease in serum phosphate. Individuals affected with primary hyperparathyroidism commonly have symptoms associated with hypercalcemia such as neuromuscular weakness and fatigue, and may first present with symptoms of renal colic as a result of renal stones or calcification of the kidneys (nephrocalcinosis). Radiographic investigation demonstrates subperiosteal bone resorption or osteopenia, especially in the diaphyses of the phalanges and clavicles. Bone resorption is also radiographically evident in the teeth. Pathologic fractures may also be present as a consequence of the softened bone matrix.

Secondary hyperparathyroidism (Fig. 2-35) represents a response to hypocalcemia, hyperphosphatemia, or hypomagnesemia. It is caused by a very complex metabolic disorder that is beyond the scope of this text and is most commonly seen in individuals with chronic renal disease. Decreased renal function leads to a loss of the kidneys' ability to produce vitamin D and compromises their ability to excrete phosphate.

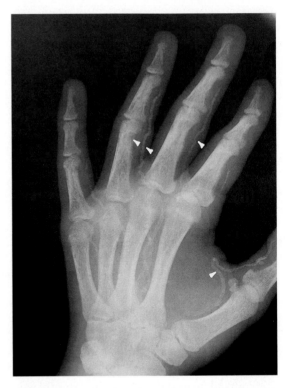

FIG. 2-35 Hand radiograph of an individual with secondary hyperparathyroidism. Notice the subperiosteal resorption of bone and calcification of the arteries of the hand.

Acromegaly

Although **acromegaly** is an endocrine disorder caused by a disturbance of the pituitary gland, it is briefly mentioned in this chapter because of its effect on the skeletal system. This disorder is caused by excessive secretion of growth hormones in the adult, which is often the result of a pituitary adenoma. Acromegaly is a slowly progressive disease that may be diagnosed years after the individual is symptomatic. An increase in growth hormone in the adult produces a thickening and coarsening on the bones because the epiphyses have closed and the bone cannot grow in length. Radiographic studies demonstrate an enlarged sella turcica and changes in the skull, often obliterating the diploë found between the inner and outer

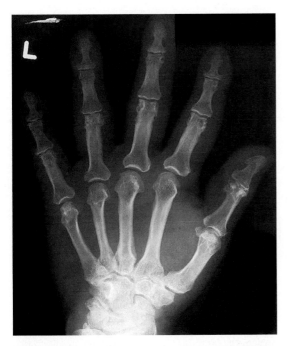

FIG. 2-36 Hand radiograph of an individual diagnosed with acromegaly. Notice the spade-like appearance of the hand.

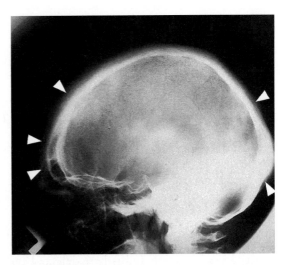

FIG. 2-37 Skull radiograph depicting the changes caused by acromegaly.

tables of the cortical bone. Individuals with acromegaly present with a prominent forehead and jaw, widened teeth, abnormally large, spade-like hands (Fig. 2-36), and a coarsening of facial features (Fig. 2-37). This disorder is frequently treated with a combination of surgery and radiation therapy to eradicate the adenoma.

VERTEBRAL COLUMN

The causes of vertebral column injuries include direct trauma, hyperextension-flexion injuries (whiplash), osteoporosis, or metastatic destruction. **Whiplash** is a broad term encompassing soft tissue neck injuries from a variety of causes. Pain in the posterior neck is a primary manifestation, either dull or sharp, and may radiate. Imaging of whiplash injuries is limited to soft tissue studies, with exclusion of fractures and dislocations the first priority. Loss of lordosis is

the most common finding on radiographs of patients suffering from whiplash.

Radiographic indications of spinal column injuries include the interruption of smooth, continuous lines formed by the vertebrae stacking on each other. Also, the vertebral bodies may lose some height, or the interspace may narrow. Muscle spasm as a result of trauma may cause a reversal or straightening of the normal spinal curvatures.

Perhaps the most common condition of the vertebral column is generalized back pain, typically in the lumbar area. Such back pain may not always result from bony involvement. Disk disease can cause muscle spasm with pain referral throughout the back. Finally, back pain may be secondary to referred pain from the hip. Conventional radiographs are the most common imaging modality utilized to assess low back pain because they can demonstrate vertebral fractures and subluxation, **spondylolysis,** or erosion of the vertebral bodies. However, they are of little value in the evaluation of disk pathologies.

Spondylolysis exists when there is a cleft, or breaking down, of the body of a vertebra between the superior and inferior articular processes (pars interarticularis). Typically, this occurs in the arch of the fifth lumbar vertebra as a result of developmental or congenital anomaly rather than as related to acute trauma. It appears radiographically as a "collar" or "broken neck" on the "Scotty dog" (Table 2-1) appearance and is demonstrated on an oblique projection of the lumbar spine (Fig. 2-38). When forward slippage of the vertebral column off a vertebra occurs because of spondylolysis, it is known as **spondylolisthesis**. The patient with this condition may present symptoms identical to those of a herniated disk. Approximately 90% of such slippage commonly occurs at the L5-S1 junction and is best detected on a lateral projection (Fig. 2-39). Conservative medical management (e.g., rest, chiropractic manipulative therapy) is the preferred choice for treatment before surgical fusion.

In cases of disk disorders, myelography may be performed. Myelographic examination, alone, can visualize the nerve roots and subarachnoid space and clearly demonstrate posture-related disk anomalies. Myelography performed in combination with CT (Fig. 2-40) adds the ability to evaluate bone detail; however, it is still an invasive procedure. MRI provides a non-invasive alternative to CT myelography. MRI demonstrates the spine in multiple planes and is unsurpassed in its ability to demonstrate the spinal cord, nerve roots, subarachnoid and epidural spaces, vertebral disks, and the para-spinal tissues (Fig. 2-41). MRI does have limi-

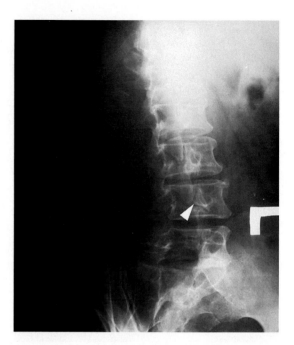

FIG. 2-38 Oblique radiograph of the lumbar spine demonstrating spondylolysis of the fourth and fifth lumbar spines on the left side. Notice the "break in the Scotty dog's neck."

tations based on patient compliance and contraindications for performing MRI examination such as pacemakers, aneurysm clips, etc. In cases of vertebral fracture, CT is the modality of choice for demonstrating bony anatomy.

NEOPLASTIC DISEASE

Many varieties of bone tumors exist and are seen in patients of all ages. The most common benign tumors are osteoma, osteochondroma, and giant cell tumor. The primary malignant bone tumors are osteosarcoma, Ewing's tumor, and multiple myeloma (discussed in Chapter 9).

The diagnosis of a bony abnormality is often made radiographically on the basis of the patient's age, pattern of bone destruction, the location of the tumor, and its position within the bone. In terms of age, benign tumors most often occur within the first three decades of life;

TABLE 2-1 ANATOMIC COMPONENTS OF THE SCOTTY DOG

Dog Part	Anatomic Component
Eye	Pedicle
Nose	Transverse process
Ear	Superior articular process
Foreleg	Inferior articular process
Neck	Pars interarticularis
Body	Lamina

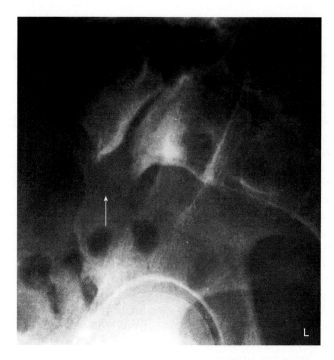

FIG. 2-39 L5-S1 spot radiograph of a woman complaining of low back pain, demonstrating spondylolisthesis of this joint.

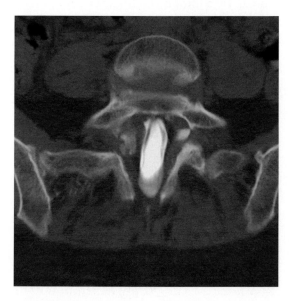

FIG. 2-40 CT myelogram demonstrating the subarachnoid space and intervertebral disks.

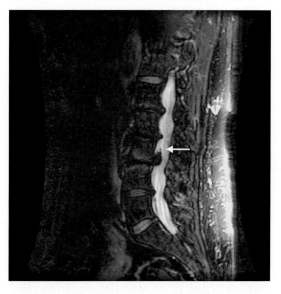

FIG. 2-41 MR image of the lumbar spine reconstructed in a sagittal plane demonstrating the spinal cord, subarachnoid space, and intervertebral disks.

a bone tumor in the elderly is likely to be malignant. The pattern of bony destruction in benign lesions is to expand the bone and demonstrate sharp, sclerotic margins. Malignant neoplasms often infiltrate, permeate, and destroy anatomic margins. The location of a tumor is also important. For example, half of all osteosarcomas appear in the distal femoral or proximal tibial metaphysis. Similarly, **chondrosarcomas** tend to involve the trunk, shoulder girdle, and proximal long bones.

Radiographic studies contribute greatly to the diagnosis and management of bone tumor patients. Plain films are used to disclose the lesions and show the growth characteristics that assist in determining their benign or malignant nature. In conjunction with CT, plain radiographs identify malignant growth patterns and the proper site for biopsy. Sometimes, seemingly unrelated examinations, such as a barium enema or chest radiograph, are ordered by the physician to rule out distant metastases.

CT plays a key role in the primary diagnosis and continued evaluation of neoplasms of the skeletal system because of its ability to produce images with excellent soft tissue and contrast resolution. Cross-sectional images of the area of interest provide physicians with the exact location and extent of the specific tumor, thus allowing the surgeon to identify the optimal surgical procedure and possibly limiting the surgical resection of the affected bone as well as assisting in the postsurgical management of the disease process. CT is also commonly used to assist during bone biopsy procedures.

As mentioned earlier in this chapter, radionuclide bone scans are helpful in assessing neoplastic diseases because the bone scan reflects the metabolic reaction of bone to the neoplastic disease process. Nuclear medicine procedures may also be performed during the initial stages of treatment planning to identify possible metastatic involvement of other anatomic sites.

Because cortical bone does not produce a signal, MRI provides the unique ability to clearly demonstrate fat and bone marrow due to their high water content. This information is helpful in differentiating between normal bone marrow and tumor tissue in the assessment of many neoplastic diseases of the skeletal system.

Osteochondroma (Exostosis)

The most common benign bone tumor is the **osteochondroma** (Fig. 2-42), typically affecting men three times more often than women. An osteochondroma arises from the growth zone between the epiphysis and diaphysis of long bones, also called the metaphysis. Most commonly, it involves the lower femur or upper tibia and is capped by growing cartilage attached to the skeleton by a bony stalk. The cortex of an osteochondroma blends with the normal bone, and the growth tends to protrude up and away from the nearest joint, most commonly the knee. **Exostoses** or excessive bone growth may appear as singular or multiple lesions and are normally diagnosed in childhood or adolescence. Multiple exostoses indicate a hereditary disorder and usually appear at an earlier age than the single-lesion osteochondroma. In addition, multiple exostoses may transform to malignant neoplasms such as chondrosarcoma. Many times, osteochondromas are asymptomatic unless the affected long

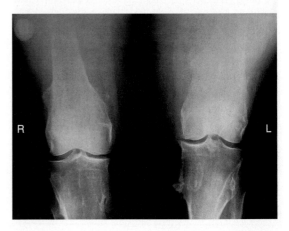

FIG. 2-42 Bilateral AP knee radiographs demonstrating osteochondroma with exostoses within the knee joint.

bone is traumatized, which results in a pathologic fracture of the diseased bone. An osteochondroma has an osteosclerotic or osteoblastic radiologic appearance.

Osteoma

An **osteoma** is a less frequent benign growth most commonly located in the skull. These lesions are composed of very dense, well-circumscribed, normal bone tissue that usually projects into the orbits or paranasal sinuses. They are generally slow-growing tumors of little significance unless they cause obstruction, impinge on the brain or eye, or interfere with the oral cavity. A term associated with osteoma of the skull is **hyperostosis frontalis interna** (Fig. 2-43).

Endochondroma

An **endochondroma** is a slow-growing benign tumor composed of cartilage. It grows in the marrow space and most commonly affects the small bones of the hands and feet in individuals between the ages of 30 and 40 years. These benign tumors do not invade the surrounding tissue as they grow; however, they do expand the cortical bone, causing thinning. Radiographically, endochondromas appear as radiolucent lesions containing small, stippled calcifications (Fig. 2-44). They are well circumscribed and appear as a "bubbly" lesion of the bone. The erosion of the cortex may cause pain and swelling and increase the incidence of pathologic fractures. Multiple growths, termed endochondromatosis, may also occur in childhood and, like multiple osteochondromas, may undergo malignant transformation.

Simple Bone Cyst

A **simple bone cyst** is a wall of fibrous tissue filled with fluid. These frequently occur in the long bones of children, most commonly in the humerus and proximal femur. Eighty percent of all simple bone cysts occur between 3 and 14 years of age, and twice as often in boys as in girls. The cyst is usually first noticed when the patient presents with pain caused by the increased tumor growth or as a result of a pathologic fracture.

Radiographically, simple bone cysts appear radiolucent with well-defined margins from the normal bone surrounding the lesion (Fig. 2-45). Occasionally, the cyst may be surrounded by a thin rim of sclerotic bone. Small cysts tend to heal and obliterate themselves; larger cysts require surgical intervention. The benign bone cyst is treated by surgical excision and packing with bone chips to obtain complete healing.

Osteoid Osteoma and Osteoblastoma

Other common benign tumors of the skeletal system are the **osteoid osteoma** and the **osteoblastoma**. Similar in histologic features, they differ in size, origin, and symptoms. Osteoid osteomas are less than 2 cm in dimension, whereas osteoblastomas are larger. Osteoblastomas more frequently involve the spine, and

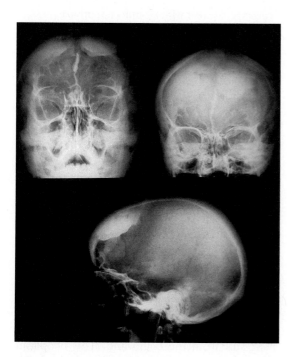

FIG. 2-43 Various skull projections demonstrating hyperostosis frontalis interna.

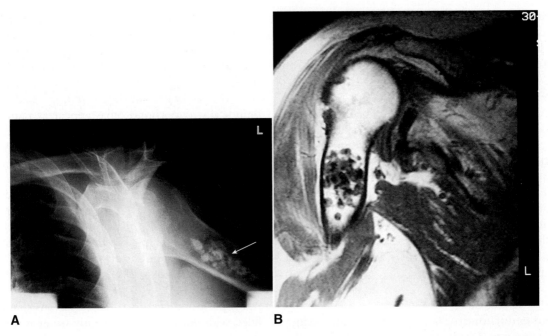

FIG. 2-44 A, Conventional shoulder radiograph in a 66-year-old man demonstrates calcification in the proximal diaphysis of the right humerus. **B,** Follow-up MRI demonstrates an intramedullary lesion without breakthrough of the cortex, consistent with an endochondroma.

pain may not be present. Further, they are not associated with a marked bony reaction or new bone production and are classified radiographically as osteolytic lesions. Osteoblastomas have a higher recurrence rate than osteoid osteomas and in rare cases may undergo malignant transformation to osteogenic sarcoma.

Osteoid osteomas occur twice as often in men as in women and almost always develop before the age of 30 years. Osteoid osteomas are most commonly found in the femur, tibia, or spine of the young adult. They arise within the cortical bone and erode the underlying bone tissue, resulting in a lytic lesion called a nidus. The area of erosion is surrounded by a zone of dense, sclerotic bone, making the radiographic appearance of osteoid osteomas very distinctive (Fig. 2-46). The radiographic appearance of an osteoid osteoma demonstrates a well- circumscribed, small radiolucent area containing a dense center (nidus). The radiolucent area is surrounded by very dense, sclerotic

bone. The nidus is comprised of osteoid or newly formed bone; thus, this tumor is classified as an osteosclerotic lesion. Radionuclide bone scans are also of value in identifying and localizing osteoid osteomas. The erosion of the surrounding tissue causes extreme pain, often at night, which is readily relieved by aspirin. Surgical removal is the treatment for both an osteoblastoma and an osteoid osteoma.

Giant Cell Tumor (Osteoclastoma)

Giant cell tumors (GCTs) are characterized by the presence of numerous, multinucleated osteoclastic giant cells. Unlike the previously mentioned neoplastic diseases, GCTs may be either benign or malignant. Approximately 50% of osteoclastomas are benign, 35% recur after surgical excision, and 15% are aggressively malignant from the beginning. This neoplasm affects the sexes equally and is found in individuals between the ages of 20 to 30 years. Anatomically, this disease tends to affect the

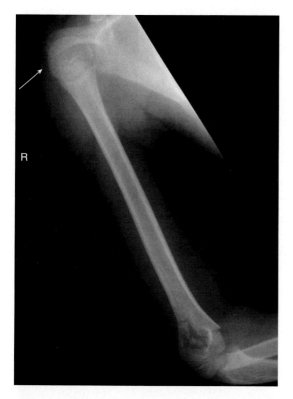

FIG. 2-45 AP radiograph demonstrating a well-circumscribed radiolucency consistent with a simple bone cyst.

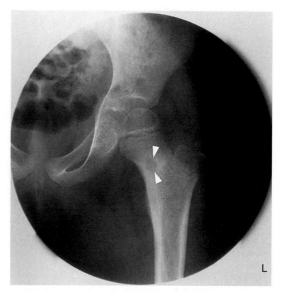

FIG. 2-46 AP hip radiograph of a 7-year-old girl who complained of a 2-month history of aching pain. The radiograph demonstrates an osteoid osteoma as evidenced by the well-defined defect in the cortical area of the femoral neck.

ends or epiphyses of long bones, especially the lower femur, upper tibia, and lower radius. It begins in the medullary canal and expands outward, producing a club-like deformity of the end of the long bone. In addition, soft tissue extensions may be present, but the GCT does not involve the joint space.

Clinical signs and symptoms of a GCT are nonspecific and include pain, tenderness, an occasional palpable mass, and an occasional pathologic fracture. Because this is an osteo-clastic disease process, bone and cartilage for-mation generally do not occur in these lesions; therefore, the technologist must decrease expo-sure factors to avoid overpenetration of the affected bone. Radiographically, a GCT pre-sents as a mass of osteolytic or cystic areas sur-rounded by a thin shell of bone, giving it the classic "soap bubble" appearance (Fig. 2-47). GCTs are usually located in the epiphysis, pro-ducing erosion and thinning of the cortical bone without new bone growth. Treatment of an osteoclastoma consists of surgical excision and bone grafting.

Osteosarcoma (Osteogenic Sarcoma)

Except for myeloma, the most common pri-mary malignancy of the skeleton is the **osteo-sarcoma**, which arises from osteoblasts. The etiology of osteosarcoma is unknown, but researchers believe it may involve genetic and environmental factors, such as exposure to radiation. This neoplasm is most frequently found in the metaphyses of long bones, with approximately 50% affecting the knee (Fig. 2-48). Osteosarcoma can occur at any age, but 75% occur in patients younger than 20 years old. It is occasionally seen in older indi-viduals with Paget's disease or following high-level radiation exposure to the bone. Clinically, the patient may present with pain and swelling.

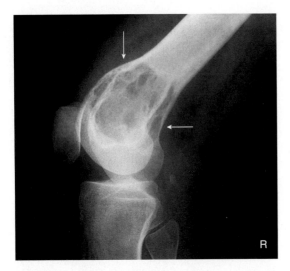

FIG. 2-47 Lateral knee radiograph of a 30-year-old man who complained of a painful knee for approximately 2 months. The radiograph demonstrates a benign osteoclastoma of the knee.

Osteosarcoma is a highly malignant disease with a poor prognosis because lung metastasis almost always occurs via the bloodstream. This metastatic lung disease may appear as multiple, rounded, calcified shadows within the lung fields on a conventional chest radiograph. If the chest radiograph is clear, high-resolution CT of the chest often demonstrates micrometastases, which are commonly present in the lungs before the primary osteosarcoma is discovered. Secondary growths or spread to other bones is very rare with osteosarcoma. In the past, treatment of osteosarcoma included amputation of the limb followed by chemotherapy. Today, most physicians place the patient on preoperative chemotherapy after the initial diagnosis is confirmed by bone biopsy. After initial chemotherapy, the patient undergoes surgical removal of the affected bone with immediate prosthesis placement. This is followed by postsurgical

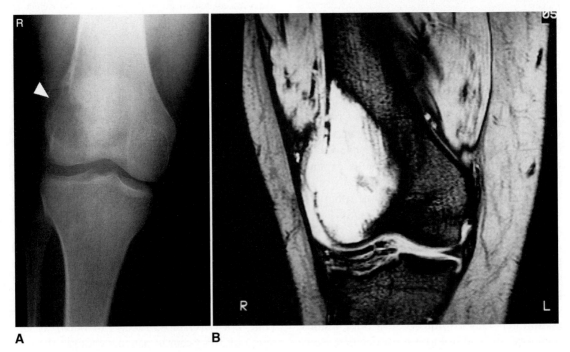

A **B**

FIG. 2-48 A, AP radiograph of the right knee demonstrates a tumor in the distal lateral femoral condyle. Interruption of the cortex and reactive sclerotic bone changes are suspect for metastatic disease or primary malignancy. **B,** Follow-up MRI of the knee reveals an osteosarcoma that has replaced the distal femoral condyle.

chemotherapy involving high doses of metho-trexate. This change in the management of osteosarcoma has increased 5-year survival rates from 20% to over 80%.

As the tumor grows from the metaphysis, it lifts the periosteum from the cortical bone and lays down spicules of new bone radiating out from the origin, which gives the radiographic appearance of a sunray or sunburst. This appearance results from the radiopaque and radiolucent changes within the newly created space between the cortex of the metaphysis and the displaced periosteum. However, radiographic findings (Figs. 2-49 and 2-50) vary greatly in appearance because some osteosarcoma tumors produce very little osteoid tissue and contain no calcifications, and others are densely opaque. In both cases, the radiograph would not display the characteristic sunray appearance. Accurate diagnosis must be made through biopsy of the questionable lesion. Blood serum analysis often shows elevated serum alkaline phosphatase as a result of the osteoblastic activity.

Ewing's Sarcoma

Another primary malignant bone tumor is a **Ewing's sarcoma**. This neoplasm occurs at a younger age than any other primary malignant bone neoplasm, usually between the ages of 5 and 15 years and rarely after age 30. It is also more common in boys than in girls and shows a predilection for whites, with blacks rarely affected.

Unlike osteosarcoma, Ewing's sarcoma arises from the medullary canal and involves the bone more diffusely, giving rise to uniform thickening of the bone. These lesions tend to be very extensive, often involving the entire shaft of a long bone. Also unlike osteogenic sarcoma, Ewing's sarcoma does not begin at the end of a long bone. It does, however, tend to affect the extremities and pelvis. Although Ewing's sarcoma is a fairly rare disease, it is extremely malignant. Increasingly effective chemotherapy has improved the prognosis to an 80% 5-year survival rate. Clinical symptoms are nonspecific

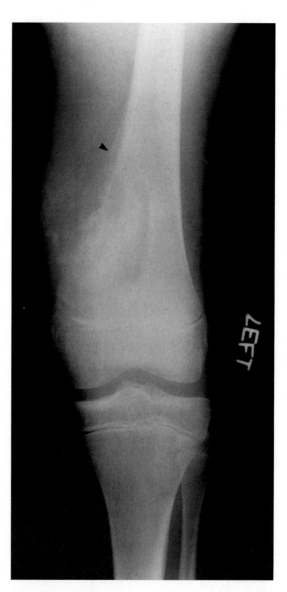

FIG. 2-49 PA projection of the knee of a 14-year-old boy with painful swelling above the left knee. The radiograph demonstrates cortical destruction along the posteromedial margin of the distal femur consistent with an osteosarcoma of the left femur.

and include pain and tenderness of the affected area. The lesions undergo a combination of bone formation in the early stages and destruction in the later stages, with new bone being formed on the surface (Fig. 2-51). This process

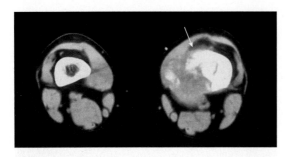

FIG. 2-50 MRI of the left femur of the patient in Fig. 2-49. MRI is helpful in determining the medullary extension of the osteosarcoma.

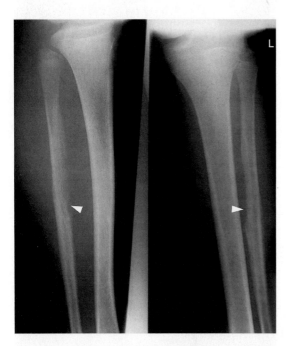

FIG. 2-51 Lower leg radiographs of a 12-year-old boy complaining of left leg pain demonstrating a Ewing's sarcoma of the tibia as indicated by the lytic defect in the proximal diaphysis of the fibula.

often gives a classic onionskin or laminated appearance radiographically.

Chondrosarcoma

A chondrosarcoma is a malignant tumor of cartilaginous origin and is composed of atypical cartilage. It is only about half as common as

osteosarcoma and comprises approximately 10% of all malignant tumors of the skeletal system. Common locations for chondrosarcoma are the pelvis, shoulder, and ribs. Men are three times more likely than women to develop chondrosarcoma, and it is more common in older adults. As mentioned earlier in this chapter, benign exostoses and multiple endochondromas may be transformed into chondrosarcomas. However, this type of change accounts for only about 10% of the cases, with approximately 90% of chondrosarcomas arising afresh without prior cartilaginous lesions. Chondrosarcomas may be bulky, and they tend to destroy the bone as they extend through the cortex into the surrounding soft tissue. These lesions have the ability to implant or seed into the surrounding soft tissue, so careful excision is a necessity. Radiographically, a chondrosarcoma shows irregular or circular radiolucencies in combination with granular areas of calcification. These tumors cause destruction and penetration of the cortex and extension into the surrounding soft tissue. Often the actual tumor may be larger than its radiographic appearance. Neither radiation therapy nor chemotherapy is particularly effective in the treatment of chondrosarcomas. Major surgery, such as amputation or chest resection, is often the treatment of choice, leading to approximately a 40% 5-year survival rate.

Metastases from Other Sites

Virtually any type of cancer can metastasize to bone; metastatic disease from carcinomas is the most common malignant tumor of the skeleton, with secondary bone tumors of any origin far outnumbering primary bone tumors. Patients presenting with skeletal metastases are usually past the fourth decade in age. Principal signs are pain and pathologic fracture.

The bones of the skeletal system that contain red bone marrow are the major bones affected by the metastatic disease because of their good vascularization. These include flat bones (such as the ribs, sternum, pelvis, and skull), the vertebrae, and the upper ends of the femora

(Fig. 2-52) and humeri. The spine is the most common site for metastasis to occur, accounting for about 40% of all metastatic lesions. Radionuclide bone scans are more accurate than conventional radiography in detection of metastasis because 3% to 5% bone destruction produces a "hot spot." Metastatic bone lesions appear as multiple, irregularly distributed areas of increased uptake that do not correspond to a single anatomic structure (Fig. 2-53). Bone scans are extremely helpful in assessing metastatic breast cancer because approximately 20% of women with breast cancer present with a solitary area of increased activity, often without pain, in the site of the metastatic tumor. Radiographically, signs of bone metastasis include alteration of bone density and architecture. These can be osteolytic, osteoblastic, or mixed. Osteolytic metastases account for 75% of all metastatic lesions, and in order to be visible radiographically, the lesions must be greater than 1 cm in diameter with a loss of about 30% to 50% of bone density. CT is often employed, especially in the spine, to clear up discrepancies where a bone scan may indicate metastatic disease that cannot be confirmed by plain

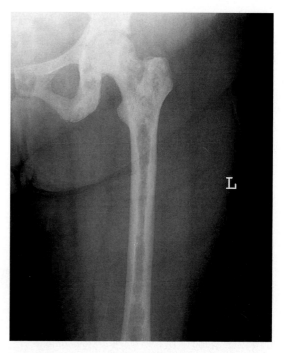

FIG. 2-52 AP hip radiograph demonstrating metastatic disease from a primary breast cancer.

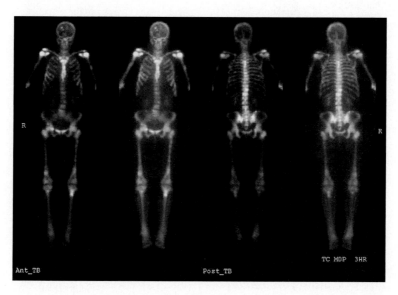

FIG. 2-53 Bone scan of the patient in Fig. 2-52 demonstrating multiple areas of metastatic disease.

radiographic analysis. MRI may also be employed to differentiate between tumor tissue and normal bone marrow.

Certain characteristics help distinguish between a primary malignant neoplasm and a secondary one. Periosteal response is much more common with primary malignant tumors. Soft tissue masses are common in primary tumors and rare in metastases. Lesions longer than 10 cm often represent a primary malignant tumor; most metastatic tumors range between 2 and 4 cm in length. Tumors that expand bone are primary in nature, with rare exception. Most primary tumors are solitary, whereas metastatic lesions are usually multiple. Definitive diagnosis is obtained through biopsy.

The most common primary sites for metastatic bone cancer are the breast, lung, prostate, kidney, thyroid, and bowel, with the tumor spreading via proximity (direct extension), the bloodstream, or the lymphatic system. Treatment of metastatic disease is dependent on the primary disease, but radiation therapy in combination with either chemotherapy or hormone therapy is commonly used to manage such patients. Bone scans are used to follow the progress of therapy; a reduction in uptake on serial scans is a positive sign.

PATHOLOGY SUMMARY: THE SKELETAL SYSTEM

Pathology	Imaging Modalities of Choice	Additive or Subtractive Pathology
Osteogenesis imperfecta	Radiographs	Subtractive
Achondroplasia	Radiographs	None
Osteopetrosis	Radiographs	Additive
Anencephaly	Ultrasound	None
Osteomyelitis	Nuclear medicine bone scans and MRI	Subtractive
Tuberculosis	Radiographs	Subtractive
Acute arthritis	Radiographs	Subtractive (early) Additive (healing)
Rheumatoid arthritis	Radiographs	Both
Ankylosing spondylitis	Radiographs	Additive
Osteoarthritis	Radiographs	Subtractive
Inflammation of joint structures	MRI	None
Gouty arthritis	Radiographs	Subtractive
Osteoporosis	Bone mineral densitometry	Subtractive
Osteomalacia	Bone mineral densitometry	Subtractive
Paget's disease	Radiographs	Both
Hyperparathyroidism	Radiographs	Additive
Acromegaly	Radiographs	Additive
Osteochondroma	CT	Additive
Osteoma	CT	Additive
Endochondroma	CT	Subtractive
Simple bone cyst	CT	Subtractive
Osteoid osteoma	CT	Subtractive
Osteoblastoma	CT	Subtractive
Giant cell tumor	CT	Subtractive
Osteosarcoma	CT	Additive
Ewing's sarcoma	CT	Both
Chondrosarcoma	CT	Subtractive
Bone metastases from other sites	Nuclear bone scans, MRI, and CT	Subtractive

QUESTIONS

1. Specialized cells responsible of the formation of bone are termed:
   a. chondroblasts
   b. osteoblasts
   c. osteoclasts
   d. both b and c

2. A freely movable joint is classified as:
   a. amphiarthrodial
   b. diarthrodial
   c. synarthrodial
   d. triarthrodial

3. Bone marrow is located anatomically within the:
   a. cortex
   b. medullary canal
   c. periosteum
   d. trabeculae

4. The end portion of a long bone is referred to as the:
   a. epiphysis
   b. diaphysis
   c. diploë
   d. metaphysis

5. The human body normally contains:
   a. 156 bones
   b. 175 bones
   c. 197 bones
   d. 206 bones

6. The most common inherited disorder that results in dwarfism is:
   a. achondroplasia
   b. Albers-Schönberg disease
   c. osteogenesis imperfecta
   d. spina bifida

7. Osteopenia is a term used to describe the radiographic appearance associated with a decrease in bone density and is associated with:
   a. craniosynostoses
   b. osteopetrosis
   c. osteoporosis
   d. scoliosis

8. The formation of extra digits is termed:
   a. adactyly
   b. polydactyly
   c. syndactyly
   d. talipes

9. An abnormal lateral curvature of the spine is referred to as:
   a. ankylosing spondylitis
   b. scoliosis
   c. spondylolisthesis
   d. spondylolysis

10. Osteomyelitis is a disease of the skeletal system that is:
    a. arthritic
    b. congenital
    c. inflammatory
    d. neoplastic

11. Osteoarthritis affects the weight-bearing joints within the body and may be treated with:
    a. exercise
    b. medication
    c. surgery
    d. all of the above

12. The type of arthritis believed to be an autoimmune disease is:
    a. bursitis
    b. gout
    c. osteoarthritis
    d. rheumatoid arthritis

13. Rickets, which affects children, is a type of:
    a. hyperparathyroidism
    b. osteomalacia
    c. osteopetrosis
    d. osteoporosis

14. The most common benign bone tumor is the:
    a. endochondroma
    b. osteoid osteoma
    c. osteoma
    d. osteochondroma

15. All of the following are malignant neoplasms of the skeletal system except:
    a. chondrosarcoma
    b. Ewing's sarcoma
    c. osteosarcoma
    d. osteoma

16. A 60-year-old patient who was discharged from the hospital following knee replacement continued to complain of generalized pain in the area of the knee for several days. If you're this patient's physician, what imaging test might you order and why?

17. A 35-year-old woman presents to her family physician with complaints of swelling that comes and goes in her hands. What might be your initial suspicion?

18. Describe the mechanism behind the development of osteoporosis.

19. A male construction worker presents to his physician with lower back pain. What might a couple of causes be that are unrelated to the bony vertebral column?

20. In diagnosing bone tumors, what are some of the characteristics taken into consideration?

The Respiratory System

UPON COMPLETION OF CHAPTER 3, THE READER SHOULD BE ABLE TO:

- Describe the anatomic components of the respiratory system.
- Distinguish between the results obtained and uses for the various projections of the chest.
- Describe the various types of tubes, vascular access lines, and catheters used in relation to the respiratory system.
- Characterize a given condition as congenital, inflammatory, or neoplastic.
- Identify the pathogenesis of the chest pathologies cited and the typical treatments for them.
- Describe, in general, the radiographic appearance of each of the given pathologies.

ANATOMY AND PHYSIOLOGY

The respiratory system distributes air for the gas exchange with the circulatory system. This system is usually subdivided into the upper respiratory tract—the nose, mouth, pharynx, and larynx—and the lower respiratory tract—the trachea, bronchi, alveoli, and lungs (Fig. 3-1). The thoracic cavity comprises the right and left pleural cavities and the mediastinum. The parietal pleura lines the thoracic cavity, and the visceral pleura adheres directly to the lung tissue.

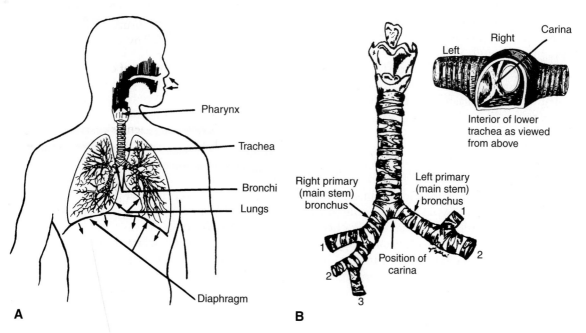

FIG. 3-1 A, The respiratory system. **B,** The trachea and its bifurcation at the carina.

Anatomically, the mediastinum is divided into anterior, middle, and posterior portions. The anterior mediastinum contains the thyroid and thymus glands. The middle mediastinum contains the heart and great vessels, esophagus, and trachea. The posterior mediastinum contains the descending aorta and spine.

The anatomic bony structures of the thorax assist in both inspiration and expiration. These bony structures include the ribs, sternum, and thoracic vertebrae.

The paranasal sinuses are lined with respiratory epithelium and communicate with the nasal cavities, hence their inclusion in this chapter. The maxillary and ethmoid sinuses are the only paranasal sinuses present at birth. The frontal sinuses generally develop shortly after birth and are fully developed by the age of 10 years. The sphenoid sinus begins to develop around the age of 2 or 3 years and is fully developed by late adolescence.

IMAGING CONSIDERATIONS

Radiography

The examination most frequently performed in any radiology department is the chest radiograph. Although this examination may seem routine, chest radiography provides important information about the soft tissues, bone, pleura, and mediastinum in addition to the lung tissue.

Exposure Factor Conditions

Correct exposure factor selection is critical because an incorrect exposure factor may hide or appear to create pathologic findings. This is particularly true for serial portable radiographs because the interpreting physician relies heavily on consistent exposure conditions to analyze the change in pathology after treatment. Institutions use various manual recording techniques for portable chest images so that different technologists can use similar exposure conditions, especially when using a film/screen imaging system. Mobile automatic exposure control (AEC) devices are available for portable situations and offer the advantage of exposure consistency associated with conventional AEC. Their use is a bit trickier in portable conditions, however, because of the reduced number of sensors. Computed radiography (CR) using indirect photostimulable phosphor imaging plates is commonly used for mobile chest radiography to eliminate exposure repeats caused by the inadequacy or inconsistency of technical factors. Although accurate technical selection is important when using indirect or direct capture digital radiography systems, both systems offer a wider latitude of error because of their wider dynamic range of useful densities.

Some sources describe pathologies, including those in the chest, as additive (harder than normal to penetrate) or subtractive (easier than normal to penetrate). In the respiratory system, any condition that adds fluid or tissue to the normally aerated chest (e.g., pneumonia) requires an increase in exposure to afford proper penetration. Similarly, any condition that increases the aeration of the chest (e.g., emphysema) reduces the amount of exposure required for proper densities to be achieved. Most experts agree that manipulation of the milliampere seconds (mAs) is the best approach for exposure adjustments when using a film/screen imaging system because kilovoltage peak (kVp) changes affect image contrast, making it more difficult for the clinician to compare films. However, when chest radiography is done using a digital system, a higher kVp may be used to decrease patient dose. The kilovoltage range should be chosen based on the energy level necessary to penetrate the part of interest, keeping in mind the presence of additive or subtractive pathologies.

The use of AEC facilitates consistent radiographic exposures but requires careful analysis of the clinical history and conscious thought about the type of disease present and its location to ensure truly optimal diagnostic-quality radiographs. Activation of the sensor, for example, over an area of significant aeration or consolidation (tissue or fluid accumulation) can result in excessive or insufficient exposure, respectively, necessitating a repeat exposure. Again, experience with AEC, combined with careful thought in selecting the proper sensor, can eliminate these mistakes.

Position and Projection

Patient position and projection are also critical exposure conditions that may distort the final image. Position refers to the arrangement of the patient's body (e.g., erect, supine, recumbent), and projection refers to the path of the x-ray beam [e.g., anteroposterior (AP), meaning entering through the body's anterior surface and exiting the posterior surface]. The standard projections for chest radiography are the erect posteroanterior (PA) and left lateral (Fig. 3-2). Each of these serves to place the heart closest to the film because it lies in the anterior part of the chest and mostly to the left side. When combined with a standard 72-inch source-to-image distance (SID), magnification of the heart is minimized.

Chest Radiographs

On a normal erect PA chest image, the costophrenic and cardiophrenic angles are demonstrated with the right hemidiaphragm appearing 1 to 2 cm higher than the left because of the liver. When a patient is radiographed in a recumbent position, the lower lung fields may be obscured because of abdominal pressure raising the level of the diaphragm (Fig. 3-3).

Other projections of the thorax are used less frequently than the erect PA and left lateral chest radiographs. The AP projection is the method of choice for portable radiography when the patient is too ill to tolerate a visit to the department and assume an erect position. As much as possible, it is important that portable or mobile chest radiographs be taken

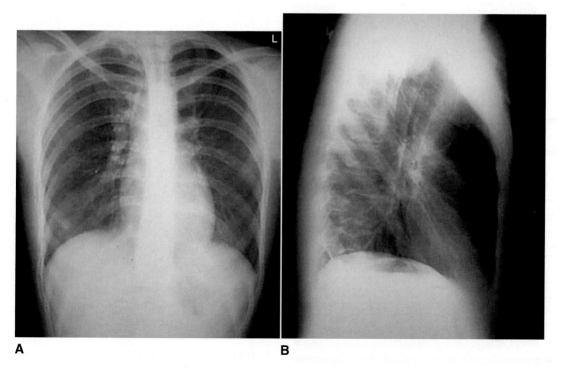

FIG. 3-2 A, Normal erect PA chest. **B,** Normal erect lateral chest.

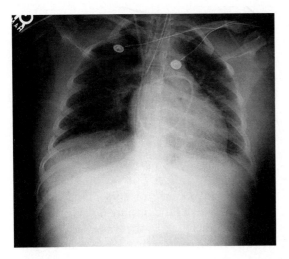

FIG. 3-3 Recumbent AP chest demonstrating obscuring of the lower lung fields.

in an erect position with the patient sitting in bed to demonstrate any air-fluid levels present. Maintenance of the beam perpendicular to the plane of the image receptor is most important to avoid any foreshortening of the heart. Further, use of the 72-inch SID is most important for portable radiography to minimize magnification of the heart, which is located further from the image receptor in the AP projection.

The AP or PA projections of the patient lying in a lateral decubitus position are also useful under specific conditions, such as diagnosing free air in the pleural space or pleural fluid. For example, for a right lateral decubitus chest radiograph, the patient lies on his or her right side. In this position, any fluid present tends to layer out along the edge of the lung field on the dependent side, which enhances its visibility, whereas the free air rises toward the left side.

For evaluation of the standard PA chest radiograph, the size and radiolucency of both lungs should be compared. Criteria for adequate inspiration and penetration of chest radiographs vary from institution to institution; however, a rule of thumb is that adequate inspiration should provide visualization of 10 posterior ribs within the lung field. Additionally, all thoracic vertebrae and intervertebral disk spaces

should be faintly visible through the mediastinum on an adequately penetrated chest radiograph. The average movement of the lungs and diaphragm between inspiration and expiration is approximately 3 cm (Fig. 3-4).

Oblique projections of the thorax are useful in separating superimposed structures such as the sternum, esophagus, and thoracic spine. A lordotic chest radiograph is useful in demonstrating the apical regions of the lung, which are normally obscured by bony structures on the standard PA projection (Fig. 3-5). Certain diseases (e.g., tuberculosis [TB]) have a predilection for the apices. Fluoroscopy of the chest is rarely performed today, but it may be used to appraise the movements of the diaphragm or to assist the physician in biopsy procedures.

CR has emerged as an imaging modality important in chest radiography (Fig. 3-6), particularly in portable situations such as the intensive care unit. Most CR applications used for mobile radiography feature indirect conversion systems utilizing photostimulable phosphor plate technology as a replacement for the typical film-screen combination. Direct radiography or direct conversion systems may also be employed in stationary chest radiography systems. Both types of digital imaging systems offer significant improvements in film latitude and image availability but offer less resolving capability than a conventional film-screen image. Precise positioning of the thorax is critical regardless of the imaging system employed, but the improvement in exposure latitude possible with CR can decrease the number of radiographs repeated for poor exposure technique—a common complaint of radiologists reading these critical films. Several advantages exist with electronic image review capabilities including the ability to maintain several days of on-line storage at the patient care site, elimination of lost films, and increased availability of the images.

Soft Tissues of the Chest

Various soft tissue densities are present on chest radiographs. They may vary with patient

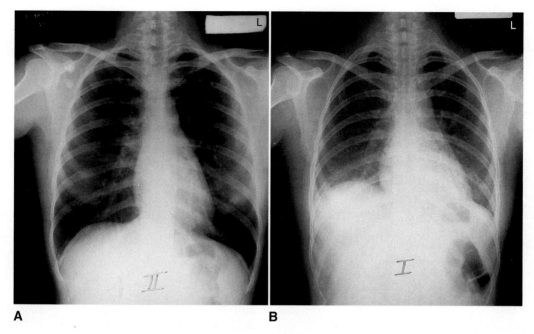

FIG. 3-4 A, Normal chest appearance on inspiration. **B,** Expiration film on the same patient demonstrates elevation of the diaphragm and a heart that is more transverse and appears larger.

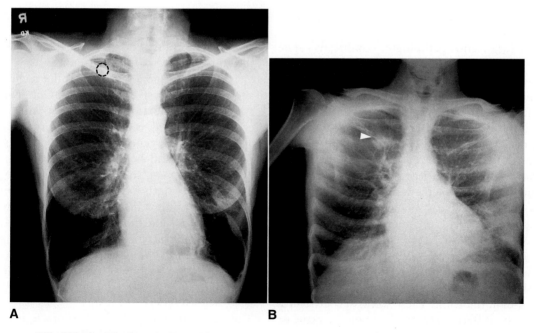

FIG. 3-5 A, PA chest radiograph reveals a suspicious density *(circled)* behind the right clavicle. **B,** Lordotic chest radiograph more clearly reveals coin lesion *(arrowhead)* previously obscured by the right clavicle, later revealed to be cancer.

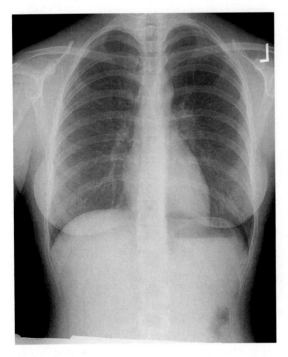

FIG. 3-6 PA chest radiograph obtained with CR.

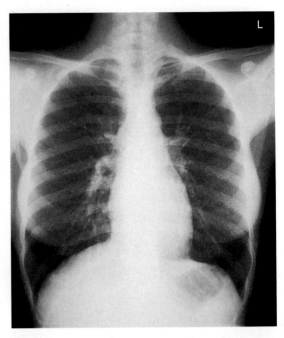

FIG. 3-7 Breast shadows are readily recognizable on the normal PA chest radiograph.

age, sex, and pathologic conditions. The pectoral muscles are normally demonstrated overlying and extending beyond the lung fields. Radiographs of both men and women demonstrate breast shadows in the midchest region (Fig. 3-7). These shadows are normally homogeneous in appearance, and female breasts may obscure the costophrenic angles. Elevation of the breasts may be necessary to better demonstrate the bases of the lungs. Surgical removal of one or both breasts is also evident on a chest radiograph; breast prostheses, which appear as well-defined, circular radiopaque densities, are also evident. Nipple shadows may be visible at the level of the fourth or fifth anterior rib spaces and may occasionally mimic nodules or masses in the chest. These soft tissue structures may be differentiated with nipple markers or oblique projections of the chest.

Bony Structures of the Chest

The ribs, sternum, and thoracic spine enclose the thoracic cavity. These structures assist the technologist in the assessment of the technical adequacy of chest radiographs. Congenital anomalies of the ribs may be demonstrated (Fig. 3-8), as well as calcified costal cartilages. This calcification generally occurs in patients in their late 20s and beyond. Rib fractures may be seen (Fig. 3-9), sometimes with an accompanying pneumothorax. A depressed sternum (pectus excavatum) may also be demonstrated, possibly displacing the heart (Fig. 3-10). The thoracic spine may be assessed for scoliosis, which can affect the chest cavity, and kyphosis or compression fractures of the vertebrae.

The Mediastinum

The mediastinum contains all thoracic organs except the lungs. The heart occupies a large

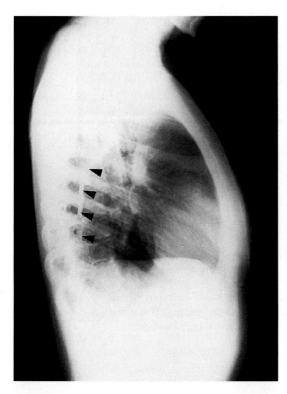

FIG. 3-8 Congenital intrathoracic rib seen as curving, tubular density in the posterior thorax. Usually, these ribs are attached at one or both ends of a posterior rib and lie extrapleurally inside the thoracic cage.

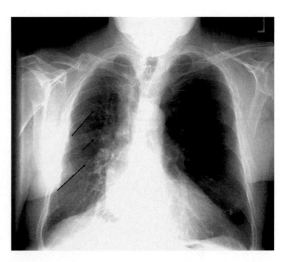

FIG. 3-9 Right-sided rib fractures *(see arrows)* in combination with a right clavicular fracture.

portion of the mediastinum, and its shape varies with age, degree of respiration, and patient position. Other organs contained within the mediastinum include the thyroid and thymus glands and nervous and lymphatic tissues.

Radiographically, the mediastinum is divided into three sections. Anterior mediastinal masses generally arise from the thyroid gland, thymus gland, or lymphatic tissue. Middle mediastinal masses are commonly lymphatic tissue, and posterior mediastinal masses usually arise from nervous or bony tissue.

In infants, the mediastinum appears wide because the thymus is normally large in a healthy infant. On frontal projections, it may extend beyond the heart borders and caudally to the diaphragm, and on a lateral projection it may fill the anterior portion of the mediastinum, which is normally radiolucent later in life. This radiographic appearance is readily visible on both PA and lateral views and is referred to as the "sail sign" because of its characteristic appearance (Fig. 3-11). Diagnosis is difficult because the width of the upper mediastinum varies greatly with the phase of respiration. A crying child may present an opportune moment for the technologist to make an exposure, but the resultant Valsalva maneuver adds to the distortion of the thymus. True mediastinal masses are rare in infants and generally represent congenital malformations or neoplasms. In the elderly mediastinum, the aorta dilates, and the aortic knob becomes much more visible.

Mediastinal emphysema (pneumomediastinum) occurs when there has been a disruption in the esophagus or airway and air is trapped in the mediastinum (Fig. 3-12). It may result from chest trauma, endoscopy, or violent vomiting. When unaccompanied by a pneumothorax, spontaneous mediastinal emphysema is usually self-limited, subsiding in a few days

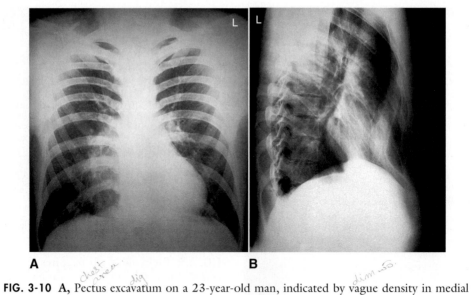

A   **B**

FIG. 3-10 A, Pectus excavatum on a 23-year-old man, indicated by vague density in medial portion of right lower lung field and obscuring of right heart margin. **B,** Lateral projection demonstrating pectus excavatum, including compression of heart toward spine.

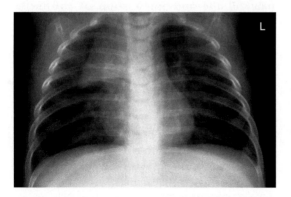

FIG. 3-11 Normal enlargement of the thymus in a 3-month-old infant demonstrates the "sail sign," evidenced by the uniform density increase in the right upper lung area.

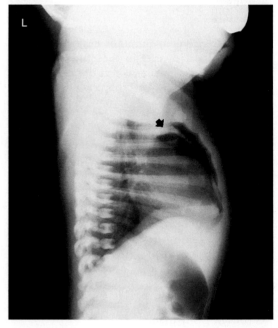

without complication. Air in the mediastinum from rupture of the esophagus (usually from vomiting) or a major bronchus (usually from trauma) is more serious and requires prompt diagnosis and surgical intervention. An esophogram may be performed with a water-soluble

FIG. 3-12 Pneumomediastinum in a lateral chest projection of a full-term newborn, evidenced by air in the normally dense retrosternal space, with sharp outlining of the heart's anterior border.

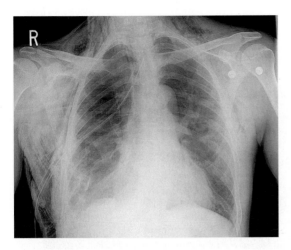

FIG. 3-13 Significant subcutaneous emphysema seen throughout the thorax, especially extending along the right border of the chest.

contrast agent to verify that a leak has not occurred.

When the pneumomediastinum is extensive, air may pass from the mediastinum into the subcutaneous tissues of the chest or neck, resulting in **subcutaneous emphysema** (Fig. 3-13). Diagnosis of this may be made by feeling air bubbles in the skin of the chest or the neck.

Glandular enlargements of the thyroid gland are demonstrated by a displacement or narrowing of the trachea. The thyroid gland is usually located superior to the lung apices, but an ectopic thyroid gland may also displace the trachea.

Clinical manifestations of an ectopic thyroid gland are often absent, and the mass may be discovered accidentally when chest radiography is performed for some other purpose. Nuclear medicine studies are the modality of choice for detecting thyroid dysfunction and location.

Computed Tomography

Computed tomography (CT) is the method of choice for evaluation of pulmonary adenopathy (Fig. 3-14). Standard radiographs are only about 50% sensitive to chest disease, typically displaying advanced pathologic conditions. On the other hand, the excellent specificity of CT can be a problem because most people have granulomatous disease, which is often benign. A rule of thumb for evaluating the character of a visualized nodule relates to its size: Those less than 1 cm in size are usually benign, and those larger than 1 cm may be malignant. Also, the presence of calcium within a nodule is a reasonable indication of benignancy, particularly in the middle of the lesion or diffusely within the nodule, but eccentric calcification may indicate malignancy.

Spiral or helical CT offers the advantage of imaging the entire chest with one breath hold, which allows better evaluation of the chest, especially the diaphragm area. These techniques have increased the sensitivity of CT to better detect emboli within the thoracic vessels (Fig. 3-15). Advances in CT software allowing high-resolution thin slice thicknesses ranging from 1 to 1.5 mm (Fig. 3-16), spiral CT, and faster scan times, in combination with dynamic scanning (Fig. 3-17), have greatly enhanced CT's role in chest imaging. Percutaneous transthoracic needle aspiration is commonly performed under CT guidance. Needle aspirations are performed to obtain cytologic specimens from lesions within the lungs (Fig. 3-18), pleural space, and mediastinum. Following the biopsy, chest x-rays should be obtained to check for a possible pneumothorax or hemorrhage.

Nuclear Medicine Procedures

Perfusion and ventilation scans, as performed in nuclear medicine, are useful in evaluating chest disease, particularly in the case of obstructive disease and pulmonary emboli. Injection of a radionuclide into the venous system for a perfusion causes it to become trapped in the pulmonary circulation, allowing for γ-camera visualization of its distribution. In a ventilation scan, the patient inhales a radioactive gas (such as xenon) and holds his or her breath while an image is taken of the gas distribution throughout the lungs (Fig. 3-19). Positron emission

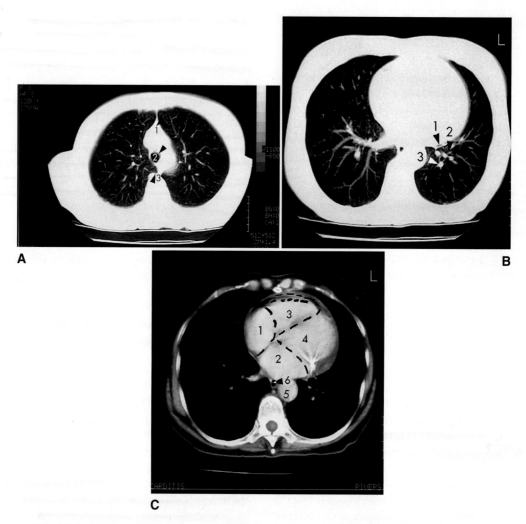

FIG. 3-14 A, Normal CT of the chest in the upper lungs with "lung windows," demonstrating *1,* the anterior junction line (sometimes seen on chest radiographs), *2,* the trachea, and *3,* the esophageal recess. **B,** CT view of the chest in the midlungs, demonstrating *1,* a pulmonary vein (distinguished from an artery because of its oval shape), *2,* bronchi, and *3,* an artery (with characteristic rounded shape). **C,** Third CT view of the same chest at the same level as **B,** with a window level adjusted to demonstrate the heart and surrounding structures. Seen are the heart's chambers, *1,* right atrium, *2,* left atrium, *3,* right ventricle, and *4,* left ventricle, as well as other structures, including *5,* the aorta, and *6,* the esophagus (fitting in the esophageal recess). The azygos vein is the small rounded density immediately inferior to the esophagus. Also seen are a small pericardial effusion immediately above the right ventricle. The star-shaped calcification in the left atrium is a mitral anulus calcification.

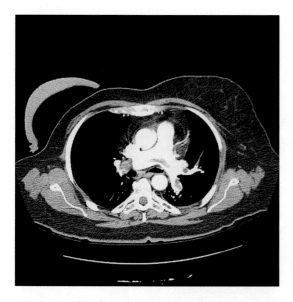

FIG. 3-15 CT of the lung demonstrating a massive embolism within the main pulmonary artery branches and smaller bronchial vessels.

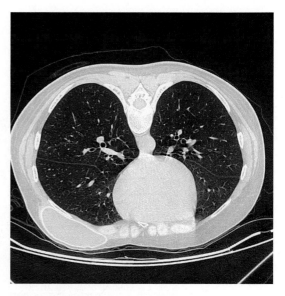

FIG. 3-16 High-resolution CT of a normal chest.

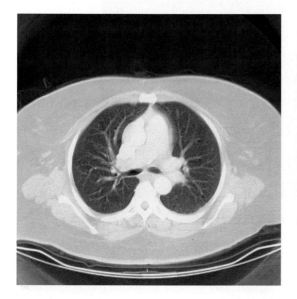

FIG. 3-17 Spiral CT of a normal chest following a bolus injection of IV contrast media.

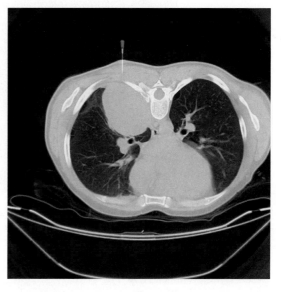

FIG. 3-18 CT-assisted core biopsy of a large right lung mass.

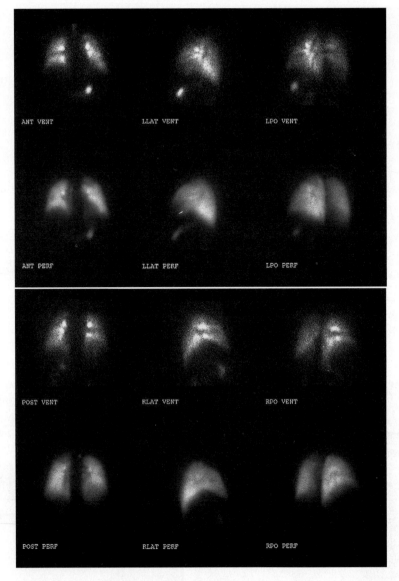

FIG. 3-19 Example of a nuclear medicine perfusion and ventilation scan performed to evaluate a possible pulmonary embolism.

tomography (PET) captures information regarding metabolic activity. The primary imaging agent used in PET of the lungs is fluorodeoxyglucose, making it useful in distinguishing benign and malignant lesions within the chest because it has the capability of imaging an increase in glucose uptake from neoplastic cells.

Because PET can image chest neoplasms before they are visible on a conventional chest radiograph, it is a promising modality for the future, especially when it is combined with CT using fusion technology. Because of cost constraints, however, PET is not currently consistently utilized in the staging of early lung cancers.

CHEST TUBES, VASCULAR ACCESS LINES, AND CATHETERS

A variety of tubes, lines, and catheters can be placed in relation to particular parts of the respiratory system. It is important for the technologist to be familiar with each of these and exercise great caution in attempting patient movement with any of these in place. It is best to have assistance from another technologist or nursing personnel to ensure that the lines and tubes are free of any obstructions before patient movement occurs. Further, the technologist who is unsure whether the patient is allowed to sit erect should always ask the patient's nurse. The x-ray tube, image receptor, and exposure technique should be established before the patient is moved. Patients in critical care units often can be erect for only a short period because of the instability of their blood pressure. Finally, it is necessary to cover cassettes

with a plastic bag to limit infection transfer and keep the cold cassette surface from touching the patient's back.

An endotracheal (ET) tube is a large plastic tube inserted through the patient's nose or mouth into the trachea. It helps to manage the patient's airway, allows frequent suctioning, and allows mechanical ventilation. Its proper position is below the vocal cords and above the carina (the bifurcation of the trachea; Fig. 3-20). Movement of a patient with an ET tube should be done with great caution because inadvertent displacement or extubation may leave the patient without a patent airway.

A chest tube is a large plastic tube inserted through the chest wall between the ribs. It allows drainage of air (e.g., pneumothorax) or fluid (e.g., pleural effusion or hemothorax) from the thoracic cavity (Fig. 3-21) and allows the lungs to inflate to help the patient breathe normally. Those placed lower on the chest wall

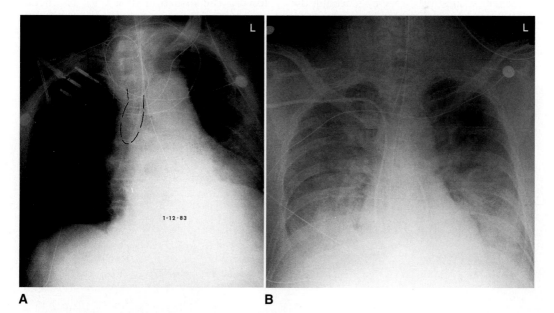

FIG. 3-20 A, Incorrect endotracheal (ET) tube placement creates shift of heart and mediastinum to the left with loss of air volume in the left lung. The ET tube tip lies in the proximal right main stem bronchus inferior to the carina. **B,** Correct placement of the ET tube demonstrating balanced lung ventilation.

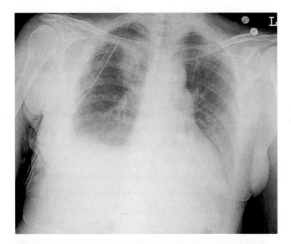

FIG. 3-21 Portable chest radiograph demonstrating proper chest tube placement in the right lung near the apex.

are usually for fluid drainage; those placed higher are usually for air removal. After open heart surgery, a chest tube may be placed in the mediastinum for proper fluid drainage. Its location is midline, just below the sternum. The collection device attached to the chest tube must be kept below the level of the chest to allow for proper drainage. The amount of time a chest tube remains in the thorax is dependent on the amount of deflation of the lung.

Central venous pressure (CVP) lines are usually inserted via the subclavian vein, but they can also be placed through the jugular vein, antecubital vein, or femoral vein. Proper insertion places the tip of the CVP catheter in the distal superior vena cava (SVC) just above the right atrium (Fig. 3-22). This catheter provides an alternative injection site to compensate for loss of peripheral infusion sites or to allow for infusion of massive volumes of fluids. In addition, it allows for measurement of CVP, which indicates the patient's fluid status and provides information about the function of the heart's right side. However, pulmonary artery catheters have largely supplanted the use of CVP lines for these purposes because they provide even greater accuracy in measurements. Chest radiographs are generally requested following the insertion of a CVP to check for proper placement and the presence of a pneumothorax or hemothorax. Improperly placed catheters can result in cardiac arrhythmias.

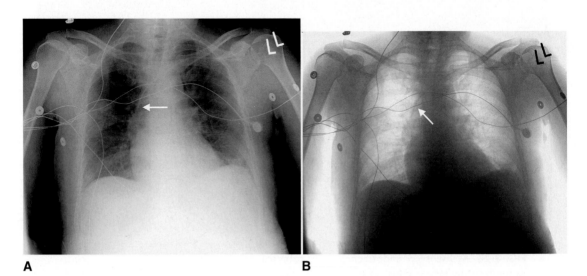

A   **B**

FIG. 3-22 A, Central venous catheter entering the left subclavian vein is positioned with the tip properly placed in the distal superior vena cava. **B,** Inverted CR image of same patient to demonstrate the advantages of CR when evaluating proper line placement.

A pulmonary artery catheter (Swan-Ganz catheter) is usually inserted via the subclavian vein, but other injection sites include the antecubital vein, jugular vein, and femoral vein. It is a multilumen catheter that serves to evaluate cardiac function. The pulmonary artery catheter measures pulmonary wedge pressure, reflecting left atrial pressure. It does not enter the heart's left side but is positioned in the pulmonary artery (Fig. 3-23). Inflation of the balloon at the tip of the catheter allows the tube to float into a smaller pulmonary artery capillary. Diagnosis and management of heart failure resulting from myocardial infarction and cardiogenic shock represent the most common use of the catheter.

Access catheters such as a Hickman catheter or a Port-A-Cath are usually inserted via the subclavian vein. Hickman catheters are open to the outside of the body with the tip of the catheter placed in the SVC (Fig. 3-24). Port-A-Cath access devices are placed under the skin, just below the clavicle. Because these devices are not open to the outside, a Port-A-Cath access device is less likely to become infected and requires little maintenance. Access catheters allow multiple tapping for injection of various agents, typically chemotherapeutics. Patients on whom these catheters are used typically have poor peripheral venous access because of the toxic effects of chemotherapeutic drugs. Location in the subclavian vein provides ready access to the venous circulation and its blood flow return to the heart. An intra-aortic balloon pump (IABP) catheter is a specialized device typically inserted in surgery or percutaneously at the bedside in critical care units. A 40-cc balloon at the distal end of the catheter allows inflation and deflation by a pump that is synchronized to the patient's cardiac cycle to provide mechanical support of the left ventricle. These devices reduce the workload of the heart and help to improve systemic blood flow including an increased blood supply to the cardiac muscle. The balloon is placed in the descending aorta below the subclavian artery and above the renal arteries (Fig. 3-25). Particular caution should be used in moving these

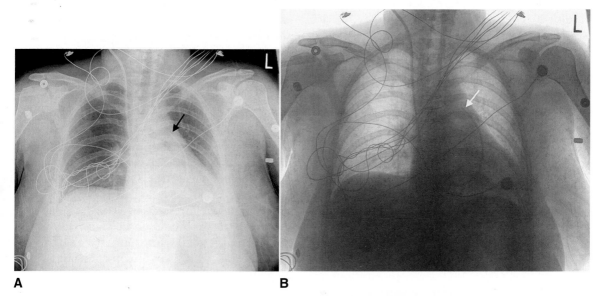

A   **B**

FIG. 3-23 A, Swan-Ganz catheter placement from the right interjugular vein (IJ) with the tip in the proximal right pulmonary artery. **B,** Inverted computed CR image of same patient to demonstrate the advantages of CR when evaluating proper line placement.

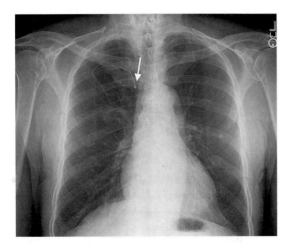

FIG. 3-24 Correct placement of a central venous access catheter inserted via the right jugular vein with the tip located within the superior vena cava.

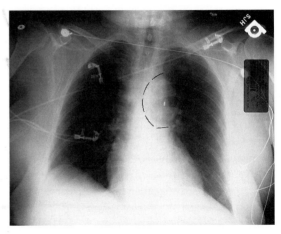

FIG. 3-25 Portable chest radiograph demonstrates proper placement of an intra-aortic balloon pump in the descending thoracic aorta of this 76-year-old woman following a myocardial infarction.

patients because movement may cause the balloon to float downward, possibly blocking the lower circulation.

Ventricular pacing electrodes may be placed for temporary or permanent purposes. Temporary pacing electrodes are inserted via the antecubital vein into the right ventricle. They provide electrical pacing of the heart in patients experiencing a very slow heart rate (i.e., bradycardia) as a result of misfiring of the heart's electrical system. Also, patients who have had open heart surgery may have these electrodes placed directly on the heart's surface and brought externally beneath the sternum at midline as a temporary precaution against heart arrhythmia problems. Permanent electrodes are used for permanent heart pacing needs. The pacemaker generator is inserted under the skin below the right clavicle, with the electrodes placed into the right ventricle (Fig. 3-26).

RESPIRATORY FAILURE

Respiratory failure is a term used to describe lack of respiratory function or the lack of

oxygen and carbon dioxide exchange. This can occur at two levels: within the lungs (intrapulmonary gas exchange) or as a result of impaired breathing (inability to move air into and out of the lungs). **Hypoxemia** denotes low oxygen levels within the arterial blood and is caused by toxic gas or smoke inhalation, high altitudes, hypoventilation, or impaired diffusion (a physical separation of gas and blood). In cases of congenital heart defects, hypoxemia can also be caused by shunting of blood from the right side to the left side of the heart without passing through the lungs. The term **hypercapnia** denotes the inability to move air into and out of the lungs, with consequent increased blood carbon dioxide content.

Respiratory failure (i.e., hypoxemia and/or hypercapnia) may be caused by an obstructed airway, insufficient respiratory drive, respiratory muscle fatigue, intrinsic lung disease, or a dysfunction of the central nervous system resulting in a defective ventilatory pump. Individuals in respiratory failure usually exhibit tachypnea, tachycardia, irregular or gasping breathing patterns, and paradoxic abdominal motion. If

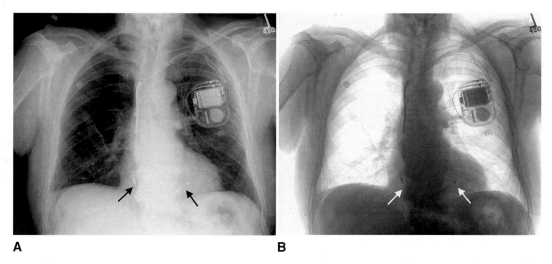

FIG. 3-26 A, Portable chest radiograph taken after pacemaker insertion demonstrating proper placement of lead wires. **B,** Inverted CR image of same patient.

the hypoxemia is acute, it may cause cardiac arrhythmias and alteration of consciousness ranging from confusion to coma.

Arterial blood gas measurement is the primary method of diagnosing respiratory failure as well as determining the severity of the failure. Chest radiographs are often obtained to help identify the cause of failure. The treatment of respiratory failure includes the administration of oxygen therapy with the use of specialized, nonventilator masks termed continuous positive airway pressure (CPAP) and bilevel positive airway pressure (BiPAP) devices. Individuals may also be intubated and placed on a mechanical positive pressure ventilator (PPV). Care must also be taken to maintain cardiac output and assist the failing circulation secondary to cardiac dysfunction.

CONGENITAL AND HEREDITARY DISEASES

Cystic Fibrosis

Cystic fibrosis is a generalized disorder resulting from a genetic defect transmitted as an autosomal recessive gene that affects the function of exocrine glands. The recessive gene responsible for the development of cystic fibrosis has been localized to 250,000 base pairs of genomic DNA on chromosome 7q. It involves many organs in addition to the respiratory system, and nearly all exocrine glands are affected in varying distribution and degree of severity. These glands and other organs affected include the salivary glands, small bowel, pancreas, biliary tract, female cervix, and male genital system. In the respiratory system, evidence suggests that the lungs are histologically normal at birth. Pulmonary damage is initiated by gradually increasing secretions from hypertrophy of bronchial glands, leading to obstruction of the bronchial system. The resultant plugging promotes staphylococcal infection, followed by more tissue damage, as well as atelectasis (collapse of lung tissue) and emphysema. Once the cycle is in motion, it is difficult to stop. The signs and symptoms of cystic fibrosis usually include a chronic cough and wheezing associated with recurrent or chronic pulmonary infections. The cough is often accompanied by sputum, gagging, vomiting, and disturbed sleep. A barrel-chest deformity, clubbing of the fingers, and cyanosis occur as the disease progresses. In adolescents and adults the pulmonary complications associated with cystic fibrosis include pneumothorax, hemoptysis, and right heart failure secondary to pulmonary hypertension.

The disease remains the most common lethal genetic disease for white children despite increasing life spans to the age of 20 years or older because of improved treatments. Its diagnosis rests largely on certain clinical and laboratory findings, most notably elevated sodium and chloride levels in sweat. Chest radiographs aid in the diagnosis of cystic fibrosis. Radiographs taken over a period of years demonstrate gradually worsening structural abnormalities. Early changes of bronchial thickening and hyperinflation (Fig. 3-27) progress to extensive bronchiectasis, cyst formation, lobar atelectasis, scarring, pulmonary artery and right ventricular enlargement, and overinflation of the lung and

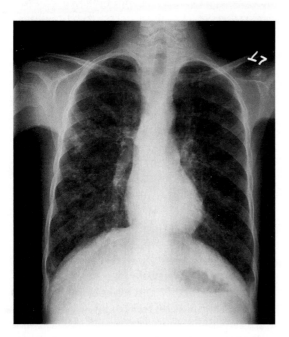

FIG. 3-27 Increased lung volume resulting from generalized obstructive disease and air trapping, which is characteristic of cystic fibrosis, as seen in this 9-year-old boy. Also seen are areas of irregular aeration with cystic and nodular densities.

chest wall. Conventional sinus radiographs and CT studies of the paranasal sinuses demonstrate persistent opacification of the paranasal sinuses.

The prognosis associated with cystic fibrosis is determined by the degree of pulmonary involvement and varies greatly. However, respiratory failure due to deterioration of the lungs is inevitable and eventually leads to death in the late 20s to early 30s. Treatment methods include antimicrobial drugs to combat infection, bronchodilators administered through inhalers, and respiratory physical therapy. The development of a pneumothorax can be treated by closed chest tube thoracostomy drainage, and massive or recurrent hemoptysis is treated by embolizing involved bronchial arteries. Expert psychological guidance is also important in helping affected patients adjust to limitations to their quality of life.

Hyaline Membrane Disease

Also known as **respiratory distress syndrome** (RDS), hyaline membrane disease affects infants and is a disorder of prematurity or infants born at less than a 37-week gestation. Incomplete maturation of the surfactant-producing system causes unstable alveoli, the structures in which gas exchanges occur in the lungs. Infants are particularly in need of a low surface tension in the alveoli, and surfactant (an agent that lowers surface tension) provides this. Its deficiency results in alveolar collapse with widespread atelectasis. The signs of RDS include rapid and labored breathing immediately or within a few hours after delivery with the atelectasis and respiratory failure progressively worsening. In severe cases, respiratory and metabolic acidosis develop because blood passing through the lungs is not adequately oxygenated and its carbon dioxide is inadequately eliminated.

Chest radiographs demonstrate severe atelectasis with an air-bronchogram sign, characterized by bronchi surrounded by nonaerated alveoli (Fig. 3-28). This is a life-threatening condition, but, if the infant's ventilation is adequately supported, surfactant production

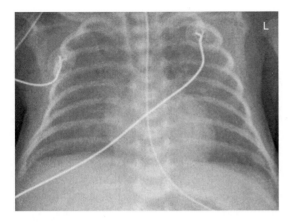

FIG. 3-28 Respiratory distress syndrome in a preterm infant. Notice the "ground glass" appearance of the lungs, especially in the right perihilar area.

should begin within a few days. Treatment consists of maintenance of a proper thermal environment and satisfactory levels of tissue oxygenation, which is monitored frequently via arterial blood gas measurements. In some instances, pulmonary surfactant may be introduced intratracheally to reduce the severity of the disease. Once the surfactant is present, RDS will resolve by 4 or 5 days.

INFLAMMATORY DISEASES

Pneumonias

Pneumonia is the most frequent type of lung infection, resulting in an inflammation of the lung (pneumonitis) and compromised pulmonary function. Pneumonia ranks sixth among the leading causes of death in the United States and is the most common lethal nosocomial infection. The main causes of pneumonia are bacteria, viruses, and mycoplasmas. In adults, bacteria such as *Streptococcus, Staphylococcus, Pneumococcus, Haemophilus influenzae, Chlamydia pneumoniae,* and *Legionella pneumophila* are the most common causes of pneumonia. A bacteria-like organism termed *Mycoplasma pneumoniae* is a common cause of pneumonia

in adolescents and young adults. Viral pathogens are most common in infants and children; however, they may also cause pneumonia in adults. Fungal infections such as *Pneumocystis carinii* may also cause pneumonia, especially in immunodepressed patients.

The inflammation may affect the entire lobe of a lung (lobar pneumonia), a segment of a lung (segmental pneumonia), the bronchi and associated alveoli (bronchopneumonia), or the interstitial lung tissue (interstitial pneumonia). Chest radiographs are important in determining the location of the inflammation, with the pneumonias appearing as soft, patchy, ill-defined alveolar infiltrates or pulmonary densities. Alveolar infiltration results when the alveolar air spaces are filled with fluid or cells. Symptoms associated with pneumonia include a cough, fever, and sputum production, usually developing over days. Individuals with pneumonia often exhibit tachypnea, and on physical evaluation, crackles may be heard in conjunction with bronchial breath sounds.

Pneumococcal (lobar) **pneumonia** is the most common bacterial pneumonia because this type of bacteria is often present in healthy throats. This infection is generally preceded by an upper respiratory infection. When the body defenses are weakened, the bacteria multiply, work their way into the lungs, and inflame the alveoli. This disease is usually accompanied by chills, a cough, and a fever. Pneumococcal pneumonia generally affects the alveoli of an entire lobe of a lung, without affecting the bronchi themselves (Fig. 3-29). Chest radiographs demonstrate a collection of fluid in one or more lobes, with a lateral view serving to identify the degree of segmental involvement. Pleural fluid can often be seen in lateral decubitus projections of the chest. Antibiotics, based on Gram stain laboratory results, patient age, and epidemiology, as well as bed rest are the treatment for pneumococcal pneumonia, which is usually resolved in approximately 1 week.

Far less frequent types of bacterial pneumonia are staphylococcal and streptococcal

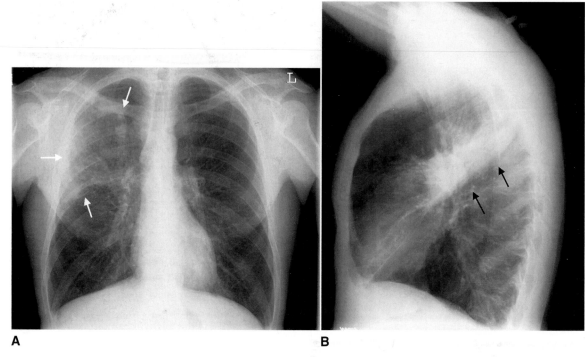

FIG. 3-29 PA (**A**) and lateral (**B**) chest radiographs demonstrating pneumococcal pneumonia infiltrates in the upper lobe of the right lung. Notice the lateral projection clearly demonstrates the segment of the lobe affected, and the PA projection shows a faint outline of the air-filled bronchi.

pneumonia (Fig. 3-30). **Staphylococcal pneumonia** occurs sporadically except during epidemics of influenza, when secondary infection with staphylococci is common. It is severe and may be fatal, especially in infants. A pneumatocele (a thin-walled, air-containing cyst) is the characteristic radiographic lesion and is more typically seen in children. These may enlarge and form abscesses in the later stages of the disease. Another characteristic sign is the spread of patchy areas localized in and around the bronchi (Fig. 3-31). Drug therapy with particular chemotherapeutic agents is the treatment of choice.

Streptococcal pneumonias are even rarer, accounting for fewer than 1% of all hospital admissions for acute bacterial pneumonia. The radiographic appearance is localized around the bronchi, usually of the lower lobes. Appropriate antibiotic therapy is the treatment of choice for this condition.

Legionnaires' disease is the name given to a severe bacterial pneumonia that became known after it caused the deaths of four people attending an American Legion convention in Philadelphia in 1976. The causative bacteria (*Legionella pneumophila*) was unknown at the time of the 1976 outbreak, and its explosive effects attracted significant attention. *Legionella pneumophila* thrives in warm, moist places and may be transmitted through heating-cooling systems. Clinically, patients complain of malaise, muscular aches, chest pain with a nonproductive cough, and occasional vomiting and diarrhea. Its radiographic appearance is similar to those of other bacterial pneumonias, with patchy

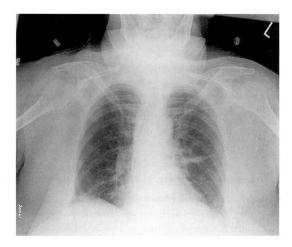

FIG. 3-30 Chest radiograph demonstrating strepto-coccal pneumonia.

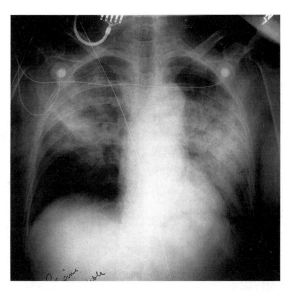

FIG. 3-32 Legionnaires' disease in a 55-year-old woman showing rounded opacities in the upper half of the right lung and lower two thirds of the left lung.

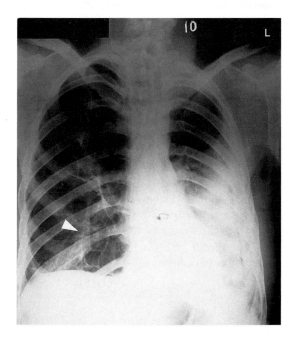

FIG. 3-31 Staphylococcal pneumonia in a 20-year-old man indicated by multiple large pneumatoceles in right lung and consolidation of the left lower lobe of the lung. An empyema in the lower left lung was later drained surgically.

infiltrates throughout the lungs (Fig. 3-32). Treatment consists primarily of antibiotic administration and oxygen therapy.

Mycoplasma pneumonia is caused by mycoplasmas, the smallest group of living organisms. They have characteristics of both bacteria and viruses. Because they do not have a typical bacterial cell wall, there was confusion among the scientific community in the past in reference to their classification. Today they are classified as bacteria-like. Mycoplasma pneumonia is most common in older children and young adults. Radiographically, this disease appears as a fine reticular pattern in a segmental distribution, followed by patchy areas of air space consolidation. In severe cases, the radiographic appearance may mimic TB. The morbidity rate associated with mycoplasma pneumonia is very low, even when the disease is not treated.

Aspiration (chemical) **pneumonia** is caused by acid vomitus aspirated into the lower respiratory tract, resulting in a chemical pneu-

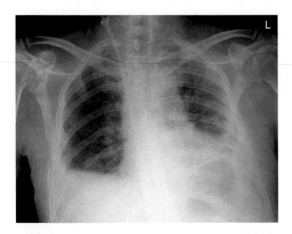

FIG. 3-33 Aspiration pneumonia caused by aspiration of gastric contents.

monitis. It may follow anesthesia, alcoholic intoxication, or stroke that causes loss of the cough reflex. Chest radiographs reveal edema produced by the irritation of the air passages (Fig. 3-33), appearing as densities radiating from one or both hila into the dependent segments. The treatment of aspiration pneumonia is strictly supportive, including correction of hypoxia, control of secretions, and replacement of fluids. Further infection is treated by antimicrobial drugs based on laboratory results.

Viral (interstitial) **pneumonia** can be caused by various viruses, most commonly influenza. It is more common than bacterial pneumonia but less severe. This disease is spread by an infected person shedding the virus to a nonimmune individual. Most cases of viral pneumonia are mild, and the radiographic findings are often minimal. The diagnosis of this disease is based on clinical findings and serologic tests. Symptoms include a dry cough and fever. Complications include secondary bacterial infections, termed superinfections, which result from a lowered resistance brought on by the inflammatory response to the virus. Otherwise, treatment of viral pneumonia usually focuses on relief of symptoms because viral infections do not respond to antibiotic agents.

Bronchiectasis

Bronchiectasis is a permanent, abnormal dilatation of one or more large bronchi as a result of destruction of the elastic and muscular components of the bronchial wall (Fig. 3-34). The basic pathogenesis is either congenital or an acquired weakness, typically following inflammation of the bronchial walls, because of a viral or bacterial infection. In the early stage of disease, the most common symptom is a chronic cough; however, some individuals may initially remain asymptomatic. As the bronchiectasis progresses, the cough becomes more productive because the weakened wall allows the bronchus to become dilated, forming a sac-like structure that is a haven for infection. As infection grows, the bronchial wall is destroyed, resulting in an abscess. These individuals may also complain of pleuritic pain and/or demonstrate recurrent fevers, wheezing, and shortness of breath upon physical examination.

Conventional chest radiographs generally demonstrate increased bronchovascular mark-

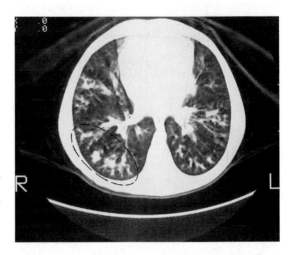

FIG. 3-34 Bronchiectatic changes are seen peripherally on this CT of the lungs from the 9-year-old patient with cystic fibrosis in Fig. 3-27. Compare the size of these bronchi with those seen in the normal chest CT (Fig. 3-14).

ings and parallel lines outlining the dilated bronchi (tram lines) because of peribronchial fibrosis and inflammation and intrabronchial secretions. Occasionally areas of honeycombing or cystic areas may be present. Bronchography is rarely performed in cases of bronchiectasis; it has been replaced by high-resolution CT of the chest obtaining 1- to 2-mm slice images. High-resolution CT with or without contrast enhancement is able to diagnose bronchiectasis better than clinical findings and conventional radiographs alone. It clearly demonstrates dilated airways (those with a luminal diameter more than 1.5 times that of the adjacent vessel in cross section), extension of the bronchi as a result of the destruction of lung parenchyma, thickening of the bronchial walls, and obstruction of the airways either by a mucus plug or by air trapping. Additional information regarding the extent of bronchiectasis and its distribution within a segment of lung may be obtained using helical or spiral CT (Fig. 3-35).

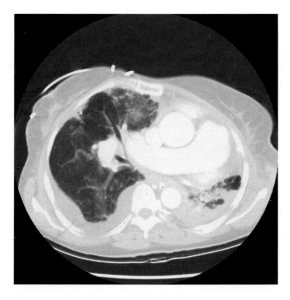

FIG. 3-35 High-resolution CT demonstrating bilateral lung bronchiectasis with associated left lung pneumatoceles.

Pulmonary Tuberculosis

Pulmonary **tuberculosis (TB)** is an infection caused by inhalation of *Mycobacterium tuberculosis*. Although *Mycobacterium tuberculosis* generally affects the lungs, it may also affect other areas of the body, such as the genitourinary, skeletal, and central nervous systems. Of great concern worldwide is an alarming increase in TB, including its rise in the United States, where it was once considered nearly eradicated. This is in part because of the development of organisms resistant to all "first-line" drugs. According to health statistics, approximately 8 out of 100,000 individuals in the United States developed TB annually in the late 1990s, primarily the elderly and those affected with human immunodeficiency virus (HIV). An estimated 1.7 billion people worldwide (including 10 million Americans) carry the TB bacteria.

Early pulmonary TB is asymptomatic almost 90–95% of the time and may be identified only with a skin test. Signs appear when the lesion or nodular scars are large enough to be seen on a chest radiograph. Lesions are most commonly seen in the apical region of the chest (Fig. 3-36); therefore, the apical lordotic projection of the chest is useful in the evaluation of TB. A positive response to intradermal injection of purified protein derivative (the Mantoux test) is the primary means of diagnosing TB. Because reading the results of this test is more art than science, further testing may be necessary to confirm the diagnosis. The most common symptom is a morning cough producing minimal mucus. As the disease progresses, the cough becomes more productive, the patient may complain of dyspnea, and a spontaneous pneumothorax or pleural effusion may develop.

If the patient is in good health, and the dose of the bacteria is fairly small, healing with scarring of the lung tissue is the most common result of infection. The presence of tuberculous scars may be demonstrated radiographically in the apex of one or both lungs. These scars result from the body's immune system

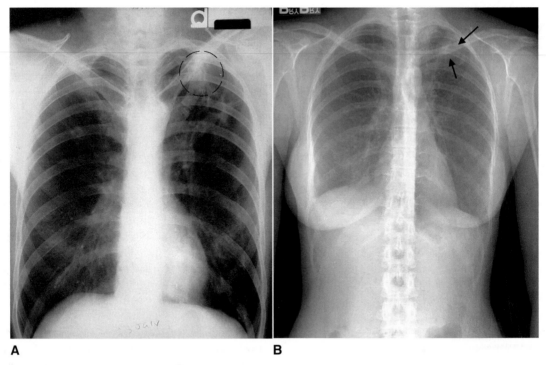

A   **B**

FIG. 3-36 A, Tuberculosis (TB) of left upper lobe in a 49-year-old man admitted with esophagitis and dull pain in the left subclavicular region. **B,** Old TB scarring evident in the left apical region just posterior to the clavicle of this female patient.

surrounding the bacilli with fibrous tissue, which invades and destroys the infectious agent. Fibrocaseous TB is usually the disease's course if the patient demonstrates active signs of TB. Necrosis is a prominent feature of the disease because its infiltration affects lung parenchyma. This infiltration may expand and produce the formation of a cavity (cavitation) (Fig. 3-37). If these cavities spread to communicate with the bronchus, the bacteria is spread throughout the lung. In elderly patients, dormant TB may reactivate and remain undiagnosed for weeks or months. Infection spreads to the lobar or segmental bronchus, causing a persistent pneumonia resistant to antibiotic therapy. As a result, these individuals are especially susceptible to **miliary TB,** which occurs when the bloodstream picks up the TB and large numbers of bacteria are carried throughout the body. Miliary refers to its characteristic resemblance

to millet seeds, which are small, white grains (Fig. 3-38). Initially the disseminated miliary pattern may not be radiographically identifiable, but when disseminated TB is suspected, chest radiographs should be repeated in a few days to better visualize the millet-sized tubercles.

In immunocompromised patients, the infection is much more aggressive. It overwhelms the immune system and progresses through the lungs at a rapid rate to cause acute tuberculous pneumonia. The body does not develop fibrous tissue to surround the bacteria, so the infection spreads quickly. Without medical treatment, acute tuberculous pneumonia may result in death within a few months. If the particular bacteria strain is resistant to drug therapy, the result is a 50% death rate within a median time of 60 days.

Patients with pulmonary TB are contagious and should be placed in respiratory isolation.

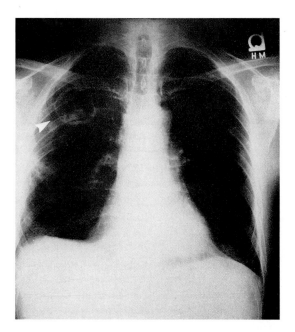

FIG. 3-37 Cavitation in the right lung resulting from expansion of tubercular lesion.

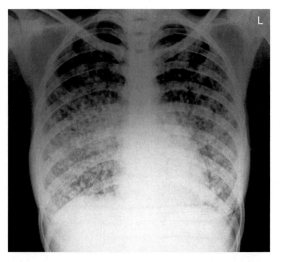

FIG. 3-38 Miliary tuberculosis (TB) resulting from hematogenous spread of TB, demonstrating small, distinct nodules throughout the lung fields.

The bacteria are spread through sputum and airborne droplets expelled on coughing. Modern treatment of TB consists primarily of various chemotherapeutic agents that are effective and usually curative if the full course is taken. TB must be treated with at least two antituberculous drugs including both bactericidal and bacteriostatic drugs that act through different mechanisms. In extreme cases where the disease shows drug resistance, surgical resection of a persistent TB may be performed to eliminate the bacteria.

Chronic Obstructive Pulmonary Disease

Chronic obstructive pulmonary disease (COPD) refers to a group of disorders that cause chronic airway obstruction. The most common forms are chronic bronchitis and emphysema, which frequently coexist and may be associated with varying degrees of asthma and bronchiectasis—two other causes of airway obstruction.

Because it may be difficult to determine whether the pulmonary obstruction is caused by bronchitis, emphysema, or a combination of the two diseases, the designation of chronic obstructive pulmonary disease is commonly used. This disease is irreversible and results in limited airflow and, in the case of emphysema, decreased elastic recoil of the alveoli. Statistics show that the mortality rate of COPD has dramatically increased over the past 20 years, and it continues to rank in the top five most common causes of death in the United States. In addition, the number of individuals diagnosed with COPD in the United States has increased over 60% since the early 1980s. The predominant risk factor associated with COPD is cigarette smoking. Air pollution, airborne chemical fumes, and inhalation of hazardous dust such as silica may also increase the risk of developing COPD but are minimal in relation to the effects of cigarette smoke.

Chronic bronchitis most often arises from long-term, heavy cigarette smoking or prolonged exposure to high levels of industrial air pollution, which irritates the mucous lining of the bronchial tree and increases susceptibility to both bacterial and viral infections. Chronic exposure to these respiratory irritants leads to hyperplasia of the mucus glands, hypertrophy of the smooth muscle, and thickening of the bronchial wall.

Persistent cough and expectoration (expulsion of mucus or phlegm from the throat) are the primary symptoms of chronic bronchitis. The effects of the disease develop slowly and progressively over months and years, gradually resulting in bronchial obstruction from excess secretion of mucus. Eventually, the lungs remain in a chronically inflated state because more air is inhaled than is exhaled. Additional signs and symptoms of chronic bronchitis include wheezing, shortness of breath, and arterial hypoxemia leading to right heart hypertrophy and failure (cor pulmonale). No dependable radiographic criteria exist for a definitive diagnosis of chronic bronchitis.

Chest radiographs may demonstrate hyperinflation of the lungs. Elimination of the causa-tive agent (e.g., cigarettes) is an important first step in treatment. Antibiotics can reduce the presence of infection; bronchodilators are used to reduce bronchospasm.

Emphysema is a condition in which the lung's alveoli become distended, usually from loss of elasticity or interference with expiration. It is characterized by an increase in the air spaces distal to the terminal bronchioles, with destruction of the alveolar walls.

The primary symptom of emphysema is dyspnea, which at first occurs only during exertion but eventually even at rest. In the early stages of emphysema, the patient may present with a normal chest radiograph. However, as the disease progresses, hyperinflation results (Fig. 3-39), and the AP diameter of the chest increases because of increased air in the lungs. Emphysema appears radiographically as a

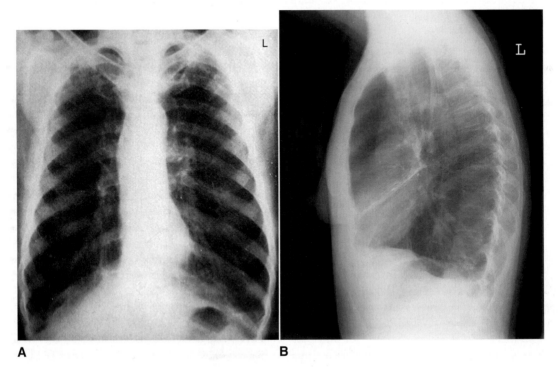

A   **B**

FIG. 3-39 A, PA chest radiograph demonstrating pulmonary emphysema, a form of chronic obstructive pulmonary disease (COPD), with its characteristic hyperinflation of the lungs, increased radiolucence, and barrel-shaped chest. **B,** Lateral chest imaging of patient with COPD demonstrating blunting of costophrenic angles.

depressed or flattened diaphragm, abnormally radiolucent lungs, and an increased retrosternal air space (barrel-shaped chest). Conventional chest radiographs help to differentiate emphysema from other lung disorders having similar symptoms such as TB or lung cancer. Large bullae (>1 cm in diameter), prominent hilar markings, or blisters filled with air may be visible on conventional chest radiographs (Fig. 3-40), but smaller lesions are best demonstrated by CT examinations of the chest. High-resolution CT using thin section cuts (1–2 mm) clearly demonstrate areas of hypovascularity and bullae associated with emphysema (Fig. 3-41).

Treatment of emphysema is much like that for chronic bronchitis. Goals are to improve symptoms, treat any reversible elements (e.g., infection), and prevent further progression of the disease as possible.

Because these two forms of COPD represent chronic deterioration of the pulmonary system, the continued problems eventually lead to heart failure. The heart begins to wear out over time in its effort to overcompensate blood flow for the decreased airflow caused by COPD. This may result in death from associated complications such as respiratory failure, pneumonia, cardiac arrhythmias, or pulmonary embolism. However, some individuals may live for many years with COPD and will eventually develop pulmonary edema and cor pulmonale. These conditions are both discussed in Chapter 8.

Pneumoconioses (Occupational Lung Diseases)

Pneumoconioses are occupational diseases in which inhalation of foreign inorganic dust from a particular work environment results in pulmonary fibrosis. The effects of an inhaled foreign material depends on its physical and chemical properties, the dose of the agent, as well as the site of deposition within the bronchial tree. The size of the dust particle inhaled is of particular importance. Most occupationally generated dusts and those occurring

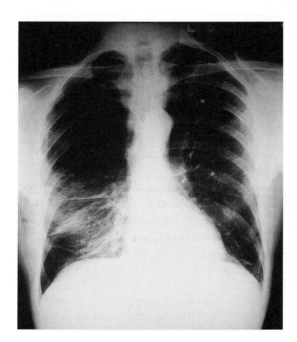

FIG. 3-40 Pulmonary emphysema with a giant emphysematous bleb occupying the upper half of the right lung.

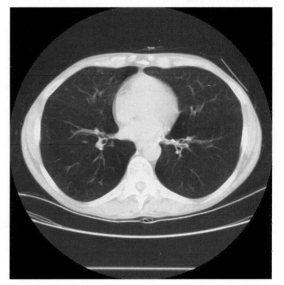

FIG. 3-41 High-resolution CT of the chest demonstrating parenchymal changes associated with emphysema.

naturally are too large to cause pneumoconioses. Dusts greater than 10 µm are filtered out in the nasal passages or the mucous lining of the tracheobronchial tree; those smaller than 1 µm generally remain suspended in air and are exhaled. Those most likely to be trapped are 1 to 5 µm. In addition to the size criterion, exposure to a substance capable of causing disease for a sufficient duration (dose) and a susceptible host are factors required to cause a pneumoconiosis. Fibrogenic inorganic dusts responsible for pneumoconiosis generally include silica, coal, asbestos, or beryllium.

Radiography assists in the detection and follow-up of this disease group. Lesions produced by the different pneumoconioses vary but may include nodules, cavitation, and pleural thickening. The three primary types of pneumoconioses are silicosis, anthracosis, and asbestosis. Treatment centers on preventing infection, relieving any respiratory symptoms, and maintaining adequate oxygenation.

Silicosis, the oldest known pneumoconiosis, results from inhaling silica (quartz) dust and is common among miners, grinders, and sandblasters. It is the most widespread and most serious type of pneumoconiosis. This disease occurs following 10 to 30 years of exposure to the silica dust. Phagocytes located within the bronchioles carry the silica dust into the septa of the alveoli. In response to the foreign dust particles, the alveoli form large amounts of fibrous connective tissue, thus destroying the normal lung tissue. This disease is clearly visible on conventional chest radiographs as multiple small, rounded, opaque nodules throughout the lungs, resulting from the creation of the fibrous tissue. Sometimes these calcifications are peripheral "eggshell calcifications" (Fig. 3-42). With the exception of a lung transplant, there is no treatment for silicosis. Therefore, prevention through protective masks and adequate ventilation is the key to controlling this occupational disease.

Anthracosis (black lung disease) results from inhalation of coal dust (Fig. 3-43) over an extended period of about 20 years. As the coal dust is deposited in the lungs, "coal macules" develop around the bronchioles and cause their dilation. This dilation does not affect the alveoli or the airflow; thus, impairment of the function of the lungs and the lung architecture is limited. Other than suppressing the coal dust, there is no real treatment for anthracosis, and usually efforts to treat this condition are futile.

Asbestosis results from the inhalation of asbestos dust, which can cause chronic injury to the lungs. Asbestos dust is found in building materials and insulation. Radiographically, diffuse, small irregular or linear opacities may be demonstrated in the lower lungs, and diaphragmatic pleural calcifications suggest asbestosis. Pleural changes in asbestosis are considered far more striking than parenchymal changes. Pleural thickening may also be present. This disease may be prevented by effectively suppressing asbestos dust in the work environment. Because of a heightened awareness of asbestosis, advances in industry, and the use of occupational face mask ventilators, the incidence of asbestosis has decreased, and further advances are likely to eliminate it in the United States. Exposure to a cumulative, extended exposure to asbestos dust has been shown to promote the chance of developing mesothelioma, a rare malignant neoplasm of the pleura. This neoplasm develops at least 15 years after a high exposure to asbestos.

Fungal Diseases

Fungi are plants without chlorophyll and are widely found in nature. Many fungi found in nature are not usually pathogenic unless they enter a compromised host. Therefore, most severe fungal infections are termed opportunistic. They are more likely to disseminate, causing severe illness in patients undergoing therapy with corticosteroids or immunosuppressants, or in individuals with acquired immune deficiency syndrome (AIDS), diabetes mellitus, bronchiectasis, emphysema, TB, lymphoma, leukemia, or serious burns.

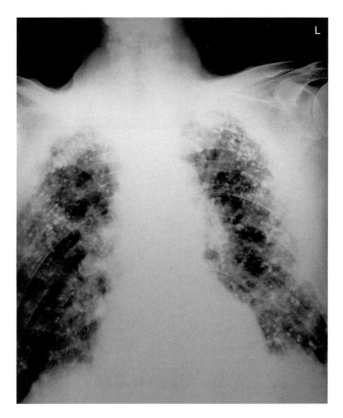

FIG. 3-42 "Eggshell calcifications" of silicosis in hilar and mediastinal lymph nodes of 70-year-old male stonecutter. Multiple small calcifications are also distributed throughout the lungs.

Histoplasmosis is a systemic fungal infection caused by a fungus that thrives in soil, especially that fueled by bird or bat excreta. Histoplasmosis is particularly endemic to the Ohio and Mississippi River valleys. Most cases are classified as acute primary histoplasmosis and are so mild that they go undiagnosed. Symptoms of acute primary histoplasmosis are nonspecific and include a fever, cough, and general malaise. However, if the immune system is not effective at controlling and overcoming the fungal infection, it can spread from the lungs. This condition is termed **progressive disseminated histoplasmosis**. This is considered an opportunistic infection for AIDS, often leading to severe acute pneumonia. Disseminated histoplasmosis that leads to cavitary formations (chronic cavitary histoplasmosis) is more serious. The cavities resemble TB, often affecting the apical portion of the lungs. Dyspnea, cough, and fatigue may persist for months or even years. Diagnosis of histoplasmosis is made by histological laboratory analysis. Chest radiographs eventually may reveal small calcifications as a late manifestation of the disease, although these do not usually appear for 4 or 5 years (Fig. 3-44).

Fewer than 1% of those who acquire histoplasmosis require treatment because most forms of the disease (acute primary histoplasmosis) are self-limiting and may evade diagnosis. If undiagnosed, however, advanced cases such as

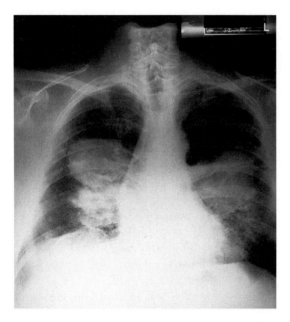

FIG. 3-43 Large perihilar nodules without eggshell calcifications. Thoracotomy revealed heavy anthracotic pigmentation, with two largest nodules containing black fluid, consistent with anthracosis.

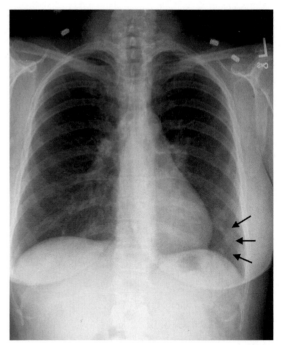

FIG. 3-44 PA chest radiograph demonstrating old histoplasmosis with calcified nodes in left lower lobe.

chronic cavitary histoplasmosis can result in death. Antifungal therapy is used to treat progressive disseminated histoplasmosis on diagnosis, and AIDS patients often receive intermittent doses of intravenous antifungal medications necessary for chronic suppression of the infectious agent.

Coccidioidomycosis is also a systemic, fungal infection. It is caused by a fungus that thrives in semiarid soil, particularly the southwestern United States and northern Mexico. Infective spores in the soil become airborne from winds, digging, or other disruption. For this reason, agriculture and construction workers are particularly at risk. Like histoplasmosis, most primary coccidioidomycosis infections are mild, usually self-limited, and may go unrecognized. The most common radiographic finding of primary coccidioidomycosis, if present, is a small area of pulmonary consolidation. Lesions may form nodules of varying size that can simulate a

malignant nodule, thus requiring biopsy or surgical excision. The typical treatment is bed rest because most occurrences are mild. However, in a few cases, progressive coccidioidomycosis may develop weeks or months following a primary infection, especially in immonosuppressed individuals. If disseminated coccidioidomycosis is not treated, it can lead to meningitis. The treatment for meningeal coccidioidomycosis must be continued for many months or years. Progressive coccidioidomycosis can also be a very deadly disease, as over 70% of individuals infected with HIV who develop this disease die from disseminated coccidioidomycosis within 1 month of initial diagnosis.

Lung Abscess

A lung abscess is a localized area of dead (necrotic) lung tissue surrounded by inflammatory debris. These abscesses may result from periodontal disease, pneumonia, neoplasms, or other organisms that invade the lungs. Lung abscess is more common in the right lung because of the vertical orientation of the right main bronchus. Clinical manifestations of a lung abscess include fever, cough, expectoration of pus, and foul sputum. Radiographically, an abscess generally appears as a lobar or segmental consolidation that becomes globular in shape as pus accumulates, or it may appear as a round, thick-walled capsule containing air and fluid. CT may be used to provide better anatomic information or to detect cavity formations. Empyemas consist of an accumulation of pus in the pleural cavity, usually caused by some primary lung infection. They may be caused by the invasion of a lung abscess, resulting in a bronchopleural fistula.

Treatment of an abscess and empyema centers on treatment of the primary condition causing it, including antibiotic therapy and possible drainage of fluids. If the abscess is resistant to the antibiotics, surgical resection of the abscess may be necessary, and in cases of multiple drug-resistant abscesses, the entire lobe may be surgically removed.

Pleurisy

Inflammation of the pleura is loosely termed **pleurisy,** a word often used to indicate inconsequential thoracic pain. True pleurisy is often indicative of serious conditions such as pneumonia, pulmonary embolism, TB, or malignant disease. Pain, varying in intensity, is usually distributed to one side or the other and along the intercostal nerve roots. Because the parietal layer of the pleura contains sensory receptors (the visceral layer does not), pain indicates that the parietal layer is involved in the inflammatory process.

Chest radiographs do not generally demonstrate pleurisy, but they are helpful in confirming the presence of pleural fluid associated with the disease. Diagnosis and treatment of any underlying condition are important in relieving the symptoms of pleurisy.

Pleural Effusion

Pleural effusion results when excess fluid collects in the pleural cavity. It is a frequent manifestation of serious thoracic disease, usually pulmonary or cardiac in origin. It should be regarded not as a disease entity but rather as a sign of an important underlying condition. Pleural effusion may be caused by inflammation, such as in the case of pleurisy, a pulmonary embolism, or neoplasm. These pleural effusions are termed **exudates.** Pleural effusions may also result from microvascular changes such as those associated with heart failure or ascites and are termed **transudates.** A pleural effusion containing blood is called a **hemothorax** and most frequently follows trauma to the thorax or thoracic surgery.

Conventional chest radiographs are commonly used in the diagnosis of pleural effusion. The radiographic signs of pleural effusion include a blunting of the costophrenic angles (Fig. 3-45), which is often best demonstrated on an erect lateral chest radiograph. The blunting occurs as part of the healing process, and the fibrous changes in the lung tissue may remain even after the pleural effusion has resolved. Lateral decubitus chest radiographs are also valuable (Fig. 3-46) because they can detect smaller amounts (<100 ml) of fluid in the pleural space than either the erect PA or lateral chest radiograph. In severe cases, an entire lung may be opacified, and the mediastinum may be shifted to the contralateral side of the chest. Because a pleural effusion is indicative of an underlying medical problem, CT may be used to evaluate the lung parenchyma in search of a neoplasm, abscess, or pneumonia hidden by the effusion. Diagnostic medical sonography is also an excellent modality for locating or localizing pleural effusion (Fig. 3-47) and assisting the clinician in performing thoracocentesis. Thoracocentesis is used to remove excess fluids for symptom alleviation and laboratory analysis and to confirm the presence and type of fluid present in the pleural cavity. In the case of a hemothorax, the

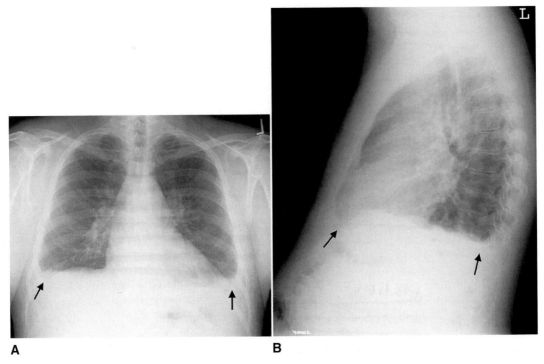

FIG. 3-45 PA (**A**) and left lateral (**B**) chest radiographs demonstrating bilateral pleural effusions.

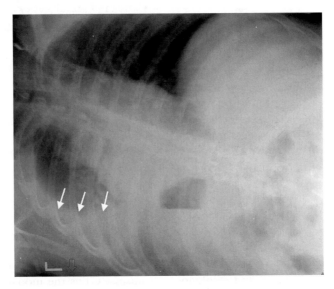

FIG. 3-46 Left lateral decubitus chest shows free pleural fluid layering out against the chest wall.

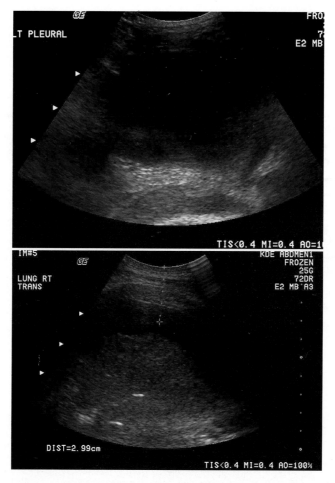

FIG. 3-47 Sonograms demonstrating pleural effusion, which help the clinician in preparation for performing a thoracentesis.

blood rarely clots within the pleural cavity, so a water-sealed chest tube drainage is placed within the pleural cavity to drain the blood, provided the bleeding has stopped.

Sinusitis

The communication with the nasal cavities subjects the paranasal sinuses to infection and inflammation called **sinusitis**. Common causes of acute sinusitis include streptococcal, pneumococcal, *Haemophilus influenzae,* and staphylococcal bacteria. Sinusitis often follows acute viral infection of the respiratory tract, and the ethmoid sinuses tend to be the most commonly affected sinuses because of their proximity to the nose. Exposure to extremes in humidity or temperature, poor oral hygiene, and/or the presence of a deviated septum may exacerbate the condition. The symptoms of sinusitis include nasal discharge, headache, tenderness over the affected area, a toothache, and/or general malaise.

Radiography is important in the diagnosis of sinusitis. CT is the modality of choice because it clearly demonstrates the swollen mucous membrane and retained exudate caused by the infection. Although upright sinus radiographs do demonstrate the increased density and possible air-fluid levels (Fig. 3-48) from both mucosal swelling and fluid accumulation, CT provides better definition of the extent and degree of the sinusitis (Fig. 3-49). Chronic sinusitis may cause nasal polyps.

Treatment of sinusitis typically involves saline nasal sprays, antibiotic therapy, and analgesics for pain relief. A deviated septum that contributes to sinusitis can be corrected surgically, if necessary.

NEOPLASTIC DISEASES

Bronchial Carcinoid

Bronchial carcinoid (adenomas) are usually considered benign but are included in the World Health Organization's classification of "lung cancer" because they tend to invade local tissues, sometimes metastasize to regional lymph nodes, and are treated much like other

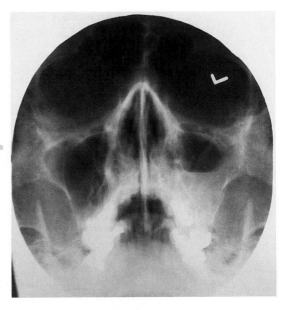

FIG. 3-48 Air-fluid level present in the left maxillary sinus reflects sinusitis in this 26-year-old woman, secondary to an oral-antral fistula.

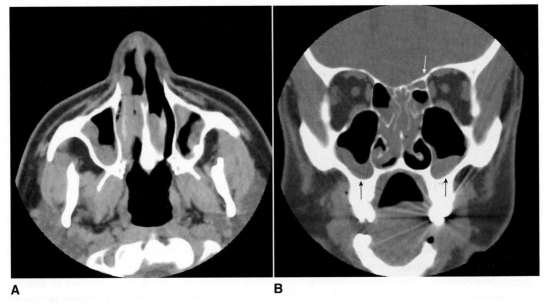

A   B

FIG. 3-49 Axial (**A**) and coronal (**B**) CTs of paranasal sinuses demonstrating bilateral mucosal thickening of the maxillary sinuses and opacification of the nasal cavity.

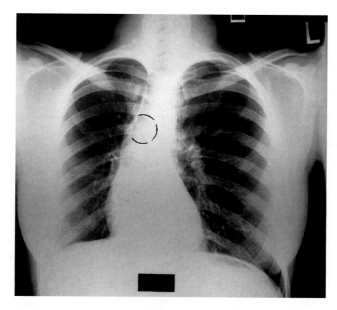

FIG. 3-50 Rounded marble-size density within the lumen of the right mainstem bronchus, along with clinical history indicative of bronchial carcinoid.

malignant neoplasms. They occur equally in both sexes and often have a prolonged course of disease. The radiographic appearance of this neoplasm shows opacity (Fig. 3- 50), bronchial narrowing and/or obstruction, and possible collapse of the affected segment of the lung. Bronchial obstruction is the most common presentation, and recurrent pneumonia within the same area of the lung in combination with pleural pain is a common occurrence in these individuals.

Bronchogenic Carcinoma

Bronchogenic carcinoma is the most common fatal primary malignancy in the United States, usually occurring in individuals between the ages of 45 and 70 years. There are four main histologic types: squamous cell, undifferentiated small (oat) cell, undifferentiated large cell, and adenocarcinoma. These tumors arise in the major bronchi near the hilar area and metastasize via lymph nodes, the bloodstream, or both. In addition to a thorough patient history, chest radiographs are essential to the diagnosis of bronchogenic carcinoma. The most common radiographic presentation of this neoplasm is airway obstruction caused by a unilateral hilar mass (Fig. 3-51); however, the lesion must be larger than 6 mm to be visualized on a conventional radiograph. As the tumor grows, it may occlude the bronchus, producing atelectasis and pneumonitis. These secondary effects provide more opacity radiographically than the actual tumor. The second most common radiographic presentation of a neoplasm consists of a solitary radiopaque lung nodule, sometimes called a **coin lesion.** Histologic confirmation is necessary to make a definitive diagnosis.

CT is essential in demonstrating nodules smaller than 6 mm that are not visualized with conventional chest radiography. It has the ability to show calcifications to help differentiate malignant and benign tumors of the lung and is useful in staging the disease by demonstrating the presence or absence of spread to the lymph nodes in the thoracic and upper

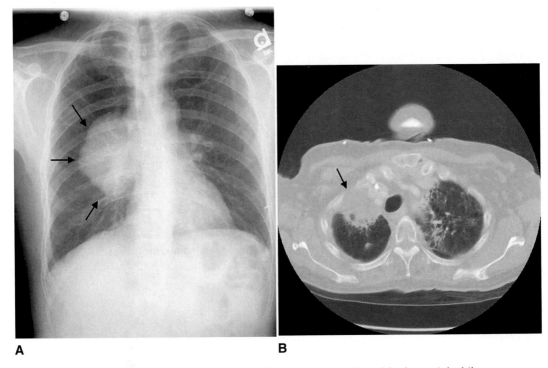

FIG. 3-51 A, Bronchogenic carcinoma on PA projection indicated by large right hilar mass. **B,** Chest CT demonstrating a large bronchogenic mass in the anteromedial aspect of the right lung with a cavitary lesion just above the level of the right mainstem bronchus.

abdominal areas. Malignant lesions are rarely calcified (Fig. 3-52), whereas benign lesions generally have a calcified center. Staging bronchogenic carcinoma is critical to the selection of treatment of the disease. CT can assist in determining metastases to the liver (Fig. 3-53), brain, and adrenal glands, so it is now a common practice to include a portion of the upper abdomen on oncologic CT examinations of the chest. Advances in technology have made possible the ability to perform virtual bronchoscopy to also assess the location and extent of the carcinoma. Thoracic magnetic resonance (MR) is of limited value, but it is helpful in assessing tissue planes and the chest wall before surgery and in cases where apical tumors invade the vertebral column. Nuclear medicine bone scans may be used to screen for bone metastases, which are often confirmed with either conventional skeletal radiographs or MR.

The patient may undergo percutaneous lung biopsy, bronchoscopy, or brush biopsy. In the latter procedure, a device with tiny brushes is introduced through a bronchoscope or bronchial catheter to procure cells and tissues under fluoroscopic guidance.

The prognosis is very poor for bronchogenic carcinoma, with a 5-year survival rate of only 12% to 14%. Fairly good results are associated with a lobectomy in individuals with peripheral nodular lesions; however, second primary lesions occur in 6% to 10% of survivors. Small cell tumors tend to be the most deadly because the cancer almost always spreads before diagnosis. Cigarette smoking is by far the most important etiologic factor, accounting for over 90% of cases in men and over 80% of cases in women. Exposure to potentially carcinogenic substances from air pollution and occupational exposure are also etiologic factors.

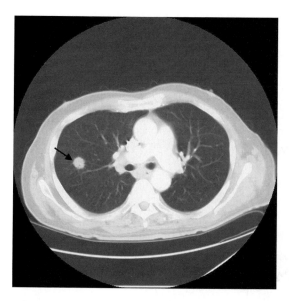

FIG. 3-52 Chest CT of a bronchogenic lesion (arrow) in the upper lobe of the right lung.

This disease process may be treated with surgery, chemotherapy, radiation therapy, or any combination of the three modalities depending on the type, location, and stage of disease. Chemotherapy and/or radiation therapy may be administered before surgical resection, and radiation therapy may also be used for palliative treatment to control the pain associated with skeletal metastasis, spinal cord compression, or brain metastasis. As mentioned earlier, CT, MR, and nuclear medicine bone scans are all vital in helping to stage the extent of the carcinoma to assist in determining the optimal treatment.

Metastases from Other Sites

Pulmonary metastases are much more common than primary lung neoplasms. Many malignancies develop pulmonary metastases, which are detectable on a chest radiograph. The most common primary sites for these tumors are the breast, gastrointestinal tract, female reproductive system, prostate, melanoma, and the kidneys.

Malignancy is spread to the lungs from a primary site via five different routes: (1) through the bloodstream in hematogenous metastases, (2) through the lymph system in lymphogenous metastases, (3) by direct extension in local invasion, (4) through the tracheobronchial system in bronchogenic metastases, and, rarely, by (5) direct implantation from biopsies or other surgical procedures. Radiographically, these metastatic lesions appear as single or multiple rounded opacities throughout the lungs (Fig. 3-54). Again, CT is more sensitive than conventional chest radiography in the detection of small metastatic lesions.

As in the case of bronchogenic carcinoma, treatment of pulmonary metastases is accomplished through surgery, chemotherapy, radiation therapy, or a combination of them, depending on the type of tumor and its likely primary site. For example, hormonal therapy of prostatic and breast carcinoma can cause pulmonary lesions to resolve. The field of oncology is growing, with new treatment options in research and ongoing development.

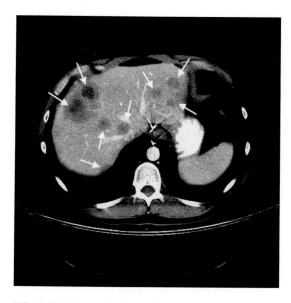

FIG. 3-53 Upper abdominal CT of patient with liver metastases from a bronchogenic carcinoma primary lesion.

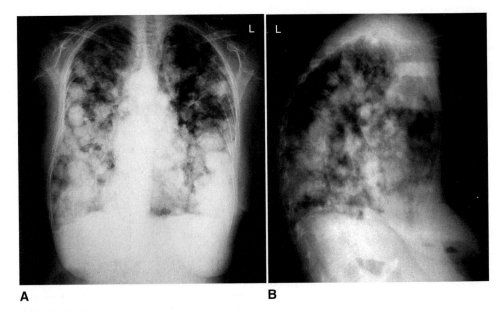

FIG. 3-54 A, Pulmonary metastases from uterine cancer demonstrate multiple lesions with characteristic "cotton ball" appearance. **B,** Lateral projection of pulmonary metastases resulting from uterine cancer.

PATHOLOGY SUMMARY: THE RESPIRATORY SYSTEM

Pathology	Imaging Modalities of Choice	Additive or Subtractive Pathology
Cystic fibrosis	Chest radiograph	Additive
Hyaline membrane disease	Chest radiograph	Additive
Pneumonias	Chest radiograph	Additive
Bronchiectasis	Chest radiograph, high-resolution chest CT	Additive
Tuberculosis	Chest radiograph, chest CT	Additive
COPD	Chest radiograph, high-resolution chest CT	Subtractive
Pneumoconioses	Chest radiograph	Additive
Fungal disease	Chest radiograph	Additive
Lung abscess	Chest radiograph, chest CT	Additive
Pleurisy	None	None
Pleural effusion	Chest radiograph, chest CT, ultrasound	Additive
Sinusitis	Sinus CT	Additive
Bronchial adenoma	Chest CT	Additive
Bronchogenic carcinoma	Chest CT	Additive
Metastatic lung disease	Chest CT	Additive

QUESTIONS

1. Bony structures such as the clavicles can be removed from the apices of the lungs by use of what radiographic position?
   a. AP
   b. lateral decubitus
   c. lordotic
   d. 45-degree oblique

2. The "sail sign" in an infant is commonly associated with enlargement of the:
   a. heart
   b. pulmonary arteries
   c. thymus
   d. thyroid

3. Posterior mediastinal masses most commonly originate from _____ tissue.
   a. lymphatic
   b. nervous
   c. thymus
   d. thyroid

4. An infant born after only 6 months of gestation may likely suffer from:
   a. cystic fibrosis
   b. hyaline membrane disease
   c. mediastinal emphysema
   d. pectus excavatum

5. A lack of respiratory function or lack of proper oxygen and carbon dioxide exchange best describes:
   a. cardiac arrest
   b. cardiac arrhythmia
   c. respiratory failure
   d. tachypnea

6. Which of the following is the most common type of bacterial pneumonia?
   a. aspiration
   b. Legionnaires'
   c. pneumococcal
   d. streptococcal

7. Loss of elasticity of the bronchial walls as a result of bacterial infection can result in:
   a. bronchiectasis
   b. bronchogenic carcinoma
   c. pneumococcal pneumonia
   d. tuberculosis

8. Pulmonary fibrosis resulting from occupationally inhaled dusts is characteristic of:
   a. atelectasis
   b. chronic bronchitis
   c. pleural effusion
   d. pneumoconiosis

9. An accumulation of pus in the pleural cavity is known as a(n):
   a. coin lesion
   b. empyema
   c. pleural effusion
   d. pleurisy

10. The most common etiologic factor in the development of bronchogenic carcinoma is:
    a. automobile emissions
    b. cigarette smoking
    c. dust
    d. iatrogenic treatment

11. Explain how technical exposure factors must be changed to compensate for additive and subtractive pathologies of the chest. Give one example of each type of pathology.

12. Specify the reasons chest radiographs should be obtained in an erect position at a 72-inch source-to-image distance.

13. What specialized radiographic projection of the chest is utilized to demonstrate tuberculosis? Why is this projection of benefit?

14. Chronic obstructive pulmonary disease (COPD) includes both emphysema and chronic bronchitis. Compare and contrast these two pathologic conditions and explain how both can be considered COPD.

15. Metastasis to the lungs from other primary tumors occurs via five routes. What are they?

The Abdomen and Gastrointestinal System

UPON COMPLETION OF CHAPTER 4, THE READER SHOULD BE ABLE TO:

- Describe the anatomic components of the abdomen and gastrointestinal system and how they are visualized radiographically.
- Compare and contrast the various imaging modalities used in evaluation of the abdomen and its contents.
- Identify the tubes and catheters related to the gastrointestinal system by type, and briefly explain their use.
- Characterize a given condition as congenital, inflammatory, neurogenic, or neoplastic.

- Identify the pathogenesis of the gastrointestinal pathologies cited and typical treatments for them.
- Describe, in general, the radiographic appearance of each of the given pathologies.

KEY TERMS

Achalasia	Gallstone ileus	Malabsorption syndrome
Adenocarcinoma	Gastroenteritis	Malrotation
Appendicitis	Gastroesophageal reflux disease	Mechanical bowel obstruction
Atresia	Hernia	Paralytic ileus
Colostomy	Hiatal hernia	Peptic ulcer
Crohn's disease	Hirschsprung's disease	Reflux esophagitis
Diverticulitis	Hypertrophic pyloric stenosis	Regional enteritis
Diverticulum	Ileostomy	Situs inversus
Dysphagia	Imperforate anus	Ulcerative colitis
Endoscopy	Intussusception	Volvulus
Esophageal varices	Leiomyoma	

ANATOMY AND PHYSIOLOGY

The Abdomen

The abdomen comprises the abdominal and pelvic cavities and is often divided into nine anatomic regions: right hypochondriac, epigastric, left hypochondriac, right lumbar, umbilical, left lumbar, right iliac, hypogastric, and left iliac (Fig. 4-1). It may also be described in terms of quadrants: right-upper (RUQ), right-lower (RLQ), left-upper (LUQ), and left-lower (LLQ) (Fig. 4-2). The abdominal cavity contains organs of the digestive system (stomach and intestines), the hepatobiliary system (liver, gallbladder, and pancreas), the urinary system (kidneys and ureters), and the circulatory system (spleen). The pelvic cavity contains the bladder, portions of the intestines, and the reproductive organs.

The abdominal cavity is lined by the peritoneum, a serous membrane (Fig. 4-3, *A*). The serous lining attached to the abdominal organs

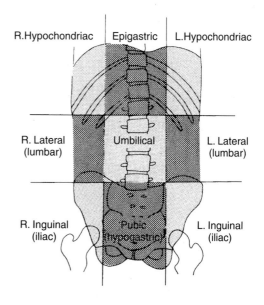

FIG. 4-1 The nine regions of the abdomen.

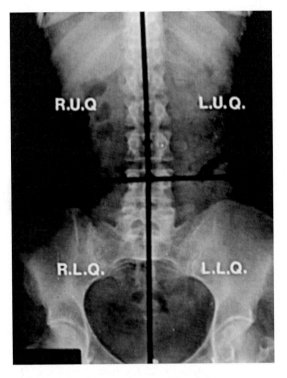

FIG. 4-2 The four quadrants of the abdomen.

is the visceral peritoneum. The peritoneum attached directly to the abdominal wall is the parietal peritoneum. The mesentery is a double fold of parietal peritoneum projecting from the posterior abdominal wall in the lumbar region (Fig. 4-3, *B*). Most of the small bowel is attached to the outer edge of the mesentery.

The greater omentum is a double fold of peritoneum that attaches to the duodenum, stomach, and transverse colon. It hangs loosely over the intestines. The lesser omentum is a fold of peritoneum that attaches the liver to the lesser curvature of the stomach and the duodenum (Fig. 4-4).

The Gastrointestinal System

A major portion of the gastrointestinal (GI) system is the alimentary tract, which serves to digest and absorb food. Extending from the mouth to the anus, the alimentary tract comprises the mouth, pharynx, esophagus, stomach, small and large bowel, and rectum.

The esophagus is the first part of the GI system. It is approximately 10 to 12 inches long and extends from the posterior pharynx to the

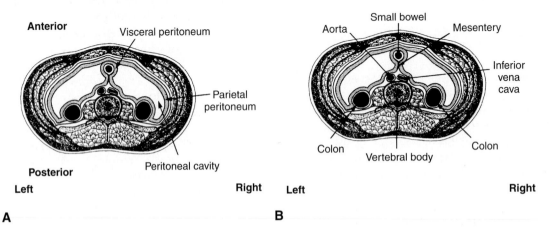

FIG. 4-3 A, A cross-sectional drawing of the abdomen demonstrates the peritoneum. **B,** A cross-sectional drawing of the lower abdomen demonstrates the mesentery.

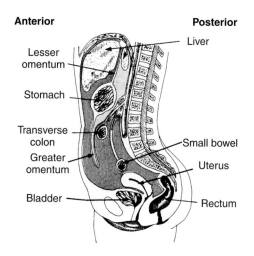

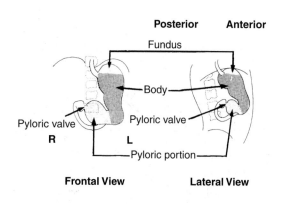

FIG. 4-6 The stomach depicted in its average orientation when empty.

FIG. 4-4 A cross-sectional drawing of the abdominal cavity demonstrates the omentum.

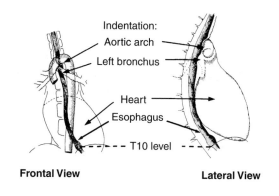

FIG. 4-5 The esophagus in the mediastinum.

stomach (Fig. 4-5). The upper esophagus is midline, but it courses to the left to pass behind the aortic arch, which indents the esophagus. Other indentations occur at the level of the left main stem bronchus and at the gastro-esophageal junction. As it passes downward, the esophagus follows the curvature of the thoracic spine and thoracic descending aorta.

The stomach occupies the body's left-upper quadrant, with the cardiac orifice at the level of the tenth or eleventh thoracic vertebra and the pyloric canal just to the right of the first or second lumbar vertebra (Fig. 4-6). Peristalsis churns the gastric content and propels it toward the pylorus. Gastric emptying of liquids is accounted for by the peristalsis initiated in the fundus of the stomach; gastric emptying of solids requires a to-and-fro action of the antrum and pylorus. In the presence of masses, inflammation, or diabetes, the peristaltic activity may be diminished. When filled with barium, the curvatures of the stomach visualize as generally smooth contours. The rugae appear as longitudinal ridges within the stomach.

The small bowel includes the duodenum, jejunum, and ileum. It arises from the stomach at the duodenal bulb and courses to the ileo-cecal valve (Fig. 4-7), over a length of nearly 21 feet. The duodenal C-loop moves posteriorly from the gastric antrum to its ending at the ligament of Treitz. The jejunum begins here and coils in the left-upper quadrant before terminating into the ileum in the right-upper quadrant. The ileum then courses through the right- and left-lower quadrants to terminate at the ileocecal junction. When filled with barium, the segments of the small bowel are distinguishable by their appearance. Duodenal mucosa is indicated by its transverse rigid appearance. Jejunal mucosa appears delicate and feathery. Ileal folds look like those of the duodenum, though not as large.

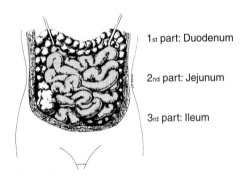

FIG. 4-7 The small bowel and its divisions.

1st part: Duodenum

2nd part: Jejunum

3rd part: Ileum

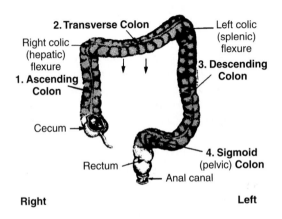

FIG. 4-8 The colon and its four parts.

The large bowel extends from the terminal ileum to the anus for a length of about 6 feet (Fig. 4-8). Its distinct regions are the cecum, the orifices for the terminal ileum and the appendix, the ascending colon and hepatic flexure, the transverse colon and the splenic flexure, the descending colon, sigmoid, rectum, and anus. The cecum is usually retroperitoneal and anterior and lies against the abdominal wall. The ascending colon is also retroperitoneal and becomes more posterior as it ascends to lie adjacent to the undersurface of the liver. The hepatic flexure, transverse colon, and splenic flexure are all intraperitoneal. They lie more anteriorly and are attached to the posterior abdominal wall by the mesocolon, a double layer of peritoneum. The descending colon is retroperitoneal, moving posteriorly as it descends. The peritoneal sigmoid colon lies in the pelvis and is quite mobile. Structures located anterior to it include the bladder and the female uterus. Posterior structures include the iliac arteries and sacral nerves. The rectum is extraperitoneal, beginning at the third sacral segment and following the sacrococcygeal curve to the anus. The valves of Houston are prominent transverse folds in the distal rectum where it dilates. The anus forms the distal 1 to 2 inches of the large bowel and contains no peritoneal covering.

IMAGING CONSIDERATIONS

Radiography

The Abdomen

Abdominal radiography is often performed for survey purposes, without contrast agents. The usual starting point is a "KUB," which refers to a supine film taken to include the kidneys, ureters, and bladder. The frequency of abnormal findings on a plain abdominal radiograph is fairly low and nonspecific, but it is of most value for patients complaining of severe abdominal tenderness and to rule out bowel obstructions and perforations. In addition, plain abdomen radiographs are invaluable in assessing the placement of various tubes and catheters, as discussed later in this chapter.

The AP projections of the abdomen are generally taken in the supine position. Such a radiograph allows an examination of the air distribution within the bowels and of the size of the viscera, serves to evaluate vascular and other types of calcifications and body or soft tissue trauma, and, finally, serves as a preliminary radiograph for other procedures.

On the initial inspection of the abdomen radiograph, the technologist should verify that the technique chosen is correct or diagnostic, that motion is nonexistent, and that the anatomy under consideration has been properly visualized. As with other body areas, an evaluation of the abdomen should be done systematically. This should include an inspection of the renal outlines, ureters, psoas muscles, spleen, liver, gallbladder, and peritoneal fat stripes.

In a normal abdomen (Fig. 4-9), varying amounts of gas and fecal material are always present in an unprepared patient. The liver, kidney, spleen, and psoas muscle shadows are variably outlined because of the lucent layer of fat surrounding them. Properitoneal fat stripes are visible as radiolucencies extending laterally from the costal margins down to the iliac crests. The aorta and pancreas are not normally seen unless they are calcified, as might be expected in an elderly patient in the case of the aorta or in a patient with chronic calcific pancreatitis. The inferior margin of the liver should lie at or

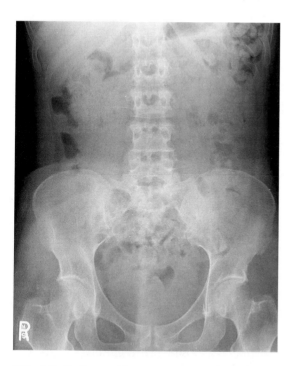

FIG. 4-9 Radiographic appearance of a normal abdomen, demonstrating kidney shadows, liver shadow, psoas muscles, and transverse processes of the lumbar spine.

above the level of the right twelfth rib. The left kidney is usually slightly higher than the right kidney because of the presence of the liver superior to it. In terms of renal size, the kidneys are generally the length of three vertebrae in children over 1 year of age. As the child becomes an adult, the kidneys are about the length of two and a half vertebrae.

Few, if any, air-fluid levels are present in the normal patient who is radiographed in the erect position. Limited fluid levels in the small and large bowel, however, may be considered normal. Fluid levels are abnormal when they are seen in dilated bowel loops or when they are numerous. The intestinal gas pattern can be confusing to the diagnostician. In infants and children, gas may be scattered throughout the bowel, but in adults gas is normally seen only in the stomach and colon. Small-bowel gas in an adult, therefore, may indicate a pathologic process. In some patients, gas may be recognizable only on erect films because of the presence of intraluminal fluid. Free air should not be visible in the peritoneal cavity and is indicative of a bowel perforation or other pathologic entities that can introduce air into the peritoneum. Erect abdominal radiographs must include the diaphragm to assess for free air and in instances where the patient is unable to stand erect, a left lateral decubitus abdomen should be obtained (Fig. 4-10).

The Gastrointestinal System

Some contents of the abdomen can be seen without contrast media, as explained. However, most of the gastrointestinal (GI) tract cannot be examined directly. The internal surfaces of both ends can be visualized through endoscopy, the use of lighted instruments with optics to visualize disease of the esophagus, stomach and duodenum, rectum and distal colon, and occasionally the terminal ileum. Endoscopy is becoming more common in health care as the instrument technology continues to improve and allows more detailed studies and improved patient comfort. Abnormal areas can be visual-

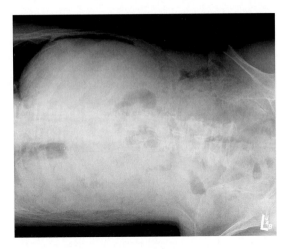

FIG. 4-10 A left lateral decubitus abdomen demonstrating free air over the dome of the liver.

ized, biopsied, and examined histologically. Those areas that cannot be directly examined are studied radiographically.

Radiographic investigation of the GI system is commonly a combination of fluoroscopy and radiography. Fluoroscopy provides dynamic information, whereas radiographs provide a permanent static record of the examination. Radiographic examination of the GI system requires positive and negative contrast agents for visualization of the body parts. Barium sulfate is generally used as the positive contrast agent but is contraindicated in cases of GI tract perforation. If a perforated bowel is suspected, a water-soluble contrast agent should be used. Although infrequently used alone, a negative contrast agent (e.g., air or carbon dioxide) may be used to distend the stomach and bowel for better visualization of the mucosal lining. A combination of both positive and negative contrast agents is commonly used so that the thicker barium sulfate adheres to the mucosa while the carbon dioxide expands the stomach or bowel, thus allowing optimal visualization of small variances in the walls of the GI organs.

Digital fluoroscopy has emerged as a substantive improvement over traditional fluoroscopy for a number of reasons. Sophisticated on-line image processing allows enhancement of selective image quality parameters relevant to diagnosis that is not possible with conventional spot-film devices. Radiologists can view the images throughout the procedure rather than waiting for film processing at the end of the study. This immediate availability has altered the practice of fluoroscopy in terms of its speed and efficiency. Hard-copy film production or transfer to a picture, archiving, and communication system (PACS) is available at the touch of a button with no interruptions for changing cassettes. Anatomic motion can be captured as it occurs instead of depending on the radiologist's synchronization of the timing of filming with, for example, esophageal swallowing. Serial filming capability further enhances this capacity and allows several images per second to be exposed. Diagnosis is often made during the fluoroscopic procedure, allowing hard copies to be produced later for historical purposes. In an environment where film is used, fewer hard copies are necessary, and film costs are consequently reduced. The radiation dose is therefore also reduced.

The Esophagus

Most upper GI studies begin with the patient in an erect position to evaluate air-fluid levels in the alimentary tract. An esophageal study may be performed to demonstrate anomalies and abnormalities of the esophagus. Transport of the food or liquid bolus through swallowing is the sole function of the esophagus. If it is studied as part of a GI tract examination, thin barium sulfate may be used. Thick barium sulfate is used if the esophagus is the single object of study. Most patients presenting for a traditional esophagram have a chief complaint of **dysphagia,** or difficult swallowing. The causes for dysphagia are numerous and are discussed later in this chapter.

Radiographs are typically taken of a barium-filled esophagus in an erect or prone position. They include a PA, right lateral, and right ante-

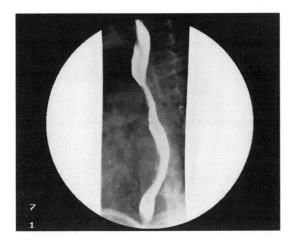

FIG. 4-11 Normal esophagus as seen on this RAO digital spot film of a 21-year-old woman.

rior oblique (RAO) (Fig. 4-11) to visualize the esophagus between the spine and the heart.

During fluoroscopy, the radiologist can visualize mechanical problems presented while the patient is swallowing the barium sulfate mixture. Esophageal studies are also used to study the contour of the heart, as described in Chapter 9. Video fluoroscopy is useful in assessing motor disorders, such as achalasia or cricopharyngeal spasms.

The Stomach

One of radiology's most common procedures is an "upper GI," in which barium sulfate flows from the esophagus and into the stomach and small bowel. Once the barium reaches the stomach, the radiologist evaluates the stomach contour, position, rugae, and the peristaltic changes occurring as the stomach fills and empties.

In the event the radiologist wishes to diminish peristalsis, glucagon is given to relax the stomach musculature. In many instances, a gas-producing substance (carbon dioxide crystals) is used with the barium sulfate to produce a double-contrast examination. The purpose is to expand the stomach and promote coating of the stomach mucosa. The duodenal bulb is

studied as it fills with barium sulfate and empties into the small bowel. Compression may be used for better visualization of specific anatomic areas of the upper GI tract.

A series of radiographs is taken after fluoroscopy, with the projections differing from one institution to another. Typical patient positions include a recumbent PA projection to demonstrate the entire stomach and duodenal bulb, RAO to highlight the pyloric canal and duodenal bulb (Fig. 4-12), right lateral to show the duodenal bulb and loop, and the LPO to demonstrate the gastric fundus. Proper positioning relates significantly to the patient's body habitus. Generally, the more hypersthenic a patient is, the higher and more transverse the stomach tends to lie. For other body habiti (i.e., sthenic, hyposthenic, and asthenic), the stomach is more J-shaped, lying lower and closer to the spine.

The Small Bowel

In some instances, the barium sulfate mixture may be followed as it progresses through the small intestines. Radiographs are exposed at set intervals to determine GI motility and to demonstrate abnormalities within the small bowel. Once the contrast agent reaches the

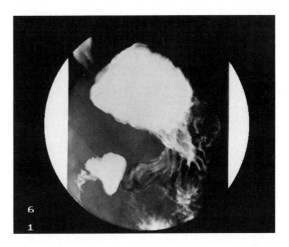

FIG. 4-12 Normal stomach as seen on this digital spot film of an 18-year-old man.

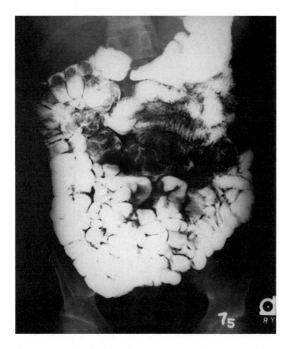

FIG. 4-13 Small bowel film taken 75 minutes after the examination began on this 18-year-old man, demonstrating passage through the ileocecal valve into the colon, with no mucosal abnormalities or dilated loops of small bowel.

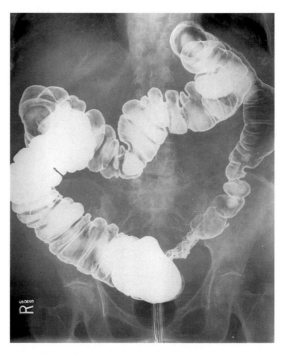

FIG. 4-14 Normal air-contrast enema as demonstrated on this AP projection.

ileocecal valve, the small-bowel study is complete, typically within 2 to 3 hours (Fig. 4-13).

The small intestines may also be studied radiographically by means of enteroclysis, a small-bowel enema. This is accomplished by advancing an intestinal tube through the patient's mouth to the end of the duodenum at the ligament of Treitz. Contrast agents, both positive and negative (barium sulfate and methylcellulose, respectively), are directly injected into the small bowel.

The Large Bowel

The lower GI tract is examined by administering a barium enema through the rectum. This examination demonstrates abnormalities of the large bowel and intraluminal neoplasms. The barium enema can be performed in a single-contrast fashion with only barium or as a double-contrast study utilizing barium sulfate in combination with a negative contrast agent (e.g., air). The negative contrast agent distends the lumen, allowing improved visualization of the mucosal lining (Fig. 4-14), especially small polyps and intraluminal tumors. In either case, the radiologist typically exposes a series of spot films with the patient in various positions to highlight certain areas of the colon (e.g., flexures). The technologist may also expose a series of radiographs per the radiologist's instructions (Fig. 4-15). Following evacuation of the barium sulfate mixture, the technologist takes a "post-evacuation" radiograph to visualize colon contraction and demonstrate mucosa.

If a patient has had a surgical enterostomy procedure, the contrast medium may be administered through the opening in the abdominal wall to the specific area of the GI system. A

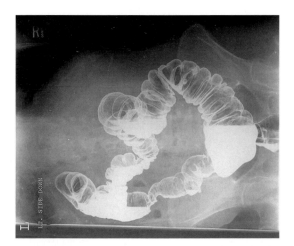

FIG. 4-15 Normal air contrast barium enema as demonstrated on this left lateral decubitus PA projection.

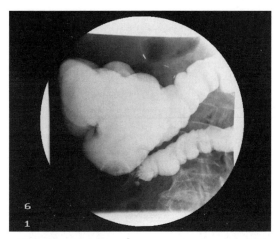

FIG. 4-16 A digital spot film of an enema through a colostomy in the descending colon on this 72-year-old man. The ostomy is clearly indicated by its circular opening into the bowel. Also visible is a small diverticulum just adjacent to the colostomy site and an inverted cecum.

colostomy is a procedure in which a stoma is surgically created to the abdominal wall to allow drainage of bowel contents into a closed pouch hung outside the body. Those in the sigmoid and descending colon are most frequently placed because of rectal or sigmoid cancer. Those placed in the transverse or ascending colon are often for indications that allow the colostomy to be placed for temporary purposes for diversion of flow of colonic contents (e.g., sigmoid diverticulitis, rectovaginal fistula, colon obstruction).

Ileostomies are similar openings but placed from the ileum, with the most common indication being ulcerative colitis. As with colostomies, patient problems with ileostomies include proper skin protection and odor control. Proper fit of the appliance for drainage is essential to prevent problems caused by excoriating digestive enzymes. Other enterostomies (i.e., jejunostomies and duodenostomies) are more rarely used, and only under very specific circumstances because of the loss of electrolytes

that occurs before their absorption through the small bowel. These patients often require total parenteral nutrition to maintain life.

If a patient has had a surgical enterostomy procedure, the contrast agent may be administered through the opening in the abdominal wall to the specific area of the GI system (Fig. 4-16).

Computed Tomography

Computed tomography (CT) is an important modality in abdominal survey examination as well as in the examination of the GI system. Because CT can visualize small differences in tissue density, it clearly demonstrates abdominal organs that are normally not apparent on conventional abdominal radiographs without the use of contrast agents. With the use of spiral or helical CT technology, small abnormalities lying within the upper abdomen that may have been missed with conventional CT methods are consistently demonstrated because one scan is obtained with one breath hold.

With conventional CT, the patient breathed between exposures, and often the depth of inspiration was inconsistent, resulting in poorer visualization of structure in the upper abdomen close to the diaphragm.

On CT examination, the liver, spleen, pancreas, and kidneys appear as homogeneous soft tissue densities, making any alteration in the density from pathologic conditions readily visible, even without contrast media. Abscesses and solid and cystic masses all have a respective range of densities between that of water and normal soft tissue densities. The CT is also quite useful in the evaluation of retroperitoneal pathologies such as lymph node enlargement resulting from neoplastic disease or infection. In combination with conventional abdominal radiographs, CT of the abdomen is recommended when a bowel obstruction is suspected. Finally, it has become the accepted modality for following the progress of GI malignancies and also plays a role in the diagnosis of inflammatory conditions (e.g., abscess). CT of the colon is commonly performed to evaluate neoplastic disease, diverticulitis, and appendicitis. It has the capability of locating the exact site of neoplasms as well as allowing the clinician to measure the size of the tumor and the presence of infiltration into surrounding tissues. It is also useful in planning radiation therapy protocols.

Routine CT examination of the abdomen requires good opacification of the bowel and vascular structures. Poorly opacified bowel loops may be mistaken for abdominal masses. Patients must be given an oral contrast agent approximately 45 minutes to 1 hour before the abdominal CT scan. This time allows the contrast agent to reach the distal ileum before examination.

Some CT scanners have the capability to perform noninvasive endoscopic procedures called virtual colonoscopy. This procedure allows the radiologist and endoscopist to view in three dimensions landmarks and structures that may not be seen during conventional colonoscopy. This in turn can reduce risk and discomfort to the patient. This application is a benefit to those who may not be able to or choose not to have a traditional colonoscopy procedure.

Magnetic Resonance Imaging

The role of magnetic resonance imaging (MRI) in the abdomen has expanded as a result of faster sequences and shorter scan times. Evaluation of the GI tract is still limited by bowel motion; however, MR is useful in demonstrating the presence of retroperitoneal masses impinging on the GI system. Breath-hold imaging in MRI allows the technologist to visualize abdominal organs in a matter of seconds (Fig. 4-17). A few different imaging sequences are used to differentiate between pathology and normal tissue. Three-dimensional contrast-enhanced magnetic resonance angiography (MRA) is also used in imaging of the arterial vessels of the abdomen.

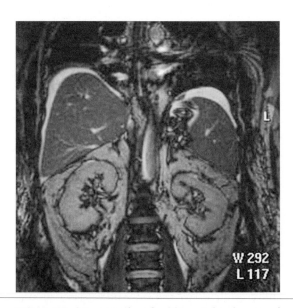

FIG. 4-17 An example of a T2-weighted coronal breath-hold MRI image of the abdomen.

Ultrasound

Ultrasound (sonography) is not useful in imaging the GI system. However, it has been used extensively to image the retroperitoneum because of the flexibility of angling the transducer to insonate that region. The aorta, kidneys, lymph nodes, and adrenal glands are subject to a variety of abnormalities, and with ultrasound, it is possible to image behind the bowel and assess for abnormalities.

Nuclear Medicine Procedures

In nuclear medicine, GI bleed scans are a quick, noninvasive procedure useful in demonstrating GI bleeding and help direct angiographers to the site of bleeding if therapeutic intervention is to be performed. This is accomplished by labeling red blood cells to identify the site of the bleed.

Gastric emptying scans are used to assess the rate food exits the stomach into the duodenum. If the patient consumes a radiolabeled meal before the scan, a high level of radioactivity within the stomach after it should normally clear indicates poor gastric emptying (Fig. 4-18).

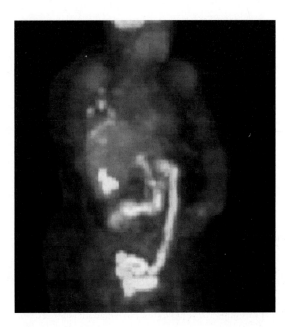

FIG. 4-19 A PET scan for staging of colon cancer demonstrates new hypermetabolic activity of metastatic disease in the liver and right hemithorax.

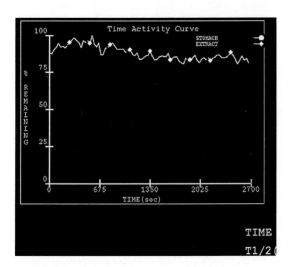

FIG. 4-18 A nuclear medicine gastric emptying scan demonstrated markedly delayed emptying of the stomach.

Urea breath tests are performed on patients with gastric ulcers to identify the presence of *Helicobacter pylori*. This bacterial infection is a common cause of gastric ulcers and can be treated quite effectively with antibiotic therapy. The procedure begins by having the patient drink radioactive urea. If the bacteria are present in the stomach, they will break down the urea, and the patient will release radioactive carbon dioxide. This is captured in the breath test.

Positron emission tomography (PET) may be used to evaluate and stage GI cancers (Fig. 4-19). PET has been proven to demonstrate approximately 20% of esophageal cancerous lesions (Fig. 4-20) undetected by CT.

Endoscopic Procedures

As earlier noted, **endoscopy** is the use of tubular fiber optic devices to look inside the GI tract and other hollow organs or cavities of the body. As its sophistication and specificity have

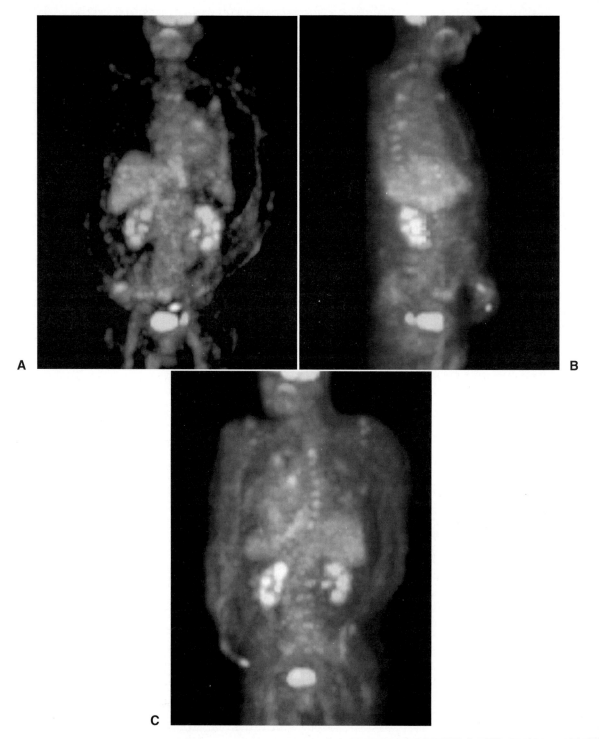

FIG. 4-20 A PET scan (**A,** frontal; **B,** lateral; **C,** oblique) on a patient with known esophageal cancer ordered for staging of the disease. Hypermetabolic focal activity is demonstrated at the level of the gastroesophageal junction designating the primary tumor and in the upper thoracic spine, right lobe of the liver, and left lung suggesting metastatic disease.

increased, it is assuming a greater role in diagnosis and therapy of the GI tract. Upper endoscopy is capable of seeing down into the esophagus, stomach, duodenum (including the ampulla of Vater), and even the proximal jejunum. Colonoscopy can allow visualization retrograde through the rectum as far as the terminal ileum. The small bowel is still largely out of reach through endoscopy. Photographic views of the interior of the body provide readily diagnosable information (Figs. 4-21 and 4-22). Therapeutic applications of endoscopy are numerous. They include polyp removal, injection and thermal methods to stop hemorrhaging, sclerosing and banding of esophageal varices, lesion biopsy, sealing of tracheoesophageal fistulas, stone removal, esophageal prosthesis insertion, and laser tumor removal (both generally for palliative purposes). In addition, enteric wall stents have been used to open colon lesions in nonoperative malignancies.

Abdominal Tubes and Catheters

As with the chest, a variety of tubes and catheters can be placed within particular portions of the abdomen. The technologist must be familiar with each type of tube and exercise great caution in attempting to move patients with abdominal tubes in place. The technologist should also ask the patient's nurse or consult the chart before altering the patient's position. In addition, some abdominal tubes and catheters allow entry into body systems that are normally sterile and require special care to avoid infection.

Gastric tubes may be placed (generally through the nose) for a variety of diagnostic and therapeutic purposes. They may be indicated for aspiration of gastric contents to help control nausea and vomiting, for decompression and removal of gastric contents because of bowel dysfunction or surgery, and for nutritional support tube feedings (gastric gavage) or

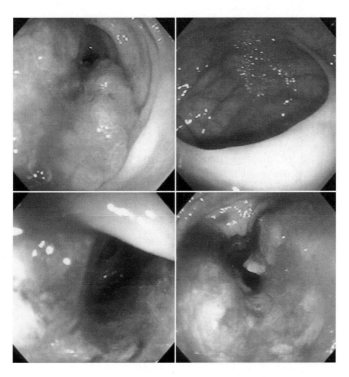

FIG. 4-21 Endoscopic image of a sigmoid colon mass in a 72-year-old woman visible as a mass bulging into the lumen of the colon.

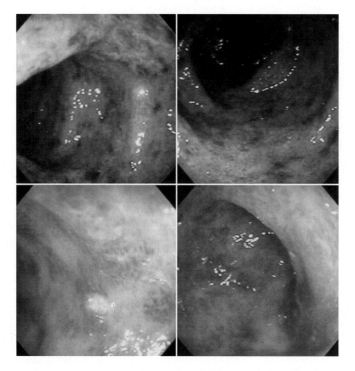

FIG. 4-22 Endoscopic image of diffuse colitis with a bacterial etiology in this 40-year-old man indicated by the splotchiness of the bowel mucosa.

medication administration. A Levin tube is the most common nasogastric tube. It is a fairly small, single-lumen tube with a plain tip, and it may be visualized radiographically. Proper placement is commonly assessed through aspiration of gastric juices and listening for proper placement within the stomach via a stethoscope. If a nasogastric tube is placed for feeding, the patient's head must remain elevated to prevent the tube from becoming displaced, leading to aspiration of the gastric contents. If an emergent condition exists that requires large amounts of gastric contents to be aspirated quickly (gastric lavage), a Ewald or Edlich tube may be used. These tubes are placed through the mouth, are wider than a Levin tube, and contain several openings that allow quicker aspiration. A Levacuator tube may also be used for evacuation of gastric contents. This is a wide, double-lumen tube placed through the

patient's mouth. The larger lumen is used for gastric lavage, while the smaller lumen allows instillation of an irrigant.

An enteral tube is a small-caliber tube used to deliver a liquid diet directly to the duodenum or jejunum. It most commonly has a weighted end to hold the tube in the proper placement. The Dobhoff tube is a common radiopaque enteral tube (Fig. 4-23). Other common types of prolonged enteral tubes include Corpak and Entriflex tubes.

Nasoenteric decompression tubes are used to remove gas and fluids in the prevention and treatment of abdominal distension. These tubes have a balloon or rubber bag at one end filled with air, mercury, or water to stimulate peristalsis and facilitate passage through the pylorus into the intestinal tract. The Miller-Abbott tube is a common type of double-lumen decompression tube. It is passed through the nose,

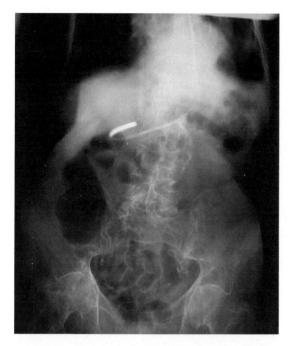

FIG. 4-23 Radiographic appearance of a Dobhoff tube being checked for placement in this 93-year-old woman. It is placed in the antrum of the stomach. Also seen are extensive vascular calcifications.

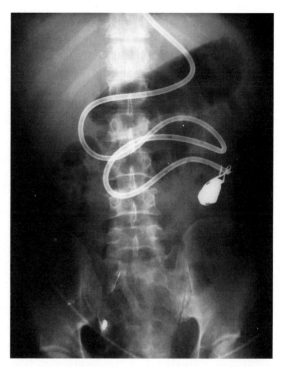

FIG. 4-24 Radiographic appearance of a Cantor tube. Placed 4 hours earlier in this 50-year-old man with a mechanical bowel obstruction, it is now advanced into the second portion of the duodenum.

pharynx, and esophagus with the balloon uninflated. Once the end of the tube reaches the stomach, the balloon is inflated, and the tube is pulled back until it stops at the cardiac sphincter. The patient is then placed on his or her right side in a semierect position, and the air is withdrawn from the balloon and replaced with mercury. Progress of the tube is assessed by taking abdominal radiographs at regular intervals. Harris and Cantor tubes are other types of decompression tubes. Unlike the Miller-Abbott tube, however, the Cantor (Fig. 4-24) and Harris tubes contain a single lumen.

Levin tubes or Foley catheters may also be surgically placed in any portion of the GI system. A gastrostomy tube indicates the tube is placed in the stomach, whereas a duodenostomy tube or jejunostomy tube is specific to that portion of the intestines. A percutaneous

endoscopic gastrostomy tube is frequently placed endoscopically. These tubes provide a direct route for administering liquid feedings.

CONGENITAL AND HEREDITARY ANOMALIES

Esophageal Atresia

Atresia is a congenital absence or closure of a normal body orifice or tubular organ. Esophageal atresia is a congenital anomaly in which the esophagus fails to develop past some point, resulting in a discontinuation of the esophagus (Fig. 4-25). The symptoms of esophageal atresia are visible soon after birth and include excessive salivation, choking, gagging, dyspnea, and cyanosis. Diagnosis of this congenital anomaly may be established by inability to pass

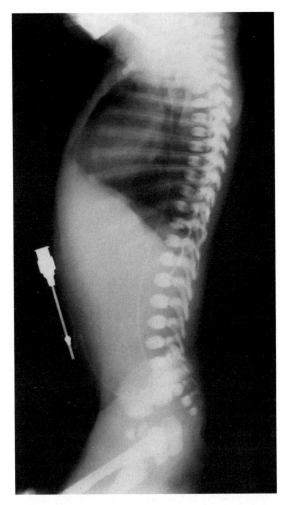

FIG. 4-25 Lack of any GI air below the diaphragm indicates an isolated esophageal atresia.

a nasogastric tube into the stomach. If a radiopaque nasogastric tube is utilized, the terminal end of the pouch may be demonstrated radiographically with a chest radiograph without the use of a contrast agent. Immediate surgery is required to alleviate the problem, and preoperative care must be taken to prevent aspiration pneumonia. The infant may not receive oral feedings, and continuous suction is necessary to prevent aspiration. Under most cir-

cumstances, this increased risk of aspiration contraindicates the use of a contrast agent to visualize the extent of the atresia.

Usually coincident with atresia is a tracheo-esophageal fistula. This consists of an atresia at the level of the fourth thoracic vertebra with a fistula—an abnormal tube-like passage from one structure to another—to the trachea (Fig. 4-26). In addition, a gastrostomy tube may be placed in the infant's stomach to prevent reflux of gastric secretions into the trachea through the fistula. Such a condition is incompatible with life for more than 2 to 3 days, but the prognosis is good if the infant is handled appropriately before surgery to prevent aspiration.

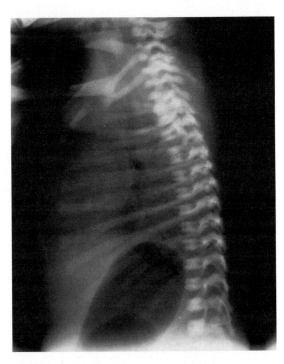

FIG. 4-26 Lateral view of the chest on a 1-day-old premature infant demonstrates distention of the distal esophagus with air and in continuity with the trachea. Marked gastric distention is also present. Appearance is consistent with esophageal atresia and a tracheoesophageal fistula.

Bowel Atresia

Ileal atresia, a congenital discontinuation of the ileum, is the most frequent type of bowel atresia, followed by duodenal atresia. This anomaly presents a few days after birth. The most common signs and symptoms of ileal atresia are abdominal distension and the inability of the infant to pass stool. Eventually the infant regurgitates feedings. Treatment consists of surgery to resect the atretic portion of the bowel and reconnect the bowel proximal and distal to the discontinuation. In some cases, the proximal ileum may be grossly dilated, requiring the surgeon to perform a double-barrel ileostomy. Once the lumen of the proximal ileum returns to a more normal size, the ileostomy is reversed, and the bowel anastomosis can be performed.

Duodenal atresia is a congenital anomaly in which the lumen of the duodenum does not exist, resulting in complete obstruction of the GI tract at the duodenum. In some cases, the atresia may be identified before the birth of the infant with the use of ultrasound. Sonographic evaluation of the fetus should demonstrate a normal stomach with amniotic fluid coursing through it. Atresia is suggested on ultrasound if a dilated stomach is noted without other fluid collections noted in the fetal abdomen. Although rare (1 in approximately 20,000 births), it is evident soon after birth when vomiting begins and the epigastrium becomes distended. A radiographic indication of duodenal atresia is the "double bubble sign." Gaseous distension of the stomach creates one bubble, and gas in the proximal duodenum creates a second bubble (Fig. 4-27). Like esophageal atresia, oral feedings should be withheld in infants with duodenal atresia. Nasogastric decompression of the stomach is indicated to

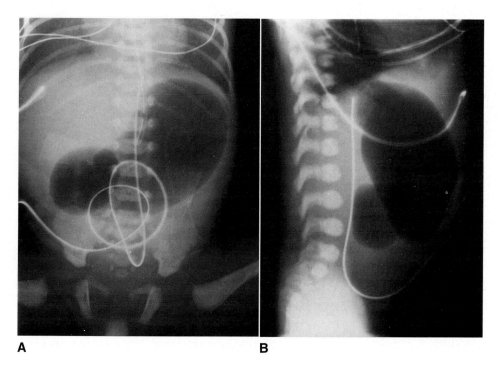

A   **B**

FIG. 4-27 A, Marked distension of the stomach and duodenal bulb with bowel gas distal to the duodenum. Visualization of the classic "double bubble sign" indicates duodenal atresia. **B,** The "double bubble sign" in a lateral projection of the same 1-day-old infant.

prevent vomiting and possible aspiration of the gastric contents. Treatment consists of surgery to open the duodenum for connection to the pylorus. During surgery, it is common to examine the other areas of the small and large bowel for other sites of atresia and malrotation, which often accompany duodenal atresia.

Colonic atresia is a congenital failure of development of the distal rectum and anus, which can occur to a variable extent (Fig. 4-28). A frequent complication is fistula formation to the genitourinary system, which often can be repaired surgically. Prognosis is excellent after surgical intervention for all three types of bowel atresia.

Imperforate Anus

Imperforate anus is a congenital disorder in which there is no anal opening to the exterior. A fistula may be present between the colon and the perineum or urethra in boys or between the colon and vagina in girls. This condition can be demonstrated radiographically with a cross-table lateral rectum projection with the patient lying prone or by performing a fistulogram. It is corrected surgically shortly after birth and may require a temporary colostomy.

Hypertrophic Pyloric Stenosis

Hypertrophic pyloric stenosis is a congenital anomaly of the stomach where the pyloric canal

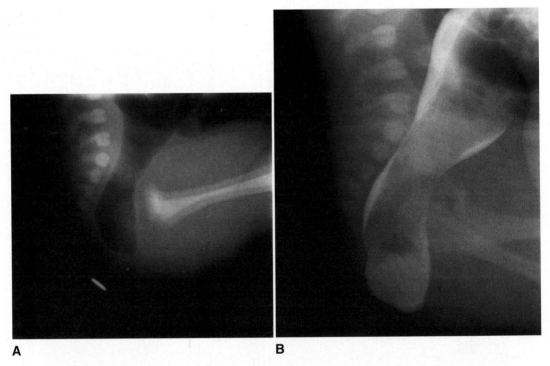

A **B**

FIG. 4-28 A, Visualization of the rectal air column extending to within centimeters of the perineum (indicated by lead marker) in a 15-hour-old newborn with abdominal distension. **B,** Transperineal percutaneous water-soluble contrast study of the rectum reveals a blind distal colon pouch, evidence of colonic atresia. No genitourinary fistulas were noted, as is common with this condition.

leading out of the stomach is greatly narrowed because of hypertrophy of the pyloric sphincter (Fig. 4-29). It is the most common indication for surgery in infants. Its exact etiology is unknown, but it seems genetically related. It occurs three to four times more often in male children and most often in the first-born boy. Typically, the first sign of the condition is projectile vomiting at 3 to 5 weeks of age. These infants often become dehydrated and fail to gain weight. Abdominal ultrasound is useful in evaluating hypertrophy of the pyloric muscle. An upper GI study demonstrates delayed gastric emptying, accompanied by a classic string sign, as the barium trickles through the narrowed, elongated pyloric canal. A surgical procedure is used to incise the hypertrophied muscle fibers and thus increase the opening of the pyloric channel. These infants generally are able to begin normal feedings within a few days after the surgical procedure.

Malrotation

Aberrations of the normal process of intestinal rotation in utero can result in the anomalous position of the small and large bowel, with abnormal fixations predisposing the patient to internal herniation and volvulus. **Malrotation** exists when the intestines are not in their normal position (Fig. 4-30), which occurs in an equal male-to-female ratio. There are varying degrees of malrotation of the intestinal tract, ranging from failure of fixation of the cecum in the right-lower quadrant to complete transposition of the bowel, a condition in which the small bowel is on the right and the colon is on the left. Malrotation of the bowel is clearly visible on a barium enema because in all cases the cecum is not located in the right-lower

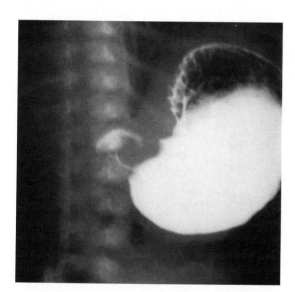

FIG. 4-29 A thin column of barium flowing from the stomach into the pylorus in this 1-month-old boy with projectile vomiting indicates hypertrophic pyloric stenosis.

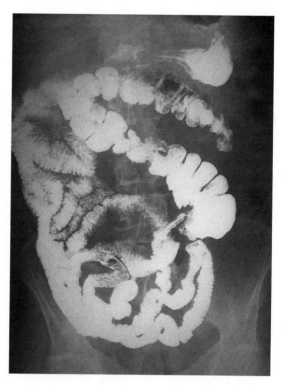

FIG. 4-30 Malrotation of the bowel indicated by the position of the small bowel in the right abdomen and the colon in the left. Note how the terminal ileum enters the cecum from the right.

quadrant of the abdomen. Such errors of fixation are often asymptomatic, but they may lead to bowel volvulus, or incarceration of bowel in an internal hernia. In some instances, the patient may present with clinical signs of bowel obstruction, as discussed later in this chapter. Surgery is the choice for correction of a volvulus or bowel incarceration, with resection of the involved bowel required to relieve the intestinal infarction. Complete reversal of all abdominal organs, although rare, is known as **situs inversus.**

Hirschsprung's Disease

Hirschsprung's disease is an absence of neurons (Meissner's and Auerbach's autonomic plexus) in the bowel wall, typically in the sigmoid colon, and is also known as congenital megacolon. Occurring in approximately 1 in 5000 births, this defect is a familial disease, primarily affecting men. The absence of neurons in the bowel wall prevents the normal relaxation of the colon and subsequent peristalsis, which results in gross dilatation to the point of narrowing and constriction.

This generally becomes apparent shortly after birth, when the affected infant passes little meconium and the abdomen becomes distended. As the patient ages, the continued effects are severe constipation and recurrent fecal impactions. It is important to diagnose this disease early because, if left untreated, it can progress to toxic megacolon. Toxic megacolon develops from bacterial overgrowth leading to fluid and electrolyte imbalances in the infant that could result in death.

Barium enemas demonstrate a transition from the narrow, distal rectum to a dilated proximal colon (Fig. 4-31). Initial treatment in an infant may consist of a temporary colostomy until surgical resection is possible later. In some cases, the surgeon may perform multiple surgeries during infancy to correct the anomaly.

Meckel's Diverticulum

Meckel's diverticulum is a congenital diverticulum of the distal ileum. This sac-like anomaly is

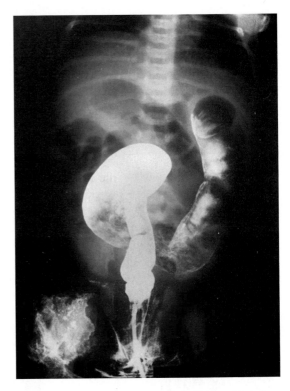

FIG. 4-31 Barium enema on a 6-day-old infant demonstrates a normal rectosigmoid leading to a distended large bowel consistent with Hirschsprung's disease.

located within 6 feet of the ileocecal valve and is a remnant of a duct connecting the small bowel to the umbilicus in the fetus. Children with a Meckel's diverticulum often develop an ulcer in the adjacent bowel, and a common sign is repeated episodes of bleeding from the ulcerated site. Symptoms in adolescents and adults include cramping, vomiting, and bowel obstruction. The symptoms mimic those of appendicitis except for the location of the pain. Diagnosis of a Meckel's diverticulum is difficult, as it may not be visible on a small bowel radiograph. However, nuclear medicine procedures are useful in diagnosing this anomaly. The treatment involves surgical resection of the diverticulum.

INFLAMMATORY DISEASES

Esophageal Strictures

Esophageal strictures can occur in varying degrees, with the symptoms displayed differing according to the amount of obstruction produced. Strictures can be secondary to the ingestion of caustic materials such as strong acids or alkalines (Fig. 4-32) or from any factor that inflames the mucosa and creates scarring. Common types of caustics include household cleansers and detergents containing sulfuric acid and sodium hydroxide. These caustic agents burn the esophagus and cause edema, swelling, and possibly perforation. Endoscopy is usually performed to assess the damage to the esophagus, and the esophageal lesions are treated with corticosteroid therapy.

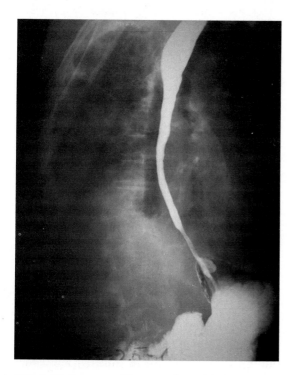

FIG. 4-32 Long-standing esophageal stricture in a 78-year-old man caused by accidental ingestion of a caustic agent at age 3.

Strictures can be differentiated radiographically from normal peristalsis by their unchanging appearance; peristalsis is transitory. The mucosa of a benign stricture appears normal with a smooth contour; the contour of a malignant stricture typically appears ragged. Esophageal strictures require repeated dilation with special, mercury-filled tubes of varying diameters to maintain proper patency. Common tubes for this purpose include Hurst and Maloney dilators and pneumatic balloon dilators that are passed over a wire.

Gastroesophageal Reflux Disease

Gastroesophageal reflux disease (GERD) results from an incompetent cardiac sphincter allowing the backward flow of gastric acid and contents into the esophagus. **Reflux esophagitis** is the primary cause of esophageal inflammation. Reflux is not necessarily abnormal. Heartburn, or symptomatic reflux, has been experienced by most people. It is only when the normal event leads to chronic symptoms and complications, such as esophagitis, a stricture, or an esophageal ulcer, that it becomes of concern.

Esophageal manometry to determine the pressure in the upper and lower esophageal sphincters, pH monitoring of the esophagus, an acid perfusion (Berstein) test, and esophagoscopy are performed, in addition to barium swallow radiographs, to help confirm the diagnosis of gastroesophageal reflux. The reflux may not be evident on a barium swallow, but ulcers and strictures caused by chronic irritation are quite visible. Treatment includes elevating the head of the individual's bed, avoiding drinks such as coffee or alcohol, that stimulate acid secretion or foods such as chocolate, that decrease sphincter competence. Smoking also must be avoided because it also lowers sphincter competence. GERD is also treated with antacids to wash gastric acids out of the esophagus for pain relief and medical therapy with a variety of medicines, such as H_2 blockers, to inhibit their production or prokinetic agents to enhance motility.

Surgery as a treatment is the last option for those whose symptoms have failed to respond to medical therapy. It is performed using video-assisted laparoscopic techniques.

Peptic Ulcer

Normally, the GI system is protected by a mucosal barrier and epithelial cells that remove excess hydrogen ions. Mucosal blood flow also helps to remove excess acid, thus maintaining a normal pH balance. A **peptic ulcer** is an erosion of the mucous membrane of the lower end of the esophagus, stomach, or duodenum. The most likely site of development of a peptic ulcer is in the duodenal bulb and on the lesser curvature of the stomach. Duodenal ulcers are found in adults of all ages and are almost always benign. Gastric ulcers can affect individuals at any age, but primarily affect those over 40 years of age.

Current studies suggest that peptic ulcers result from disruption of the normal mucosal defense and repair mechanisms. Nonsteroidal antiinflammatory drugs (NSAIDs), and the bacteria *Helicobacter pylori (H. pylori)* alter the mucosa, making it more susceptible to the effects of acid normally residing in the GI tract. *Helicobacter pylori* is a gram-negative, spiral-shaped bacillus identified in 1983. Researchers are uncertain exactly how this bacteria injures the mucosal lining, but many believe it produces ammonia and cytotoxins, making the mucosa more susceptible to acid damage. NSAIDs inflame the mucosa because they are able to diffuse through the mucosa into the epithelium and damage the epithelial cells.

The main symptom of a gastric ulcer is pain, usually above the epigastrium and radiating to all parts of the abdomen. Food ingestion or antacids provide temporary relief, but the pain usually returns when the stomach is empty. In some patients, food may actually increase pain as it stimulates peristalsis, which irritates the ulcer. Symptoms of a duodenal ulcer are more consistent, and pain generally begins midmorning. The pain subsides with food ingestion but returns 2 to 3 hours later.

Diagnosis is made primarily via endoscopy. However, double-contrast radiographic GI studies may be performed. Intermittent healing in the midst of continuing inflammation leads to considerable scarring at the base of the ulcer. Gastric ulcers generally display as radiating, spike-like wheels of mucosal folds that run to the edge of the crater (Fig. 4-33). Seen en face, the edge of this ulcer appears round and regular (Fig. 4-34).

With recent understanding of the cause of ulcers, the treatment has changed dramatically over the past 10 years. Ulcers are commonly treated with, and should respond to, antibiotic treatment. The drug regimen currently used is a combination of two or three medications, both antibiotics and acid-blocking drugs. The most common drugs used to eradicate *H. pylori* include bismuth, metronidazole, and tetracycline, and they are effective in curing 80% of infections within 2 weeks. Dietary adjustments were required to minimize irritating food substances in the past, but there is no current evidence this is effective in healing the ulcer or preventing its recurrence. Surgery is rarely performed and primarily is required only for complications of ulcers, such as bleeding or perforation. The complications can include pneumoperitoneum or peritonitis if the ulcer perforates into the abdomen. Perforations are generally confirmed by CT evaluation or conventional erect abdominal radiographs. Ulceration into an artery can produce life-threatening hemorrhage, and this is the most common complication associated with ulcers. Finally, the edema, spasm, and scarring produced by ulceration can result in bowel obstruction.

Gastroenteritis

A number of inflammatory disorders of the stomach and intestine fall into the general grouping of **gastroenteritis,** inflammation of the mucosal lining of the stomach and small bowel (Fig. 4-35). Erosive gastritis appears to be a precursor to gastric ulcer formation and results from a compromised mucosal barrier

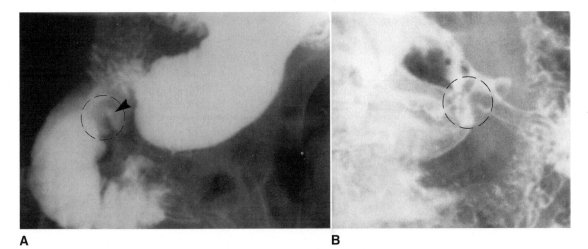

A   **B**

FIG. 4-33 A, Prone RAO projection of the duodenal bulb demonstrates a dense collection of barium in an ulcer crater, suggesting that it is on the anterior duodenal wall. **B,** Persistent collection of barium in the middle portion of the duodenal bulb indicating a superficial ulcer crater, with radiating folds extending from the ulceration. An incisura (fold) along the lower bulb margin points toward the ulcer.

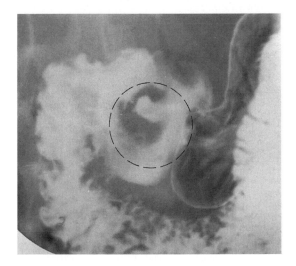

FIG. 4-34 A duodenal ulcer in a 25-year-old man, evidenced by an ulcer crater surrounded by edema represented by the radiolucent halo.

within the stomach. Causes of erosive gastritis include the ingestion of aspirin and other NSAIDs, alcohol, and steroids; physical stress, trauma; and viral or fungal infections. Acute gastric erosions heal rapidly once the cause is withdrawn. Gastric erosions may be identified on double-contrast examinations of the stomach. Complete erosion appears as slit-like collections of barium surrounded by radiolucent halos of swollen, elevated mucosa. In some cases, scalloped or nodular antral folds may also be visualized. Antral gastritis appears to result from alcohol, smoking, and *H. pylori* infection. Radiographically, it is demonstrated by decreased distensibility of the antrum in combination with thickened mucosal folds within the antrum, which tend to be oriented on its longitudinal axis and result in a narrowed antrum.

Ingestion of foods contaminated with *Salmonella* and other types of bacteria—most commonly poultry, meat, dairy products, and eggs—may also result in gastroenteritis. Because of the methods used in the mass production of eggs, there was a dramatic increase in *Salmonella* infections in the 1980s. Diarrhea results from mild mucosal ulcerations within the small bowel and the ability of the *Salmonella* bacteria to produce a secretory factor. This is a threat to the normal electrolytic balance of the body, with the diarrhea lasting

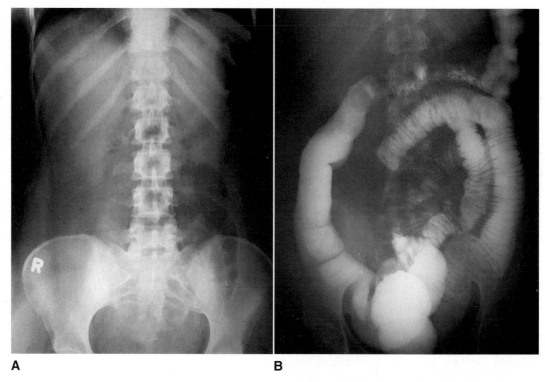

A   **B**

FIG. 4-35 A, Air-filled, dilated small-bowel loops seen on this abdominal plain film are suggestive of an obstruction in this 30-year-old patient with abdominal pain, nausea, and vomiting. **B,** Barium readily refluxes from a barium enema into the distal ileum, demonstrating dilatation without obstruction. The dilatation was secondary to inflammation caused by gastroenteritis.

3 to 4 days. A good patient history can often point out the offending agent, and treatment consists of proper fluid management and relief of nausea and vomiting.

Malabsorption Syndrome

Malabsorption syndrome is a group of diseases of various causes in which there is interference with normal digestion and absorption of food through the small bowel. Common symptoms of malabsorption syndrome include diarrhea, flatulence, weight loss, and abdominal distension. In addition, patients often present with nutritional deficiencies specific to the primary disease and the area of the GI system affected by the disorder.

The best-known small-bowel malabsorption disorder is celiac disease, which occurs as a result of sensitivity to the gliadin fraction of gluten, an agent found in wheat and rye products such as bread. The gliadin acts as an antigen and combines with antibodies within the intestinal mucosa, which promotes the aggregation of K lymphocytes. These lymphocytes cause mucosal damage in combination with an increase in crypt cells within the mucosa. With such a condition, the bowel dilates, mucosal folds atrophy, and peristalsis slows or stops. Radiographic changes generally seen with malabsorption syndrome are segmentation of the barium column, flocculation (resembling tufts of cotton), and edematous mucosal changes (Fig. 4-36). Laboratory tests demonstrate low albumin, calcium, potassium, and sodium levels in combination with elevated alkaline phosphatase and prothrombin time. Diagnosis is usually confirmed by biopsy of the small bowel. Treatment of celiac disease consists of avoidance of substances containing gluten and dietary substitution of other products. Vitamin therapy is also used to ensure adequate amounts of nutrients not available because of the malabsorption in the small bowel.

Lactase insufficiency is another form of the malabsorption syndrome, affecting about 60% of the nonwhite population and 20% to 30% of the white population. With this condition, the small bowel lacks enough of the enzyme lactase, which is used to digest lactose into simple sugars that can be absorbed. The result

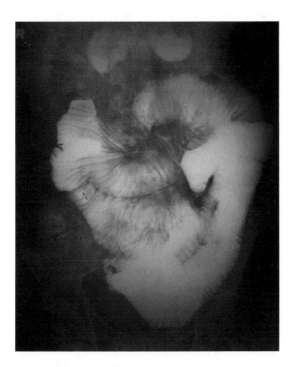

FIG. 4-36 Celiac disease in a 15-year-old patient with a history of diarrhea, indicated on this small bowel study by dilated bowel loops, thickened folds, a grayish appearance of the barium (because of excess fluid in the bowel), and a delayed transit time.

is that lactose stays in the bowel and acts as an osmotic agent, causing fluid to weep into the colon lumen from the wall and creating cramping and diarrhea. The diarrhea also leads to other nutritional deficiencies because the nutrients are purged before they can be absorbed through the intestinal mucosa. Lactose mixed with barium shows the barium moving quickly through the bowel and becoming diluted in the distal ileum and colon (Fig. 4-37). Patients affected by this condition avoid symptoms through avoidance of dairy products.

Regional Enteritis (Crohn's Disease)

Regional enteritis, also known as **Crohn's disease** or granulomatous colitis, is a chronic inflammatory disease of unknown etiology. Research indicates that these individuals have a genetic predisposition of an unregulated intestinal immune response to various agents such as food or environmental factors. Crohn's disease typically occurs in the lower ileum but may be seen anywhere throughout the bowel. Over half of all cases involve the colon. This disease typically affects young adults of both sexes between the ages of 14 and 24 years, with symptoms suggestive of appendicitis or acute bowel obstruction. Family history of Crohn's disease and emotional stress are thought to be important causative factors of bowel dysfunction.

Regional enteritis starts as inflammation of the crypt cells with ulceration of the bowel wall. It eventually affects all layers of the bowel wall. The bowel wall thickens in response to the inflammation and may form fistulas to adjacent loops of bowel, skin, or other abdominal viscera. Subsequent fibrotic scarring may give rise to mechanical obstruction of the bowel. The combination of mucosal edema and crisscrossing fine ulcerations gives the bowel a "cobblestone" radiographic appearance. The string sign (Fig. 4-38) is demonstrated where the terminal ileum is so diseased and stenotic that the barium mixture can only trickle through a small opening that looks like a string. Presentation of the disease in two or more areas with normal

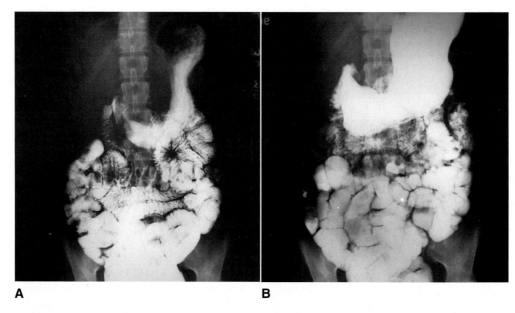

A　　　　　　　　　　　　**B**

FIG. 4-37 A, Abdominal distension, pain, and diarrhea led to this small-bowel examination, diagnosed as normal for this 35-year-old patient. **B,** Mixing of lactose with barium on a repeat study led to mild bowel dilatation, rapid transit time, and dilution of barium in the distal small bowel, indicative of lactase insufficiency.

intervening bowel between is identified as "skip areas" (Fig. 4-39), thus the designation "regional" enteritis. Most cases involve both the ileum and cecum (45%); however, it may be present in the ileum only (35%) or in the colon only (20%), and in rare cases it may affect the entire small bowel. Regional enteritis is a chronic disease characterized by periods of exacerbation interspersed with periods of inactivity. In addition, these patients tend to have an increased chance of developing carcinoma of the bowel with a very poor prognosis. Crohn's disease is classified as early stage, intermediate stage, or advanced stage, and the progression of the disease can be demonstrated radiographically by performing a small bowel series, enteroclysis, or a double-contrast barium enema. CT is not helpful for the initial diagnosis but may be used to assess fistulas or abscesses resulting from the disease.

Treatment of regional enteritis centers on decreasing inflammation, relief of diarrhea, and treatment of infection. Bowel resection to remove the involved section of the intestine is necessary approximately 70% of the time, particularly if perforation or hemorrhage is present. Recurrence of the disease in other areas of the bowel, however, is common. The disease is rarely cured, but rarely fatal.

Appendicitis

Appendicitis is an inflammation of the vermiform appendix, resulting from an obstruction caused usually by a fecalith (Fig. 4-40) or rarely by a neoplasm. It is the most common abdominal surgical emergency in the United States. Appendicitis is most frequent in the late teens and 20s and has a fairly equal distribution between the sexes. Complications, usually resulting from gangrenous or perforated appendicitis, occur in about 3% to 5% of all cases. Delayed diagnosis and treatment of appendicitis account for much of the morbidity and mortality associated with this disease.

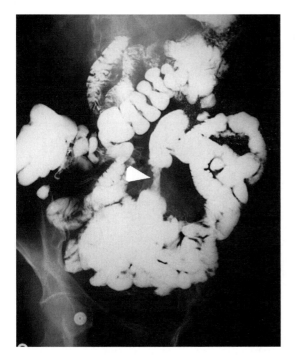

FIG. 4-38 The string sign, demonstrating a diseased, stenotic terminal ileum.

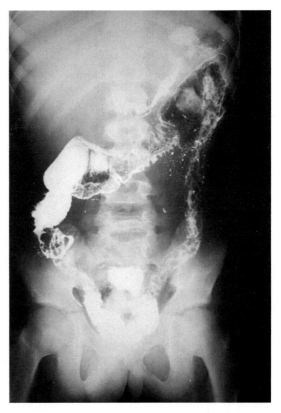

FIG. 4-39 Regional enteritis in an 11-year-old patient demonstrated by the "cobblestone" appearance of the cecum and left colon, with "skip" areas of normal bowel between.

The obstruction leads to inflammation and distension and affects the blood supply to this portion of the bowel. Venous blood return is decreased, which in turn results in deoxygenation of the tissue. All of these factors leave the appendix susceptible to infection from bacteria, such as *Escherichia coli,* which is normally found within the intestinal tract. Poor blood supply can also lead to gangrene, perforation, and possible rupture. Once the vermiform appendix ruptures, the infection spreads to the peritoneum, leading to general peritonitis that could result in death.

The signs and symptoms of appendicitis include initial pain in the epigastrium that moves to the right-lower quadrant and becomes persistent. Nausea and vomiting may occur as a reflex symptom because the vagus nerve supplies both the stomach and appendix. Individuals also carry a low-grade fever, have a sudden onset of constipation, and present with an elevated white blood cell count. The elevation of white blood cells helps to distinguish appendicitis from other colicky abdominal disorders.

Medical imaging is of little value in assessing early appendicitis, so the diagnosis is generally made from clinical information. CT is helpful in identifying abscess formation, and ultrasound has been used with some success as a means of imaging the appendix. The most successful diagnostic cases have been those where the appendix was swollen and fluid filled.

Surgical removal of the appendix is the most common treatment, and, in cases of early surgi-

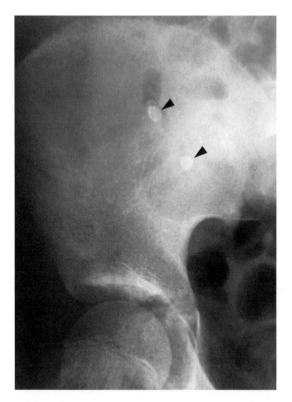

FIG. 4-40 Spot film of a fecalith within the appendix, a common cause of appendicitis.

cal intervention, the mortality is low. However, complications such as abscess formation or perforation and peritonitis place the individual at a greater risk and greatly increase the recovery period.

Ulcerative Colitis

Ulcerative colitis is an inflammatory lesion of the colon mucosa. Its etiology is unknown, but it is thought to be an autoimmune disease. It is four times more common in whites, especially Jewish persons, than in nonwhites. Typically, it affects 15- to 25-year-olds. They present with symptoms of excessive diarrhea with blood, pus, and mucus in the stools. The disease generally starts in the rectum and spreads to the sigmoid, sometimes involving the entire colon.

Its clinical course is highly variable in severity and prognosis.

Inflammation of the mucosa and submucosa (reticulin fibers beneath the mucosal epithelium) causes abscesses to form in the crypt cells, separating them from their blood supply and leading to epithelial necrosis and mucosal ulceration. Gradually, the mucosa is replaced by fibrous tissue whose crevices give a rough, cobblestone appearance to the involved colon (Fig. 4-41).

Symptoms include intermittent spells of bloody diarrhea and abdominal cramping. Colon strictures are a rare complication of ulcerative colitis. Another complication of ulcerative colitis is toxic colitis or megacolon, an acute dilatation of the colon from colonic paralytic ileus (Fig. 4-42). The dilated bowel is particularly susceptible to rupture; a barium enema is absolutely contraindicated. People

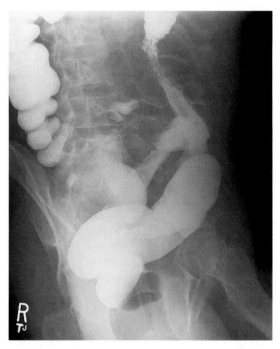

FIG. 4-41 A left posterior oblique barium enema after film demonstrating ulcerative colitis in the proximal colon.

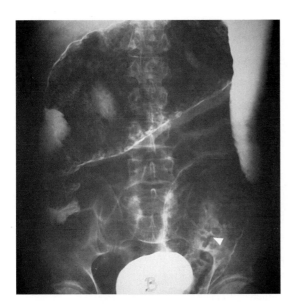

FIG. 4-42 Barium enema on a 61-year-old man demonstrates toxic megacolon secondary to ulcerative colitis. Pseudopolyps are seen in the descending colon.

with ulcerative colitis have a greatly increased incidence of colon cancer, especially if the entire colon is affected for over 10 years.

Sigmoidoscopy and colonoscopy are the usual means of diagnosing ulcerative colitis because 90% to 95% of the cases involve the distal colon or rectum. Barium enemas are used to support the clinical diagnosis and to assess the progression of the disease and its complications. When filled with barium, the normally smooth colon outline becomes irregular because of the ulceration present. Pseudopolyps are islands of unaffected mucosa that become visible when surrounded by affected mucosa. Another radiographic indication of ulcerative colitis is an easily recognized loss of colon haustration and mucosal edema.

Certain characteristics of ulcerative colitis distinguish it from regional enteritis (Crohn's disease). Ulcerative colitis is a disease of the mucosa of the colon, whereas regional enteritis affects all layers of the bowel wall. Also, ulcerative colitis typically begins at the anus and

ascends, often results in megacolon and bowel perforations, and frequently progresses to cancer; by contrast, regional enteritis usually begins in the terminal ileum and cecum and descends through the bowel, often with skip areas. It rarely produces megacolon or bowel perforations.

Treatment of ulcerative colitis is initially medical in nature and often involves dietary restrictions. Steroid therapy is used to treat ulcerative colitis, and it may be administered either orally or rectally. Development of an obstruction or neoplasm may require surgical intervention. This involves removal of the colon from cecum to sigmoid with establishment of an ileostomy or ileorectal or ileoanal anastomosis.

ESOPHAGEAL VARICES

Varicose veins are abnormally lengthened, dilated, and superficial veins; those in the esophagus are referred to as **esophageal varices.** They occur in the esophagus because of portal hypertension. Conditions that cause resistance to the normal blood flow through the liver (such as cirrhosis) cause a bypass of the normal venous drainage mechanism. Instead, the blood is directed through the esophageal and gastric collateral veins. The increase in blood flow through these channels results in venous dilatation.

Esophageal varices are best demonstrated in a recumbent position because gravity causes poor visualization in an erect position. A thin barium mixture radiographically demonstrates the varices as worm-like defects within the column of barium (Fig. 4-43). Use of thick barium may be counterproductive because it can cover the varices. Esophageal varices may also occasionally be visualized as a retrocardiac posterior mediastinal mass on a plain chest film obtained with the patient in a recumbent position.

Patients with esophageal varices are subject to their rupture and hemorrhage, which may be massive and often is fatal. Statistics show that

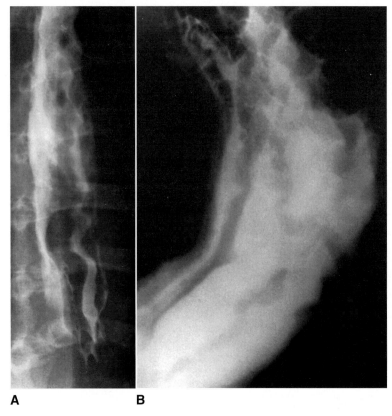

A   **B**

FIG. 4-43 A, Long, serpentine filling defects in the esophagus of a 41-year-old with chronic alcoholism, indicative of esophageal varices. **B,** Similar filling defects seen in the cardia of the stomach of the same patient, indicative of gastric varices.

ruptured varices have accounted for approximately one third of all deaths from cirrhosis. An erect film taken for this situation should be done with great caution because the patient's blood loss may be significant. The resultant reduced blood pressure along with the elevation may cause the patient to faint.

Treatment for esophageal varices may consist of endoscopic sclerotherapy, banding ligation, or infusion of vasopressin, a natural hormone useful in stopping hemorrhage. Compression of the varices through balloon tamponading may be occasionally used. Shunts such as transjugular intrahepatic portosystemic shunts (TIPS),

applied via interventional radiology or in surgery, may be used to help redirect liver blood flow, thus reducing portal hypertension and easing venous pressure in the esophageal and gastric collateral circulation. Sonography has been helpful in these patients over time to access the direction of flow with the TIPS shunt. Occasionally, the shunt can become blocked and clinically there may be concern that the shunt is not functioning correctly. Doppler interrogation of the shunt with ultrasound can give quantitative analysis about the direction and magnitude of the flow of blood within the shunt.

DEGENERATIVE DISEASES

Herniation

A **hernia** is a protrusion of a loop of bowel through a small opening, usually in the abdominal wall. Popularly referred to as a rupture, it occurs because of an anatomic weakness. As the bowel loop herniates, it pushes the peritoneum ahead of it. An inguinal hernia, which is common in men, occurs when a bowel loop protrudes through a weakness in the inguinal ring (Fig. 4-44) and may descend downward into the scrotum. Femoral and umbilical herniation (Fig. 4-45) occur in both sexes.

If a herniated loop of bowel can be pushed back into the abdominal cavity, it is said to be reducible. If it becomes stuck and cannot be reduced, it is an incarcerated hernia. As described previously, this can result in a bowel obstruction (Fig. 4-46). If the constriction through which the bowel loop has passed is tight enough to cut off blood supply to the bowel, it is called a strangulated hernia. Prompt

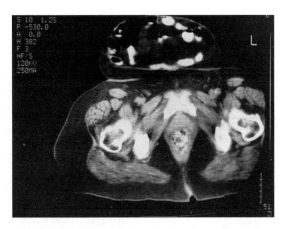

FIG. 4-45 CT demonstration of a large anterior abdominal hernia containing multiple loops of small bowel and possibly some large bowel, without evidence of obstruction in this 70-year-old man.

surgical intervention is required in this case to avoid necrosis of that portion of the bowel. Bowel that has already necrosed can generally be surgically resected.

Hiatal Hernia

A **hiatal hernia** is a weakness of the esophageal hiatus that permits some portions of the stomach to herniate into the thoracic cavity. Hiatal hernias occur in about half of the population over age 50. In its early stages, a hiatal hernia is reducible. Chronic herniation may be associated with GERD.

A direct, or sliding, hiatal hernia occurs when a portion of the stomach and gastroesophageal junction are both situated above the diaphragm (Fig. 4-47). This type of hernia comprises the outstanding majority (about 99%) of all hiatal hernias. A Schatzki's ring is often visible with this condition (Fig. 4-48) and consists of a mucosal ring that protrudes into the lumen. Such a ring has traditionally been thought to be congenital but may be related to gastric reflux. It is, however, generally of no clinical significance unless it produces narrowing sufficient to cause dysphagia, usually less than 13 mm in diameter.

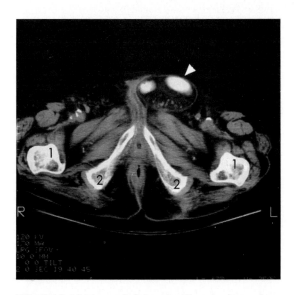

FIG. 4-44 Moderate left inguinal hernia *(arrow)* on this CT image of a 96-year-old man. Also well defined are *(1)* the femurs, showing the lesser trochanters projecting posteriorly, and *(2)* the ischial tuberosities.

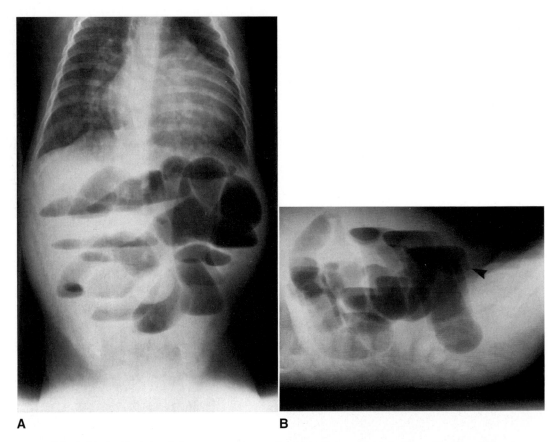

A   **B**

FIG. 4-46 **A,** Upright abdomen on a 3-month-old indicates multiple dilated loops of bowel with air–fluid levels present, suggesting a mechanical bowel obstruction. **B,** A prone cross-table lateral view shows the small bowel forming a beak-like projection at the point of obstruction at the internal inguinal ring in this incarcerated hernia.

A far less common type of hiatal hernia is the rolling, or paraesophageal, hiatal hernia. This occurs when a portion of the stomach or adjacent viscera herniates above the diaphragm while the gastroesophageal junction remains below the diaphragm (Fig. 4-49). If all of the stomach slides above the diaphragm, an intrathoracic stomach (Fig. 4-50) results. Unlike the sliding hiatal hernia, a paraesophageal hernia is potentially life threatening because of the risk of volvulus, incarceration, or strangulation of the hernia.

Most hiatal hernias are asymptomatic, but some are accompanied by reflux. Most patients experiencing reflux complain of a full feeling in the chest, particularly after meals. Some reflux of gastric contents leads to complaints of heartburn. An upper GI examination can pinpoint the herniation. Treatment of hiatal herniation is generally conservative to minimize discomfort.

BOWEL OBSTRUCTIONS

Both the small and large bowels of the normal patient are nearly always active in peristalsis. Many lesions of various types (e.g., inflammatory, degenerative) can interfere with this action and cause an obstruction of either small

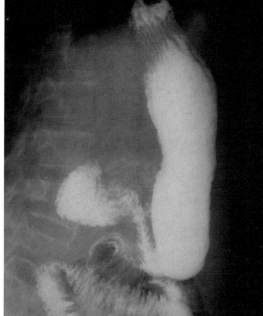

A

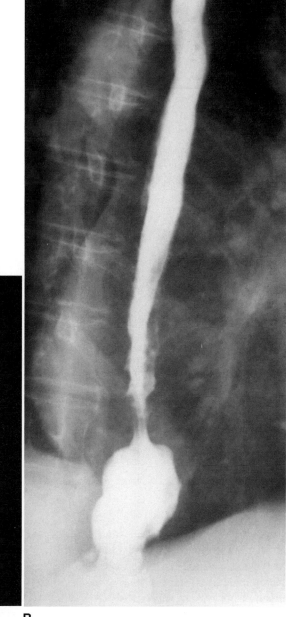

B

FIG. 4-47 A, Demonstration of contrast material above the hemidiaphragm on an upper GI series of this 51-year-old woman. **B,** The esophagus narrows to the stomach, which is seen to empty passively, above the hemidiaphragm in this sliding hiatal hernia.

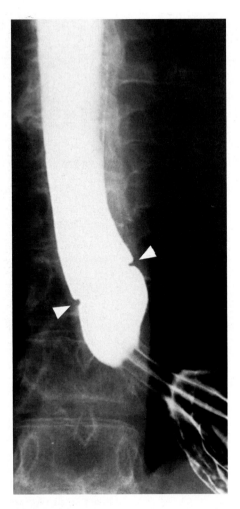

FIG. 4-48 Schatzki's ring as demonstrated in the case of a sliding hiatal hernia.

graphs over 12 to 24 hours help to determine the diagnosis and to locate the level of the obstruction in individuals with mechanical obstructions. Most commonly, gas confined to the small bowel with multiple air-fluid levels visible on an erect abdominal radiograph indicates a mechanical obstruction, whereas gas distributed throughout both the large and small bowel is indicative of paralytic ileus. The small bowel tends to be more distended in cases of mechanical obstruction. Physical signs are also helpful in distinguishing the type of obstruction present. Bowel sounds, the normal sounds of a bowel in motion as heard on auscultation, are absent with an ileus; they are present with a mechanical obstruction and are often hyperactive and high-pitched. Emesis containing bile may also indicate a mechanical obstruction.

Mechanical Bowel Obstruction

A mechanical bowel obstruction (Fig. 4-51) is one in which the lumen of the bowel becomes occluded, as might occur for a variety of reasons such as hernias, tumors, or, most often postoperatively, from adhesions. A simple mechanical obstruction does not involve the blood supply to the bowel, whereas a strangulating obstruction can lead to bowel infarction. Nearly half of all strangulating mechanical bowel obstructions are caused by an incarcerated (i.e., trapped) hernia, a condition discussed earlier in this chapter as a degenerative disease. Entrapment of a hernia, usually involving the small bowel, causes impairment of blood flow and swelling of the affected tissues. The resultant edema affects the arterial blood flow to the bowel and may lead to ischemic necrosis, perforation, and peritonitis. Prompt surgical intervention and reduction are required to relieve an incarcerated hernia.

Gallstone ileus is another cause for a mechanical bowel obstruction. In this condition, a gallstone can erode from the gallbladder and create a fistula to the small bowel. This leads to an obstruction, usually when the gallstone reaches the ileocecal valve. Radiographic signs of this include air–fluid levels or air in the

or large bowel. The resultant obstruction can be either a **mechanical bowel obstruction,** as occurs from a blockage of the bowel lumen, or a paralytic ileus, which results from a failure of peristalsis. There are gradations of each, and both may be present at the same time. Initial diagnosis of a small bowel obstruction by use of a plain abdominal radiograph may be difficult because of the frequency of vomiting and the use of nasogastric decompression.

General signs and symptoms of a bowel obstruction include vomiting, abdominal distension, and abdominal pain. Sequential radio-

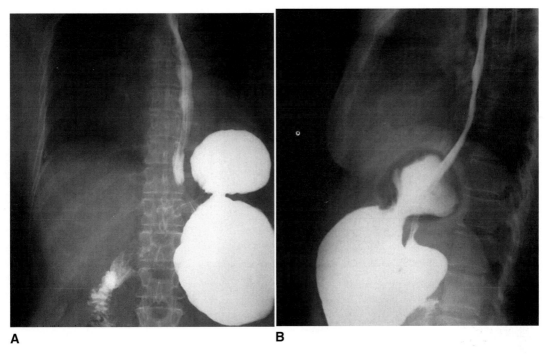

A   **B**

FIG. 4-49 **A,** Paraesophageal hiatal hernia, demonstrating narrowing in the fundus. **B,** Lateral view of the same patient demonstrates the cardioesophageal junction in its normal place below the hemidiaphragm. The fundus is highlighted by the radiolucency of the lung.

biliary tree (Fig. 4-52). The gallstone itself may also be visible, often in the terminal ileum where it causes the obstruction.

A **volvulus** is a twisting of a bowel loop about its mesenteric base, usually at either the sigmoid or ileocecal junction (Fig. 4-53). This most commonly occurs in the elderly and is identifiable on a plain abdomen radiograph as a collection of air conforming to the shape of the affected, dilated bowel. Some twists resolve spontaneously; however, bowel that is twisted more than 360 degrees requires surgical intervention. Surgical untwisting and resection are necessary to prevent necrosis and perforation of the bowel caused by a lack of blood supply.

An **intussusception** occurs when a segment of bowel, constricted by peristalsis, telescopes into a distal segment and is driven further into the distal bowel by peristalsis. Recall that the bowel is connected to the mesentery, so as the bowel telescopes into itself, the mesentery

(with its rich blood supply) is also involved. Intussusception is responsible for approximately 5% of all mechanical obstructions and most frequently affects the ileocecal valve (Fig. 4-54). It is more common in children and infants than in adults. Its presence in an adult generally signifies an accompanying intraluminal mass and is generally reduced surgically so that the physician can search for the cause of the intussusception and correct the condition. In children and infants, an intussusception can often be reduced by an enema, sparing a surgical intervention. Other causes of small bowel obstruction include Crohn's disease, and appendicitis.

Diagnosis is made based on clinical signs and symptoms including abdominal distension, abdominal cramps, and vomiting. Conventional supine and erect abdominal radiographs often confirm the diagnosis with air–fluid levels clearly visible in the erect position. In cases of a cecal volvulus, an abdominal radiograph will

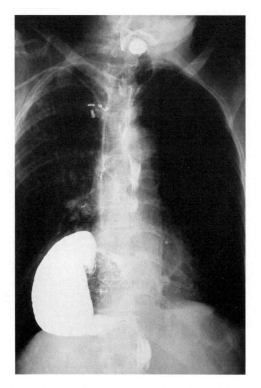

FIG. 4-50 Intrathoracic stomach indicated by the presence of the entire stomach above the diaphragm, also with malrotation of the stomach.

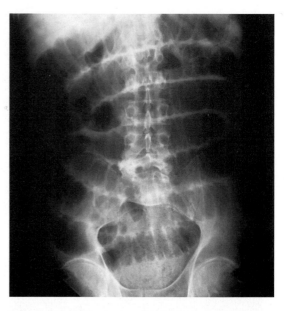

FIG. 4-51 Abdominal radiograph demonstrating a mechanical bowel obstruction, with numerous loops of dilated bowel seen within the midabdomen. The patient had an acute onset of abdominal pain, nausea, and vomiting.

reveal a large air bubble within the midabdomen. Generally, mechanical obstructions require surgical intervention.

Paralytic Ileus

Paralytic ileus or adynamic ileus is a failure of normal peristalsis that may result from a variety of factors. The most common causes are following surgery, especially that requiring manipulation of the bowel (postoperative ileus), and intraperitoneal or retroperitoneal infection. It may also be associated with bowel ischemia, certain drugs, electrolyte imbalance, pancreatitis, or simply as a reaction to any stressful medical illness. Paralytic ileus generally lasts no longer than 3 days with proper medical treatment.

Signs and symptoms of paralytic ileus include distension of the abdomen, abdominal cramp-

ing, and vomiting. The absence of peristalsis causes the lumen of both the small and large intestines to fill with gas and fluid, with the resultant dilatation extending to the rectum (Fig. 4-55). Radiographically, gas will be visible in the colon. Treatment for paralytic ileus generally consists of nasogastric suction and medical stimulation of the bowel to restore peristalsis. In some cases colonscopic decompression may be required.

NEUROGENIC DISEASES

Achalasia

Achalasia is a neuromuscular abnormality of the esophagus that results in failure of the lower esophageal sphincter of the distal esophagus to relax, leading to dysphagia. It occurs equally in men and women and most commonly affects individuals between the ages of 20 and 40. Clinically, these patients present with a slowly progressive dysphagia in swallow-

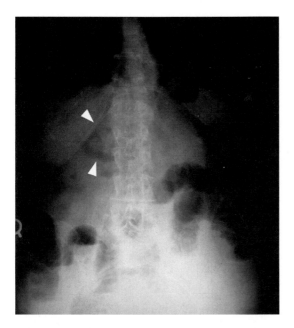

FIG. 4-52 Abdominal radiograph of a 43-year-old woman demonstrating air within the biliary ductal system and an overall density (gallstone) in the right lower abdomen.

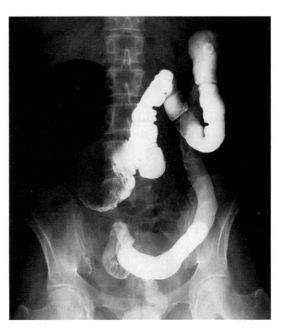

FIG. 4-53 A barium enema radiograph depicting a cecal volvulus. Note how the column of barium stops at the level of the volvulus.

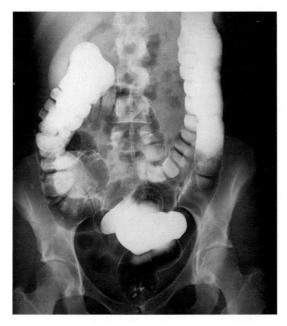

FIG. 4-54 Pediatric barium enema demonstrating intussusception at the ileocecal junction.

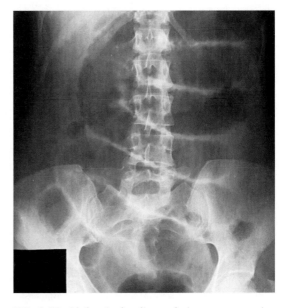

FIG. 4-55 Abdominal radiograph on a postoperative patient demonstrating paralytic ileus. Note the dilated bowel loops extending through the large intestine.

ing both solids and liquids. Patients may also experience regurgitation, chest pain, and moderate weight loss.

Radiographically, the condition demonstrates as a dilated esophagus with little or no peristalsis. The distal esophagus itself is often described as having a "beaked" appearance (Fig. 4-56). Because the distal esophagus opens only intermittently, when the pressure is high enough, food residue may be seen in the distal esophagus or even on a chest radiograph. Because the esophageal contents act as a water seal, the normal gastric gas bubble may be absent.

Initial treatment of achalasia is to reduce the pressure and obstruction at the cardiac sphincter. Esophageal dilatation is effective in about 85% of patients affected by achalasia. Medications, such as nitrates and calcium channel blockers, may be used to reduce the sphincter pressure and reduce the frequency of repeated dilatations. Botulinum toxin may also be injected

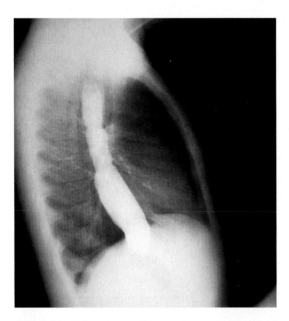

FIG. 4-56 Dilated esophagus in a 10-year-old patient that demonstrated no normal peristalsis on filling, indicating achalasia. The distal esophagus terminates into a beaked appearance.

into the sphincter to create chemical denervation, but this is effective for only 1 year. Patients not responding to dilatation and medication protocols may require surgical myotomy (cutting of the sphincter muscle fibers).

DIVERTICULAR DISEASES

Esophageal Diverticula

A **diverticulum** is a pouch or sac of variable size that occurs normally or is created by herniation of a mucous membrane through a defect in its muscular coat. Esophageal diverticula occur when mucosal outpouchings penetrate through the muscular layer of the esophagus. The two primary types of esophageal diverticula are pulsion and traction.

A pulsion diverticulum involves the mucosa only and results from a motility disorder of the esophagus, which allows the mucosa to herniate outward. This type of diverticulum appears radiographically as a rounded projection with a narrow neck and occurs more frequently in the upper and lower thirds of the esophagus. A Zenker's diverticulum is a pulsion type found at the pharyngoesophageal junction at the upper end of the esophagus (Fig. 4-57). An epiphrenic diverticulum is another pulsion type, but it is found in the distal esophagus just above the hemidiaphragm (Fig. 4-58).

A traction diverticulum involves all layers of the esophagus and results from adjacent scar tissue that pulls the esophagus toward the area of involvement (Fig. 4-59). Such a diverticulum occurs more frequently in the middle third of the esophagus at the carina and appears radiographically as a triangle whose apex points toward the disease.

Usually, diverticula are asymptomatic until they reach a relatively large size, at which time complications may occur. For example, food and secretions can collect in the diverticulum and cause a mechanical obstruction of the esophagus. Such contents can also be aspirated by a recumbent patient, resulting in a chemical pneumonia. Failure to control the effects of

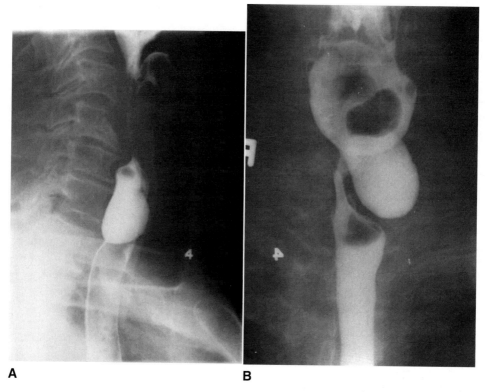

A   **B**

FIG. 4-57 A, Large Zenker's diverticulum in the esophagus of a 67-year-old man with complaints of difficulty in swallowing over the past 6 months. **B,** Zenker's diverticulum in the same patient on a magnified view.

diverticula through diet modifications may result in the need for surgical removal, depending on the amount of food retention in the diverticulum.

Colonic Diverticula

Diverticulosis, the presence of diverticula without inflammation, is seen in all parts of the colon, most frequently in the sigmoid colon, and particularly among adults over the age of 40 years (Figs. 4-60). Diverticula are associated with hypertrophy of the muscular layer of the bowel. They generally occur where the terminal branches of the mesenteric vessels pierce the bowel wall and are present in 35% to 50% of patients over age 50. Factors contributing to the development of diverticula include a pres-

sure gradient between the lumen and serosa of the bowel and areas of weakness within the bowel wall. The most common site for diverticula (95%) is the sigmoid colon, the narrowest portion of the colon, which generates the highest intrasegmental (between haustra) pressures.

Inflammation of a diverticulum, termed **diverticulitis,** occurs in approximately 10% to 20% of patients with known diverticulosis, especially the elderly. The inflammation is exacerbated by feces lodging in the diverticulum. Signs and symptoms include lower-left quadrant pain and tenderness, fever, and an increased white blood cell count. Because of these symptoms, sigmoid diverticulitis has been termed left-sided appendicitis. This condition can lead to bowel obstruction, perforation, and fistula

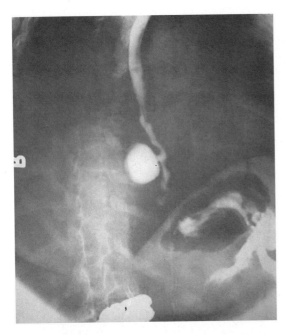

FIG. 4-58 An epiphrenic diverticulum shown as a large collection of barium connected and adjacent to the lower esophagus.

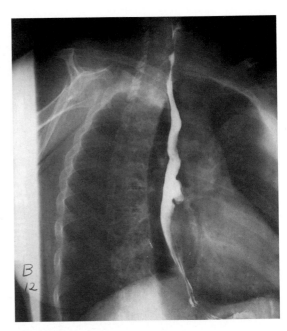

FIG. 4-59 Traction diverticulum indicated by the outpouching of the esophagus at the level of the carina seen in an esophagram of a 47-year-old woman with a history of ulcer disease.

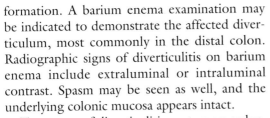

formation. A barium enema examination may be indicated to demonstrate the affected diverticulum, most commonly in the distal colon. Radiographic signs of diverticulitis on barium enema include extraluminal or intraluminal contrast. Spasm may be seen as well, and the underlying colonic mucosa appears intact.

Treatment of diverticulitis centers on reduction of inflammation and infection. Mild cases are treated with antibiotic therapy. Complications such as peritonitis can result if perforation of a diverticulum occurs, and these, of course, must be treated. Surgical resection of the bowel may be used to remove the diseased portion in more severe cases.

NEOPLASTIC DISEASES

Tumors of the Esophagus

Although benign and malignant tumors can occur anywhere in the esophagus, tumors of the lower third are the most common. Benign

tumors are almost always **leiomyomas,** which are smooth muscle tumors, although these have an incidence of less than 10% that of malignant tumors of the esophagus. Many are discovered on x-ray examination for complaints not related to esophageal problems. These benign lesions present as intramural defects in the barium-outlined esophageal wall (Fig. 4-61). The exact location of a leiomyoma, which appears as a homogeneous soft tissue mass, may be determined on CT. Treatment of a leiomyoma consists of surgical removal through a thoracic or abdominal incision that spares esophageal resection.

Cancers of the esophagus constitute approximately 7% of cancers of the GI system but carry a poor prognosis with an overall 5-year survival rate of less than 10%. Squamous cell carcinomas most commonly arise in the body of the esophagus; those at the gastroesophageal junction are typically **adenocarcinomas.** These two types of esophageal cancers have different clinical and

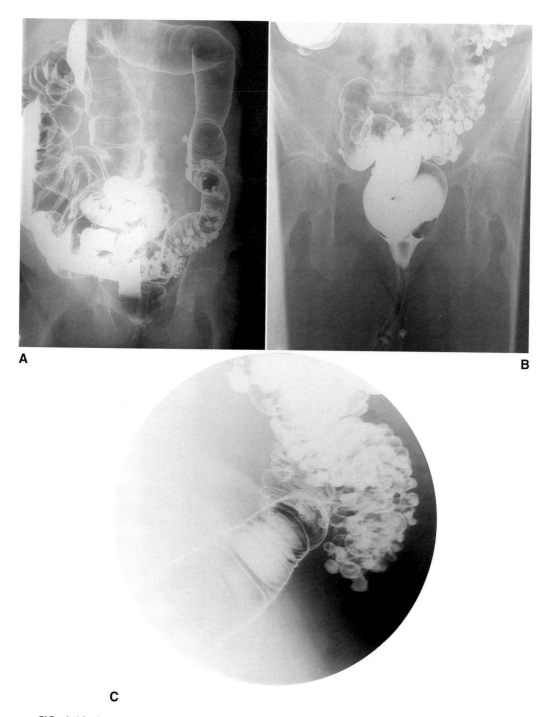

FIG. 4-60 An air-contrast barium enema demonstrating diverticulosis in various projections (**A,** right lateral decubitus projection; **B,** PA axial sigmoid projection; and **C,** digital spot film).

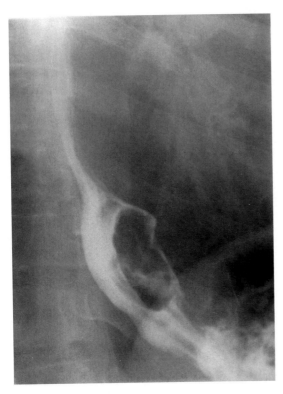

FIG. 4-61 Sharply defined filling defect in the distal esophagus indicative of a benign, esophageal leiomyoma.

radiographic features. Diagnosis is made by endoscopic biopsy of the lesion. Regardless of the type of esophageal cancer, however, CT of the neck, chest, and abdomen is helpful to stage the spread of the disease by demonstrating tumor size, lymph node involvement, and metastases. Endoscopic ultrasonography is very accurate in detecting disease but less available in many medical institutions.

Chronic irritation of the esophagus is thought to be a predisposing factor to squamous cell carcinomas, with such irritation caused by particular agents, including reflux, alcohol, and smoking, and disorders such as achalasia and esophageal diverticula. The primary symptom of esophageal cancer is dysphagia. However, dysphagia may not become significant until the tumor has narrowed the lumen to 50% to 75%

of its normal circumference, allowing metastatic spread to the adjacent lymph nodes and mediastinal structures to occur before diagnosis. Surgery is used as a treatment, with the goal to excise the tumor and regional metastasis. Chemotherapy and/or radiation therapy may be used as an adjunct to surgical intervention. The rapid spread of esophageal cancer, however, requires the goal to be palliation in many cases. The radiographic appearance of a malignant squamous cell tumor may include mucosal destruction, ulceration, narrowing, and a sharp demarcation between normal tissue and the malignant tumor.

As mentioned earlier, adenocarcinomas usually occur in the lower esophagus around the gastroesophageal junction. Many believe these begin as primary gastric carcinomas, which invade the lower esophagus. Others believe there is a direct link between a disorder termed Barrett's esophagus and the development of adenocarcinoma of the esophagus. Barrett's esophagus involves progressive columnar metaplasia of the distal esophagus as a result of chronic gastroesophageal reflux. More than 90% of adenocarcinomas of the esophagus have been found to arise from Barrett's mucosa. Similar to squamous carcinomas, adenocarcinomas spread via the lymph nodes; however, unlike squamous carcinomas, they also spread below the diaphragm. Metastasis to mediastinal structures and hematogenous spread to the liver, lung, and bone occur readily (Fig. 4-62). Radiographically, early adenocarcinomas appear as plaquelike lesions or as sessile polyps, and advanced tumors appear as infiltrating lesions with irregular narrowing of the lumen with abrupt, asymmetric borders.

Tumors of the Stomach

Benign tumors account for fewer than 10% of all stomach tumors. Those that are clinically significant are quite rare. Most stomach tumors are malignant, and the outstanding preponderance (about 95%) of these are adenocarcinomas. The incidence of gastric cancer varies strikingly by geographic area, race, diet, hered-

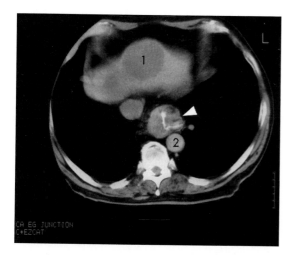

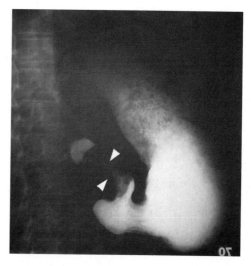

FIG. 4-62 A CT scan with contrast demonstrates an increased thickening of the esophageal wall and distortion of the lumen *(arrow)*, compatible with a gastroesophageal junction malignancy. Also seen are *(1)* a large metastatic lesion in the superior portion of the liver and *(2)* the aorta.

FIG. 4-63 Adenocarcinoma of the stomach in a 66-year-old woman, resulting in gastric outlet obstruction. Note the area of narrowing and the abrupt transition between normal stomach and the acutely narrowed area.

ity, and sex. For example, the rate is nearly five times greater in Japan than in the United States. Like esophageal cancers, gastric carcinoma has a poor prognosis, with overall 5-year survival rates less than 20%.

Most gastric carcinomas develop in the pyloric and antrum regions, particularly along the lesser curvature, although they can be present anywhere (Fig. 4-63). Gastric carcinomas may also be polypoid with a plaquelike, lobulated appearance. Most gastric carcinomas are diagnosed at an advanced stage because early stomach cancers do not result in specific symptoms. They invade other structures by a variety of routes. These tumors metastasize fairly readily outside the stomach to involve the omentum, liver, pancreas, and colon. Liver involvement creates the possibility of discharge into the bloodstream and dispersal throughout the body. Because of the abundance of lymphatics in the stomach, approximately 75% to 85% of these patients also demonstrate metastases via the lymphatic system.

Patients who complain of persistent GI pain should have a thorough workup, with the primary diagnostic study upper endoscopy with biopsy, often followed by a GI series. Symptoms of gastric tumors are often vague but include bleeding, vomiting, loss of appetite, weight loss, and early satiety. Tumors are radiographically indicated by a relative rigidity of peristalsis and filling defects on compression. Filling defects demonstrate as areas of total or relative radiolucency within the barium column. Polypoid tumors are clearly visible on CT examination. By identifying lymphatic involvement and extragastric spread of the cancer, CT is also useful in the staging of gastric cancers.

Surgical removal of gastric cancer has been the only successful treatment; a subtotal gastrectomy is the usual procedure. Resection of the stomach to attach to the jejunum via a gastrojejunostomy usually accompanies this procedure. Radiation therapy and chemotherapy treatments for stomach carcinoma have been less effective.

Small-Bowel Neoplasms

Small-bowel tumors represent fewer than 5% of all benign and malignant GI neoplasms. The incidence of malignancy for this small amount is about 50%. The low overall incidence is surprising, considering that the small bowel composes 75% of the entire GI tract, with an enormous mucosal surface. Also, it is in constant contact with enteric carcinogenic substances. Reasons for this low incidence of tumors are not entirely known or understood. Most small-bowel cancers occur in the duodenum and proximal jejunum.

One predisposing factor for small-bowel neoplasms seems to be the degree of polyposis in other areas of the GI tract, a condition frequently determined by heredity. Another predisposing factor is Kaposi's sarcoma, most common in patients with AIDS. Up to 60% of these patients have GI involvement, with the tumors arising anywhere in the stomach, small bowel, or distal colon. Intermittent abdominal pain sometimes described as cramps is the most common symptom. Endoscopy with biopsy is the most common means of identifying small-bowel neoplasms, but small-bowel barium studies may assist in the diagnosis. Surgical resection is the primary means of treating small-bowel neoplasms, both benign and malignant.

Colonic Polyps

Colonic polyps are small masses of tissue arising from the bowel wall to project inward into the lumen (Fig. 4-64). An adenomatous polyp is a tumor of benign neoplastic epithelium that can undergo dysplastic changes to become malignant. It consists of a saccular projection into the bowel lumen and is either sessile, that is, attached directly to the bowel wall with a wide base, or pedunculated, that is, attached by a narrow stalk (Fig. 4-65). Polyps are more frequently noted in the left colon, and particularly in the rectosigmoid areas. Other types of polyps are inflammatory, hyperplastic, and juvenile.

Although most polyps are asymptomatic, all should be removed, especially adenomatous

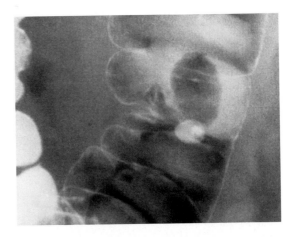

FIG. 4-64 Filling defect in the transverse colon near the splenic flexure indicates a polyp projecting into the lumen. A barium-filled diverticulum is seen immediately above it in this patient, who presented with blood in his stools.

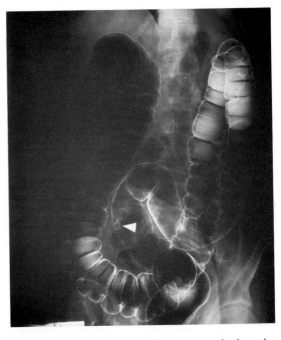

FIG. 4-65 Pedunculated polyp seen attached to the wall of the sigmoid colon by a long stalk on an air-contrast barium enema.

polyps, which have a greater chance of malignancy (Fig. 4-66). Those over 2 cm in size have a malignancy rate over 50%. Most never reach this size, however. The complications of polyps include ulceration from chronic irritation or bowel obstruction from inflammation. Most cancers of the colon and rectum arise from previously benign polyps. Patients with polyps may present with rectal bleeding, constipation, diarrhea, or flatulence, but most are asymptomatic. Radiographically, an air-contrast barium enema is the examination of choice, with the polyps demonstrating as rounded filling defects or contour defects in the barium shadow. Although pedunculated polyps are easily recognized and often considered benign, size is a better indication of malignancy versus benignancy, as noted. At times, it is difficult to discriminate between fecal material and a polyp. In general, fecal material is mobile, whereas a polyp stays fixed to the stalk. Proctosigmoidoscopy and colonoscopy are critical in evaluation and removal of polyps. Patients with polyps are followed closely after discovery.

Colon Cancer

Carcinoma of the colon is one of the most common malignancies in the United States and the second most common cause of cancer mortality. The incidence of colon cancer rises significantly after age 40 and doubles with each decade, reaching a peak at about age 75. American adults have a 1 in 20 chance of developing colorectal cancer in their lifetime and a 1 in 40 chance of dying from this disease. Predisposing factors include a family history of familial polyposis and ulcerative colitis. Environmental factors also seem to correlate with colorectal cancer, as countries with higher intakes of sugar and animal fats (e.g., the United States) have a higher incidence than countries with a higher fiber intake.

Adenocarcinoma is the most common type of colorectal cancer and is derived from the glandular epithelium of the colon. It begins as a benign adenoma that undergoes a slow malignant transformation. Although the transformation may take up to 7 years to complete, all polypoid lesions larger than 1 cm should be removed from the colon. Adenocarcinoma is characterized by infiltration of the colon wall, as opposed to being a bulky, intraluminal mass.

Although the incidence of proximal colon cancers is increasing, nearly 50% still occur below the middescending colon. Most of these (70%) occur in the rectosigmoid area and are detectable by flexible sigmoidoscopy. Right colon lesions differ considerably from left colon

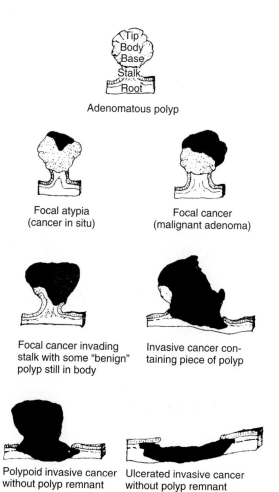

Adenomatous polyp

Focal atypia (cancer in situ)

Focal cancer (malignant adenoma)

Focal cancer invading stalk with some "benign" polyp still in body

Invasive cancer containing piece of polyp

Polypoid invasive cancer without polyp remnant

Ulcerated invasive cancer without polyp remnant

FIG. 4-66 Adenomatous polyp transformation.

lesions in terms of symptoms produced. Lesions in the right colon, on the one hand, may produce no early symptoms, often becoming quite large, ulcerating, and even bleeding without significant symptoms. They also tend to penetrate and extend into surrounding tissues without causing obstruction. Such patients often present initially with anemia and blood in their stools. Left colon lesions, on the other hand, present more often with obstruction and bleeding, largely because of a smaller lumen and an annular (ring-like) growth pattern.

The evaluation of colon cancer includes fecal blood testing, proctosigmoidoscopy, colonoscopy, and the barium enema. A double-contrast enema has been noted to produce more accurate diagnoses than the traditional single-contrast study. The radiographic appearance of adenocarcinoma has led to its designation as the "napkin-ring" carcinoma or the "apple-core" lesion, as the edges of the lesion tend to overhang and form acute angles with the bowel wall (Fig. 4-67). Although it may be difficult to distinguish between carcinoma and an inflammatory lesion (e.g., regional enteritis or ulcerative colitis), a carcinoma generally has a more clear-cut transition between malignant and normal mucosa. In addition, the length of involved bowel is usually shorter with carcinoma than with an inflammatory lesion.

Without treatment, invasion of local tissue spreads the cancer via the lymphatics to the mesenteric nodes and on to the liver (Fig. 4-68) and lungs. Fortunately, the lesion does not metastasize early, leading to a good prognosis. The primary means of treatment are surgical excision of the primary tumor and its margins and resection of the bowel as possible. A colostomy may be required, depending on the site of the tumor. Radiation therapy is generally given before and after surgery for rectal cancers. For inoperable tumors, the radiation therapy is given to reduce the tumor size and its resultant complications (e.g., obstruction) and also to provide pain relief. Chemotherapy is given when the cancer has metastasized.

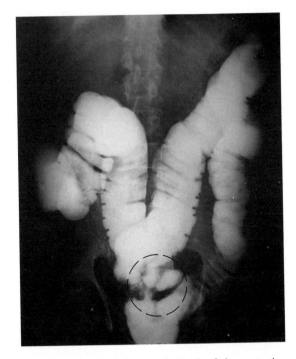

FIG. 4-67 The "apple core lesion" of the rectosigmoid colon consistent with adenocarcinoma, with characteristic appearance of abrupt change from normal to abnormal colon and shelf-like appearance of overhanging edges caused by the mass.

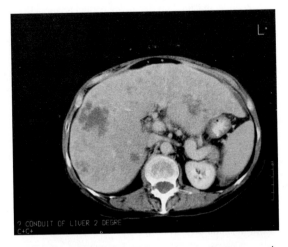

FIG. 4-68 CT demonstration of extensive metastatic disease from the colon to both lobes of the liver, ranging from punctate to up to 5 cm in this 50-year-old woman.

PATHOLOGY SUMMARY: THE GASTROINTESTINAL SYSTEM

Pathology	Imaging Modalities of Choice	Additive or Subtractive Pathology
Esophageal atresia	Radiographs	None
Bowel atresia	Radiographs in the infant, ultrasound in the fetus	None
Imperforate anus	Radiographs	None
Hypertrophic pyloric stenosis	UGI and ultrasound	None
Malrotation	Small bowel and BaE	None
Hirschsprung's disease	BaE	None
Meckel's diverticulum	Nuclear medicine Meckel's diverticulum study	None
Esophageal strictures	Ba swallow and endoscopy	None
GERD	Endoscopy	None
Peptic ulcer	Endoscopy, double-contrast UGI, nuclear medicine urea breath test	None
Malabsorption syndrome	Small bowel	None
Regional enteritis (Crohn's disease)	Small bowel and double-contrast BaE	None
Appendicitis	CT	None
Ulcerative colitis	Sigmoidoscopy and colonoscopy	None
Esophageal varices	Ba swallow	None
Bowel obstruction	Supine and erect abdominal radiographs	Subtractive
Achalasia	Ba swallow	Additive if food is present
Diverticular disease	Double-contrast Ba studies—diverticulosis CT—diverticulitis	None
Polyps	Colonoscopy and double-contrast BaE	None
Neoplastic disease of the GI system	Colonoscopy, double-contrast BaE, and CT	None

QUESTIONS

1. Esophageal atresia is classified as a(n) _____ condition of the GI system.
   a. congenital
   b. degenerative
   c. inflammatory
   d. neurologic

2. An outpouching of the bowel wall caused by a weakening in its muscular layer is a(n):
   a. atresia
   b. carcinoma
   c. diverticulum
   d. polyp

3. The radiographic string sign is associated with which disease?
   a. achalasia
   b. adenocarcinoma
   c. regional enteritis
   d. ulcerative colitis

4. Celiac disease is a type of:
   a. atresia
   b. herniation
   c. malabsorption syndrome
   d. ulcerative colitis

5. The appearance of a Schatzki's ring is associated with a(n) _____ hernia.
   a. inguinal
   b. rolling
   c. sliding
   d. umbilical

6. A congenital, neurogenic disease of the GI system characterized by an absence of neurons in the bowel wall is:
   a. achalasia
   b. diverticulosis
   c. Hirschsprung's disease
   d. toxic megacolon

7. The fewest GI tumors, both benign and malignant, occur in the:
   a. colon
   b. esophagus
   c. large bowel
   d. small bowel

8. Which of the following statements are true of colon cancer?
   1. The majority of adenocarcinoma of the colon occur in the rectosigmoid area.
   2. The appearance of the "apple core" lesion is indicative of colon cancer.
   3. Adenomatous polyps can develop into adenocarcinoma of the colon.
   a. 1 and 2
   b. 1 and 3
   c. 2 and 3
   d. 1, 2, and 3

9. A twisting of bowel about its mesenteric base best refers to a(n):
   a. ascites
   b. intussusception
   c. incarcerated hernia
   d. volvulus

10. The condition in which a gallstone erodes from the gallbladder and creates a fistula to the small bowel is:
    a. gallstone ileus
    b. intussusception
    c. incarcerated hernia
    d. volvulus

11. Describe the differences both clinically and radiographically between a mechanical bowel obstruction and paralytic ileus.

12. Explain the connection between colonic polyps and the development of colorectal cancer.

13. Describe the role of CT in the staging of various GI cancers.

14. Explain the physiologic alteration that causes esophageal varices and describe the radiographic appearance of this disorder.

15. Compare and contrast the various gastric tubes in terms of their uses and radiographic appearance.

The Hepatobiliary System

UPON COMPLETION OF CHAPTER 5, THE READER SHOULD BE ABLE TO:

- Describe the anatomic components of the hepatobiliary system and how they are visualized radiographically.
- Discuss the role of other imaging modalities in imaging of the hepatobiliary system, particularly ultrasound, MRI, and CT.
- Characterize a given condition as inflammatory, metabolic, or neoplastic.
- Identify the pathogenesis of the pathologies cited and the typical treatments for them.
- Describe, in general, the radiographic appearance of each of the given pathologies.

ANATOMY AND PHYSIOLOGY

The hepatobiliary system is composed of the liver, gallbladder, and biliary tree (Fig. 5-1). The pancreas is closely related and shares a portion of the biliary ductal system, hence its inclusion here.

The Liver

The liver is the largest organ in the body and is sheltered by the ribs in the right-upper quadrant of the abdomen. It is kept in position by peritoneal ligaments and intraabdominal pressure from muscles of the abdominal wall. The functions of the liver are multiple, including metabolism of substances delivered via its portal circulation, synthesis of substances including those concerned with blood clotting, storage of vitamin B and other materials, and detoxification and excretion of various substances.

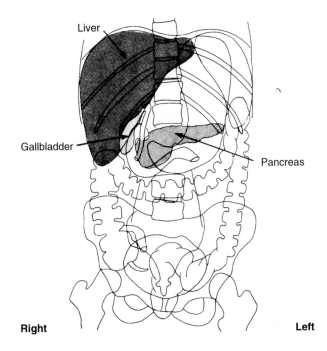

FIG. 5-1 The hepatobiliary system and the pancreas.

The liver has a double supply of blood, coming from the hepatic artery and the portal vein. The hepatic artery usually originates from the celiac axis and takes oxygenated blood to the liver. The portal vein is formed by the union of the superior mesenteric and splenic veins. It is located within the liver and serves to return venous blood from the abdominal viscera to the inferior vena cava (IVC). Any interference with blood flow, such as might occur with liver disease, results in consequences elsewhere in the abdominal viscera and spleen.

The Biliary Tree

A system of ducts acts to drain bile produced in the liver into the duodenum (Fig. 5-2). Bile from the liver's two main lobes is drained by the right and left hepatic ducts. These unite to form the common hepatic duct, which is joined usually in its midportion by the cystic duct from the gallbladder. Together, the cystic duct and the common hepatic duct form the common bile duct.

The common bile duct descends posterior to the descending duodenum to enter at its pos-teromedial aspect. Before its entrance into the duodenum, the common bile duct may be joined by the pancreatic duct from the head of the pancreas. The short part of the common bile duct, after joining the pancreatic duct, is known as the hepatopancreatic ampulla or, more commonly, the ampulla of Vater.

The flow of both bile and pancreatic juice into the duodenum is regulated by the hepato-pancreatic sphincter, more commonly known as the sphincter of Oddi. The release of bile into the duodenum is triggered by chole-cystokinin, a hormone released by the presence of fatty foods in the stomach. The purpose of bile is to emulsify fats so that they may be absorbed.

The Gallbladder

The gallbladder is a pear-shaped sac located on the undersurface on the right lobe of the liver. Normally, the walls are quite thin, but they often thicken in the presence of inflammation. The sole function of the gallbladder is to store and concentrate bile that has been produced in the liver.

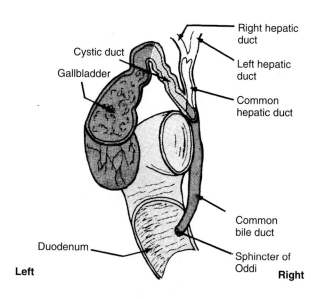

FIG. 5-2 The biliary system.

The Pancreas

The pancreas is an elongated, flat organ that obliquely crosses the left side of the abdomen behind the stomach; it is a powerful digestive organ. Its functions are both exocrine and endocrine. Exocrine function is concerned with production of digestive enzymes. These are discharged through the pancreatic duct into the duodenum. The endocrine portion of the pancreas consists of multiple clusters of specialized cells, the islets of Langerhans. Their function is to produce insulin and glucagon, which are discharged directly into the blood from the pancreas. Insulin and glucagon regulate carbohydrate metabolism.

IMAGING CONSIDERATIONS

Radiographs

A conventional abdominal radiograph may contain information about the hepatobiliary system through the demonstration of faint calcifications that might otherwise be obscured by contrast media. A plain radiograph of the gallbladder may demonstrate **milk of calcium** as a semiliquid sludge (Fig. 5-3) composed of calcium carbonate mixed with bile in the gallbladder. The hazy radiopacity results from a settling of bile as a result of an obstruction at the neck of the gallbladder, or it can develop in patients who have been fasting or have been on hyperalimentation.

Gas may occasionally be seen in the wall or lumen of the gallbladder because of the presence of gas-forming organisms in the gallbladder walls. This is most generally seen in patients with poorly controlled diabetes. Gas visualized in the biliary tree may also be a result of a spontaneous fistula, as might be seen in gallstone ileus, or postoperative biliary anastomosis.

Contrast Studies

Oral Cholecystogram

An examination formerly widely used to study the biliary system is an oral cholecystogram (OCG), although it has been largely replaced

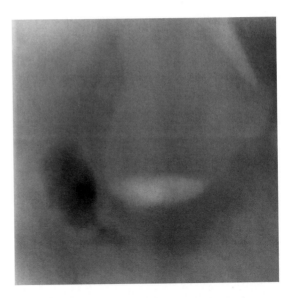

FIG. 5-3 Milk of calcium bile as seen in the bottom of this gallbladder in an erect spot film.

by ultrasound. An OCG is a functional examination in that the contrast medium is absorbed in the small bowel and passes through the portal vein to the liver. The contrast agent is excreted from the liver with bile and is stored in the gallbladder. About 25% of all patients' gallbladders fail to visualize on the first attempt at oral cholecystography. The most common causes of nonvisualization are an obstruction of the cystic duct secondary to a stone and chronic cholecystitis, with poor concentration of the contrast agent.

Percutaneous Transhepatic Cholangiography

A percutaneous transhepatic cholangiogram (PTC) is used to visualize the biliary tree and involves insertion of a needle into the biliary tree by puncture directly through the wall of the abdomen. With the use of a flexible, 22-gauge, skinny needle (Chiba), this procedure is safe and fairly easy to perform. The subsequent injection of contrast medium (Fig. 5-4) is useful in distinguishing **medical jaundice,** caused by hepatocellular dysfunction, from **surgical jaundice,** which results from biliary

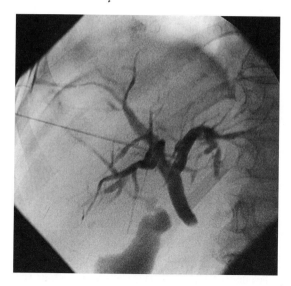

FIG. 5-4 Demonstration of the biliary system via a percutaneous transhepatic cholangiogram (PTC).

obstruction. Also, the examination is useful for detecting the presence of calculi or a tumor in the distal common bile duct. It has a high success rate in imaging the biliary ductal system, is less expensive than an endoscopic retrograde cholangiopancreatogram, and has a low complication rate of approximately 3.5%. It also may be immediately followed by a therapeutic procedure such as a biliary drainage, stone removal or crushing via contact lithotripsy or laser fragmentation, stent placement, or biopsy. This procedure is preferred in the evaluation of proximal obstructions involving the hepatic duct bifurcation, which is difficult to image with the retrograde approach via an ERCP.

Endoscopic Retrograde Cholangiopancreatogram

The endoscopic retrograde cholangiopancreatogram (ERCP), an imaging procedure performed by a gastroenterologist, is a means of visualizing the biliary system and main pancreatic duct, which provides drainage for the pancreatic enzymes into both the digestive tract and the common bile duct. A fiberoptic endo-

scope is passed through the duodenal C-loop to visualize the ampulla of Vater. A thin catheter is then directed into the orifice of the common bile duct or pancreatic duct, followed by an injection of contrast medium (Fig. 5-5). In many cases, the ERCP is preferred over the transhepatic cholangiogram and is often preceded with an ultrasonic examination or CT investigation of the pancreas. Although an ERCP is more expensive than a PTC, it is often used to visualize nondilated ducts, distal obstructions, patients with bleeding disorders, and the pancreas. The complication rate (2% to 3%) is similar to that of PTC and also offers the ability to perform therapeutic procedures such as sphincterotomy, stone extractions, stent placement, and biliary dilatation. Cytology and biopsy may also be performed.

Operative Cholangiography

Operative cholangiography is performed during surgery at the time of a cholecystectomy to detect biliary calculi and the need for common bile duct exploration (Fig. 5-6). A needle is placed directly into the cystic duct or common bile duct by the surgeon, and a small volume (5 ml) of contrast material is injected, followed by a radiograph. A second injection of 5 ml is made, followed by a second radiograph. The resulting images are reviewed for possible areas of concern before completion of the surgery. It is imperative that no air bubbles be injected

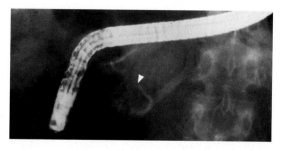

FIG. 5-5 An endoscopic retrograde cholangiopancreatogram (ERCP) showing abrupt termination of the pancreatic duct about 4 cm from its opening.

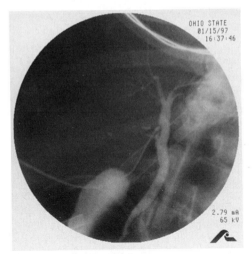

FIG. 5-6 A digital image of an operative cholangiogram taken during surgery.

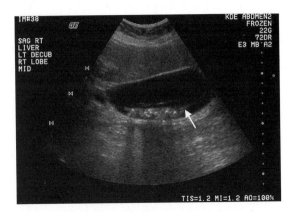

FIG. 5-7 A sagittal sonographic view of the gallbladder demonstrating stones.

into the ductal system with the contrast agent during this procedure because they can mimic stones.

T-Tube Cholangiography

T-tube cholangiography is used after a cholecystectomy to demonstrate patency of the common bile duct and to check for calculi. With a T-shaped tube already inserted surgically into the common bile duct, contrast medium is injected to verify removal of all calculi. The radiologist must take care not to inject air bubbles because they may give the radiographic appearance of radiolucent calculi.

Diagnostic Medical Sonography

Real-time diagnostic medical sonography is now the modality of choice for evaluating the gallbladder (Fig. 5-7) and biliary tree. This procedure is noninvasive, and the gallbladder can be satisfactorily imaged in almost all fasting patients regardless of the body habitus or clinical condition of the patient. When sonography is performed by a skilled sonographer, it has been proven to be almost 100% accurate in detecting gallstones, which are demonstrated as echogenic areas within the echo-free gallbladder. Thickening of the gallbladder wall is

also easily identified. It is also an excellent tool for determining the presence of common bile duct obstruction, evaluation of the intrahepatic biliary ductal system, and identification of abscesses. The liver may also be evaluated by sonography because of its ideal location in the right-upper quadrant and broad contact with the abdominal wall. Hepatic lesions of 1 cm or greater are easily identified with cystic lesions appearing echo-free and solid masses appearing echogenic, allowing excellent guidance for aspiration and biopsy of these lesions.

Doppler flow technology enhances the diagnostic capabilities of ultrasound to allow for clear analysis of the circulatory dynamics, including portal blood flow and hepatic artery thrombosis following liver transplantation. Doppler sonography can also differentiate between vessels and biliary ducts based on flow characteristics.

Computed Tomography

The role of computed tomography (CT) in the hepatobiliary system is similar to its role in the GI tract. It is the accepted modality for following malignancies and assessing masses, particularly of the gallbladder, liver, and pancreas. It is also helpful in evaluating complications of cholecystitis, such as perforations and abscess formations. The use of spiral or helical CT ensures that the entire liver is imaged in one breath, eliminating respiratory artifact and in many cases demonstrating the liver parenchyma and associated structures better than sonography. In addition to the excellent contrast resolution offered by CT, the use of large-bolus IV injections during dynamic CT examination has also improved evaluations of the hepatobiliary ductal system and blood flow via three-phase imaging of the liver to capture the arterial and portal venous blood flow (Fig. 5-8). If a biliary

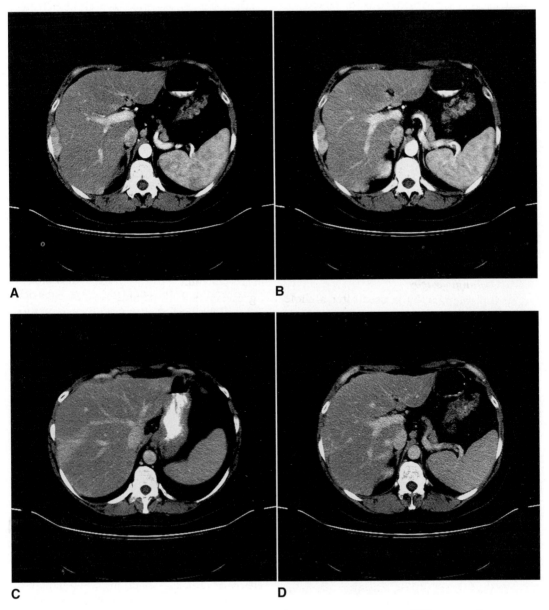

FIG. 5-8 A, B, Three phase CT of the liver following a bolus injection of IV contrast demonstrating the arterial circulation. **C, D,** Three-phase CT of liver delayed images demonstrating the portal venous flow.

obstruction is not visible on sonographic examination, CT can generally identify the location and extent of the obstruction. Lacerations of the liver and resultant abdominal bleeding are readily detected on CT (Fig. 5-9), as well as metastatic lesions within the liver. CT also demonstrates good visualization of pancreatic tumors and pseudocysts. In addition, CT-guided biopsy procedures for the liver (Fig. 5-10), pancreas, and kidney allow for analysis and drainage and offer significant advantages over conventional surgical biopsy and drainage.

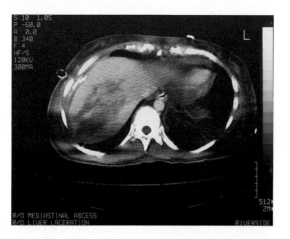

FIG. 5-9 CT of this 39-year-old woman after a car accident reveals large lacerations to the liver.

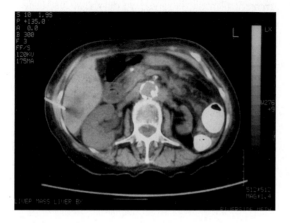

FIG. 5-10 CT of needle biopsy in this 87-year-old woman clearly demonstrates the needle in the liver.

Nuclear Medicine Procedures

Single-photon emission computed tomography (SPECT) examinations provide excellent detection of hepatobiliary lesions, especially those located deep within the liver parenchyma. SPECT provides a noninvasive method of evaluating hepatic function as well as hepatic and splenic perfusion. Because nuclear medicine imaging provides information regarding physiologic function, these scans can often provide information before any anatomic changes become visible with CT. White cells labeled with radioactive indium are useful in locating sites of infection for treatment.

Cholescintography scans performed in nuclear medicine are very useful to confirm cholecystitis, and they may be useful for distinguishing acute from chronic cholecystitis (Fig. 5-11). Radioactive technetium is cleared from the blood plasma into the bile, demonstrating the physiologic function of the liver, excretion into the biliary ductal system, and visualization of the gallbladder about 1 hour postinjection. Delays in visualization or nonvisualization of the gallbladder indicates pathology. In addition, it is a noninvasive method of

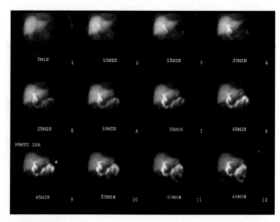

FIG. 5-11 Nuclear medicine hepatobiliary scan demonstrates ready ejection of the radionuclide from the gallbladder through sequential images into the duodenum.

evaluating biliary drainage, hepatobiliary leaks following trauma or surgery, and segmental obstruction.

Magnetic Resonance Imaging

The role of magnetic resonance imaging (MRI) of the hepatobiliary system has improved greatly as a result of shorter scan times, which allow the acquisition of several images of the abdomen in a single breath. MRI is often used in conjunction with CT to evaluate pathologies and anomalies of the peritoneum, especially the liver and pancreas. MRI may also be used to identify retroperitoneal bleeds following trauma (Fig. 5-12). Contrast-enhanced three-dimensional dynamic scans of the liver imaged at timed intervals help to differentiate certain tumors from hemangiomas.

The magnetic resonance cholangiopancreatography (MRCP) is an imaging procedure that utilizes MR to visualize the gallbladder and biliary system. The MRCP is non-invasive and does not require the use of a contrast agent (Fig. 5-13). A heavily T2 weighted sequence is used to suppress the tissues around the biliary system allowing the gallbladder and bile ducts to show up bright enabling visualization of stones or other obstructions. The MRCP usually accompanies other imaging sequences

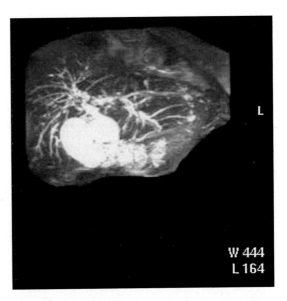

FIG. 5-13 MRI is capable of imaging the biliary system without the use of contrast agents.

of the liver but takes only about 15 seconds to acquire.

INFLAMMATORY DISEASES

Cirrhosis

Cirrhosis is a chronic liver condition in which the liver parenchyma and architecture are destroyed, fibrous tissue is laid down, and regenerative nodules are formed. In its early stages, it is usually asymptomatic, as it can take months or even years before damage becomes apparent. Cirrhosis affects the entire liver and is considered an end-stage condition resulting from liver damage by chronic alcohol abuse, drugs, auto-immune disorders, metabolic and genetic disease, chronic hepatitis, cardiac problems, and chronic biliary tract obstruction. It is the third leading cause of death in the United States in individuals between the ages of 45 and 65, with one third of the deaths secondary to hemorrhage from esophageal varices.

The scarring and formation of regenerative nodules associated with cirrhosis can have

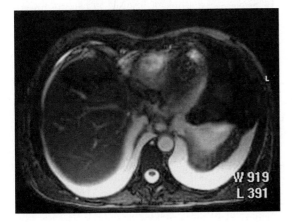

FIG. 5-12 T2 Tru-Fisp axial MR image of the abdomen demonstrating a retroperitoneal hemorrhage.

serious complications for the afflicted individual. The two functional impairments caused by cirrhosis are impaired liver function resulting from hepatocyte damage, generally resulting in jaundice, and portal hypertension. Because of interference of portal blood flow through the liver, portal hypertension may lead to development of collateral venous connections to the venae cavae. Most commonly, such connections involve the esophageal veins, which dilate to become esophageal varices, as described in the preceding chapter. These are best evaluated with endoscopy but may be seen on an esophagram. Also, the patient with cirrhosis has a tendency to bleed because the liver is unable to make the necessary clotting factors found in plasma or as a result of an esophageal variceal rupture. Such hemorrhaging may be, in fact, the first indication of portal hypertension.

Ascites, the accumulation of fluid within the peritoneal cavity (Fig. 5-14), is also seen as a result of portal hypertension and the leakage of excessive fluids from the portal capillaries. Much of this excess fluid is composed of hepatic lymph weeping from the liver surface. It is associated with approximately 50% of deaths

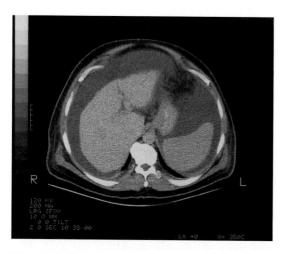

FIG. 5-14 Cirrhosis of the liver as indicated on this CT scan showing a shrunken liver with significant ascites around it within the abdomen.

from cirrhosis. Ascites may also result from chronic hepatitis, congestive heart failure, renal failure, and certain cancers. Abdominal ultrasound is commonly used in the detection or confirmation of ascites. Diagnostic and therapeutic paracentesis may be conducted with sonographic guidance in order to locate a site that will allow fluid to be removed and avoid damage to the floating bowel loops. A diagnostic paracentesis involves removal of 50 to 100 ml of peritoneal fluid for analysis. Patients with ascites generally complain of nonspecific abdominal pain and dyspnea. Medical treatment of ascites includes bed rest, dietary restrictions of sodium, use of diuretics to avoid excess fluid accumulation, and treatment of the underlying cause.

It is important for the technologist to be aware of the clinical diagnosis of ascites because the fluid accumulation can make it difficult to adequately penetrate the abdomen. An increase in exposure factors is necessary to obtain a diagnostic-quality radiograph. Radiographically, large amounts of ascitic fluid give the abdomen a dense, gray, ground-glass appearance. With the patient in a supine position, the fluid accumulates in the pelvis and ascends to either side of the bladder to give it a dog-eared appearance. Gradually, the margins of the liver, spleen, kidneys, and psoas muscles become indistinct as the volume of fluid increases. Loops of bowel filled with gas float centrally, and a lateral decubitus radiograph demonstrates the fluid descending and the gas-filled loops of bowel floating on top.

Conventional radiographic signs of cirrhosis are few and not specific. Morphologic changes in the liver from cirrhosis may cause displacement of other abdominal organs such as the stomach, duodenum, colon, gallbladder, and kidney. The primary means of evaluating the complications arising from cirrhosis is CT. Fatty infiltration of the liver, an initial feature in alcoholic liver disease, is well visualized by CT. The most characteristic finding in cirrhosis is an increase in the ratio of the caudate lobe and the right lobe because with cirrhosis the right lobe and medial segment of the left lobe atrophy while the caudate lobe and the lateral segment of the left lobe hypertrophy. Because of its dual arterial blood supply, the caudate lobe of the liver is usually spared in cirrhosis. Studies show that individuals with cirrhosis have an increased risk of developing hepatic carcinoma, so CT is also of value in assessing the presence of complications of cirrhosis, such as ascites and hepatocellular carcinoma.

Diagnostic medical sonography is helpful in suggesting the presence of liver cirrhosis and enlargement of the liver and spleen. Doppler is utilized to detect portal hypertension and evaluate portosystemic collateral circulation. It is used to measure the vessel size of the portal vein, which ranges from 0.64 to 1 cm in a normal adult. A portal vein larger than 1.3 cm in diameter is indicative of portal hypertension. In addition, the portal vein should distend with deep inspiration, but in patients with portal hypertension, the vein lacks distensibility. Doppler integration of the portal vein allows tracing of the flow of blood within the vessel. Normal portal vein flow is toward the liver; however, during portal hypertension, the flow is shunted away from the liver because of the diseased liver's inability to accept the flow of blood. As a result, the splenic vein commonly tries to handle this resistance by diverting the flow toward the spleen. In many cases, these patients develop splenic varices from the increased flow from the portal vein. Sonographic evaluation of venous structures such as the superior mesenteric and splenic veins adds additional information for the clinician. However, final diagnosis of cirrhosis is generally accomplished by biopsy of liver tissue, often performed under ultrasonic guidance.

Treatment of cirrhosis depends on the extent of liver damage and the involvement of other organs (e.g., the esophagus and stomach). The primary goal of treatment is to eliminate the underlying causes of the disease and to treat its complications. Surgical treatment of portal hypertension may be achieved by diverting blood from the portocollateral system into the lower-pressure systemic circulation. This is accomplished by placing a shunt, eliminating the chance of variceal bleeding. A distal splenorenal shunt, in which the splenic vein is divided, with the distal portion anastomosed to the left renal vein, is most commonly used. If the patient is not a candidate for this type of shunt, a total shunt, either portocaval or mesocaval, must be placed. A palliative procedure, the transjugular intrahepatic portosystemic shunt (TIPS), may also be used to divert the pressure of portal hypertension. The TIPS procedure is commonly performed in the cardiovascular interventional area of radiology. A catheter is placed in the right internal jugular vein and pushed through the right atrium into the IVC. The needle end of the catheter is punched into the closest portal vein in the liver. Commonly, the needle is inserted into the right portal vein. Using angioplasty, the tract is enlarged such that a shunt can be placed in order to reroute the flow of portal blood through the liver and into the IVC. Sonography is invaluable at assessing the long-term effect of this shunt. Typically Doppler tracings are taken at the portal end, the midshunt, and the hepatic vein end of the shunt to insure that flow through it allows the flow of blood to proceed through the liver to the IVC. However, all of the aforementioned shunts have a tendency to thrombose, requiring patency to be assessed by angiography, CT, or ultrasound. The prognosis for patients with associated complications of cirrhosis such as ascites is poor, but advances in liver transplantation have changed the long-term outcome for many patients.

Viral Hepatitis

Hepatitis is a relatively common liver condition, with an estimated 70,000 cases reported annually. At least six types of viral agents have been identified that cause acute inflammation of the liver. This inflammation interferes with the liver's ability to excrete bilirubin, the orange or yellowish pigment in bile. Evidence of the disease is seen clinically by nausea, vomiting, discomfort, and tenderness over the liver area, and laboratory results indicate a disturbance in liver function. Additional signs and symptoms include fatigue, anorexia, photophobia, and general malaise. Jaundice may also develop within 1 or 2 weeks because of the disturbance of bilirubin excretion. If the liver inflammation lasts 6 months or more, the condition is classified as chronic.

Hepatitis A (HAV) is a single-stranded RNA picornavirus. It is excreted in the GI tract in fecal material and is spread by contact with an infected individual, normally through ingestion of contaminated food, such as raw shellfish, or water. It is the most common form and highly contagious. The incubation period of the disease is relatively short (15 to 50 days), and its course is usually mild. HAV does not lead to chronic hepatitis or cirrhosis of the liver.

Hepatitis B (HBV) is transmitted parenterally in infected serum or blood products. Its incubation period is much longer (50 to 160 days), and its effects are more severe than those of HAV. The etiologic make-up of the hepatitis B virus is very complex, consisting of a viral core of DNA that replicates within the cells of the liver. The viral core is covered with a surface coat. HBV can result in an asymptomatic carrier state, acute hepatitis, chronic hepatitis, cirrhosis, and hepatocellular carcinoma. Most health care workers are now required to receive a HBV vaccine. Vaccination has dramatically reduced the incidence of infection, and the vaccines are safe with very few side effects.

Hepatitis C (HCV) is caused by a parenterally transmitted RNA virus. Type C accounts for 80% of the cases of hepatitis that develop after blood transfusions. A routine test for anti–HCV antibody has been developed, so transmission via transfused blood has been significantly decreased. HCV can cause either acute or chronic hepatitis, with 10% to 20% of these patients eventually developing cirrhosis of the liver.

Hepatitis D (HDV) is caused by an RNA virus and only occurs concurrently with acute or chronic HBV. It cannot occur alone. Hepatitis E virus (HEV) is also an RNA viral agent. It is most commonly responsible for outbreaks of waterborne epidemic acute hepatitis in developing countries. Although the infection may be severe, it does not progress to a chronic state. Hepatitis G (HGV) has been recently isolated and can also be transmitted by blood products. It can also result in chronic hepatitis.

The diagnosis of viral hepatitis is usually made through laboratory testing because the disease is carried in the bloodstream during the acute phase. Evidence of hepatitis may be seen radiographically on a plain film of the abdomen that demonstrates **hepatomegaly,** or enlargement of the liver, although this is a nonspecific finding. Cellular necrosis can be confirmed through nuclear medicine scanning of the liver, CT, or a liver biopsy. Ultrasound is also useful in distinguishing the characteristics of the liver.

HAV is usually mild; the majority of patients recover without complications. Treatment generally consists of bed rest and medication to fight nausea and vomiting. In a healthy individual, the liver regenerates after hepatitis damage, and complete recovery is gained. Patients with type B, type C, type D, and type G generally progress into chronic hepatitis. In some, the disease may become progressive and lead to liver failure.

Cholelithiasis

The incidence of **cholelithiasis** (gallstones) is fairly common, with at least 20% of all persons in the United States developing them by the age of 65 years. Women are more likely than men to have them. Their occurrence is also greater in diabetics, the obese, the elderly and in individuals eating a Western diet. Heredity plays a role in their development. Although most commonly found in the gallbladder, they can be located anywhere in the biliary tree. Symptoms associated with cholelithiasis may be vague, including bloating, nausea, and pain in the right-upper quadrant. Sludge can develop within the gallbladder and may be identified sonographically. Sometimes the sludge develops in patients who have been fasting or who have been on hyperalimentation and is a normal variant from underutilization of the bile in the gallbladder; in other cases the sludge may be a precursor to the development of gallstones.

The characteristics of gallstones are quite varied. They may occur as a single stone or as multiple stones. About 80% of all stones comprise a mixture of cholesterol, bile pigment (bilirubin), and calcium salts. The remaining 20% are composed of pure cholesterol or a calcium-bilirubin mixture. Most stones are radiolucent because only about 10% of all stones contain enough calcium to be radiopaque. Those that are radiopaque may be difficult to distinguish from renal stones, but oblique radiographs help separate the two structures (kidney and gallbladder) from each other, demonstrating the gallbladder anterior to the kidney. As noted before, sonography readily demonstrates the presence of cholelithiasis (Fig. 5-15). The best image is obtained when the gallbladder is distended and filled with bile; therefore, patients should fast 8 hours before sonographic examination. The three major sonographic criteria for gallstones include (1)

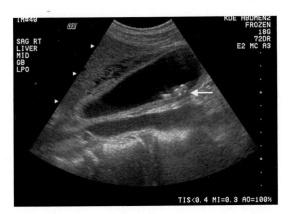

FIG. 5-15 A sagittal sonographic image of a dilated gallbladder containing stones.

an echogenic focus, (2) acoustic shadowing below the stone, and (3) gravitational dependence. Gallstones can be the size of a pinhead to the size of a large marble. The small stones tend to travel into the biliary tree and may result in obstruction. Obstruction of the bile duct causes pain and jaundice and may result in cholangitis.

Surgical removal of the gallbladder (cholecystectomy) is usually the treatment of choice with over 500,000 performed annually in the United States. Since its introduction in 1988, laparoscopic cholecystectomy has replaced many traditional open cholecystectomies. This technique allows a less traumatic entry, excision, and removal of the gallbladder, with a shortened hospitalization and reduced costs. Radiographers are commonly called to the operating environment to film injections of contrast medium into the exposed biliary duct to determine if all stones have been removed. If additional stones are suspected but not visualized, a T-tube may be inserted to allow for later study, as noted earlier.

Cholecystitis

Cholecystitis is an acute inflammation of the gallbladder. It is characterized clinically by a sudden onset of pain, fever, nausea, and vomiting. It is common in individuals with chronically symptomatic cholelithiasis. Its diagnosis is clinically suspected and supported through an ultrasound examination or radionuclide cholescintigraphy. A radiopharmaceutical comprised of ^{99m}Tc in combination with disopropyliminodiacetic acid (DISIDA) allows visualization of the biliary ductal system and results in a highly sensitive examination with consistently reliable results. Nonvisualization of the gallbladder is a good indicator of acute cholecystitis. Repeated attacks of acute cholecystitis cause damage to the gallbladder, thickening of the walls (Fig. 5-16), and decreased function.

Complications of untreated gallbladder disease include infarction and a possible gangrenous state, prompting a rupture of the walls. Perforation of the gallbladder occurs in approximately 5% to 15% of all patients with acute cholecystitis and can be diagnosed in several ways. Cholescintography provides the best images of perforation; however, stones may be visible outside the gallbladder on plain abdominal films, CT images, or sonographic images. Ultrasound and CT often also demonstrate a nonspecific pericholecystic fluid collection. If a rupture does occur, bile peritonitis may result and require immediate treatment.

Occasionally, a stone can erode through the wall of the gallbladder in cases of chronic cholecystitis and create a fistula to the bowel, most frequently the duodenum. If the stone becomes impacted in the small bowel and causes an obstruction, the condition is referred to as **gallstone ileus.** Gallstone ileus is characterized by air in the biliary ductal system, clearly visible on a conventional abdominal radiograph. The radiopaque gallstone may also be visible within the bowel surrounded by intestinal gas. Surgical removal of the stone is necessary to relieve the obstruction. Treatment of chronic cholecystitis also includes laparoscopic removal of the inflamed gallbladder.

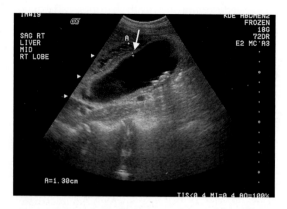

FIG. 5-16 Sonogram demonstrating a thickened wall of the gallbladder, often indicative of cholecystitis.

Pancreatitis

An inflammation of the pancreatic tissue is known as **pancreatitis.** It is one of the most complex and clinically challenging disorders of the abdomen and is classified as acute or chronic, according to clinical, morphologic, and histologic criteria. Acute pancreatitis resolves without imparing the histologic make-up of the pancreas and most often results from biliary tract disease. However, chronic pancreatitis does impair the histologic make-up of the pancreas, resulting in irreversible changes in pancreatic function. Its causes include excessive and chronic alcohol consumption and obstruction of the ampulla of Vater by a gallstone or tumor, and even the injection of contrast media during an ERCP has been known to cause pancreatitis. Once activated by any of these causes, trypsin, the pancreatic enzyme that is normally excreted through the ducts into the duodenum, begins to autodigest the organ itself. This can be quite serious and carries a high mortality rate. Hemorrhagic pancreatitis is a complication of pancreatitis and consists of erosion into local tissues and blood vessels, with subsequent hemorrhaging into the retroperitoneal space. A **pseudocyst** is a fluid collection caused by pancreatitis. It is readily visualized by sonographic or CT examination (Fig. 5-17).

Symptoms of pancreatitis vary from mild abdominal pain, nausea, and vomiting to severe pain and shock. Radiographic indications of pancreatitis are subtle and previously centered on displacement of the duodenal C-loop or the stomach by the diseased pancreas or calcified stones within the pancreatic or biliary ducts. However, CT has made a major contribution to the diagnosis and staging of acute pancreatitis. It adequately demonstrates not only the pancreas itself but also the retroperitoneum, the ligaments, the mesenteries, and the omenta. The infected pancreas is usually enlarged, with a shaggy and irregular contour. In advanced cases, fluid collections are demonstrated within

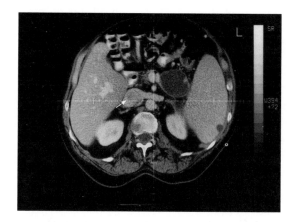

FIG. 5-17 Pancreatitis with demonstration of a 5-cm pseudocyst in the tail as seen on CT.

the pancreas, as well as within the retroperitoneum. An ERCP is of value in determining the reasons for acute recurrent pancreatitis, chronic pancreatitis, or the complications associated with pancreatitis. Because pancreatic disease is often asymptomatic in the early stages of disease, ultrasound is good for assessing the texture and size of the organ. The pancreas is routinely imaged as part of the right upper quadrant sonogram. In most ultrasound examinations, the head and body of the pancreas can be measured and compared to normal values for the age of the patient. Pancreatitis is suggested on a sonogram by the decreased echo texture and an associated enlargement in the size of the organ (Fig. 5-18). In addition, recent advances in MR allow for noninvasive, contrast-free imaging of the biliary tree. Laboratory testing is the most common way to diagnose pancreatitis, through evaluation of serum and occasionally the urine amylase level.

Management of patients with pancreatitis consists of a pain-relieving drug in mild cases and maintaining proper fluid levels to prevent shock, a frequent occurrence in acute pancreatitis. Proper dietary restrictions (e.g., abstinence from alcohol) are also important. The role of surgery in chronic pancreatitis remains controversial in regard to the effectiveness of results. The prognosis is excellent in patients with mild pancreatic inflammation and edema. However, a swollen pancreas with extravasation of fluid within the retroperitoneum or pancreatic necrosis, as demonstrated by CT, results in a more severe prognosis. Although most CT examination are performed with the use of IV contrast agents, research has shown that use of contrast agents during the onset of acute pancreatitis may cause necrosis in areas with poor blood supply. Pancreatric necrosis increases the mortality and incidence of infection, so patients should be well hydrated before a contrast-enhanced CT examination is performed. Chronic pancreatitis also increases the risk of developing pancreatic cancer, so most patients are continuously monitored for malignancy.

METABOLIC DISEASES

Jaundice

Jaundice, the yellowish discoloration of the skin and whites of the eyes, is not a disease itself but rather a sign of disease. The accumulation of excess bile pigments (i.e., bilirubin) in the body

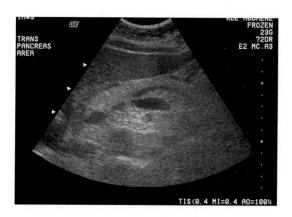

FIG. 5-18 Transverse sonographic image of the pancreas.

tissues "stains" the skin and eyes this yellowish color. Normally, bile and its pigments are secreted into the bowel and eliminated. Bilirubin is a type of bile pigment that is produced when hemoglobin breaks down. Normal serum bilirubin levels are equal to or less than 1 mg per 100 ml but must exceed 3 mg per 100 ml to be visible to the observer.

Medical (nonobstructive) jaundice occurs because of hemolytic disease in which too many red blood cells are destroyed or because of liver damage from cirrhosis or hepatitis. Its most common appearance is transient in the first few days after birth, when more bile pigments are released than can be handled. A liver that is damaged from disease simply cannot excrete the bilirubin in a normal fashion, and it enters the bloodstream.

Surgical (obstructive) jaundice occurs when the biliary system is obstructed and prevents bile from entering the duodenum. A common cause of this obstruction is blockage of the common bile duct caused by stones or masses. The longer the obstruction persists, the more likely it is that complications (e.g., liver injury, infection, or bleeding) will arise.

The jaundiced patient often undergoes an ultrasound examination of the liver, biliary tree, and pancreas to determine if the jaundice is obstructive (Fig. 5-19) or nonobstructive. The common bile duct is readily identified, and, generally speaking, a normal size implies nonobstructive jaundice and a dilated common bile duct suggests an obstruction. A variety of other methods may be used to diagnose the cause of jaundice, including ERCP, MRCP, and CT. An ultrasound or CT-directed needle biopsy may be used if an intrahepatic cause of the hepatitis is suspected. Treatment of jaundice centers on diagnosis and treatment of its underlying cause. In the case of obstructive jaundice, surgical excision of the obstructing body may be necessary. Endoscopic removal of common duct stones is frequently done, and endoscopy also offers the opportunity to stent or bypass a tumor.

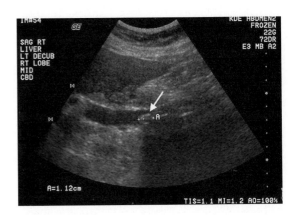

FIG. 5-19 A sagittal sonographic image demonstrating a stone *(arrow)* lodged in the distal portion of the common bile duct close to the ampulla of Vater *(A)* resulting in dilation and obstruction of the common bile duct.

NEOPLASTIC DISEASES

Hepatocellular Adenoma

A **hepatocellular adenoma** is a benign tumor of the liver. Most are asymptomatic, but the incidence of this disease has increased over the past few years. Hepatocellular adenomas occur most often in women using oral contraceptives, which play a role in the development of these benign lesions. In terms of imaging, both CT and ultrasound are useful in demonstrating hepatic lesions.

Hemangioma

A **hemangioma** is the most common tumor of the liver. It is a benign neoplasm composed of newly formed blood vessels, and these neoplasms can form in other places within the body. For instance, a port-wine stain on the face (a superficial purplish red birthmark) is an example of a hemangioma elsewhere in the body. Hemangiomas are generally well-circumscribed, solitary tumors. They can range in size from microscopic to 20 cm. They are more common in women than in men, especially postmenopausal women.

Normally the texture of the liver is homogeneous on sonographic evaluation, but occasionally an area of increased echogenicity may be demonstrated. When this appears as a solitary, round lesion, the diagnosis is usually a hemangioma. These lesions generally do not become malignant; however, ultrasound may be used to assess the lesion if there is suspicion that it has changed in size or character. In most cases, a hemangioma is insignificant, but it can present symptoms such as right-upper quadrant pain as a result of tissue displacement or bleeding. Diagnosis can be complicated when it occurs with a known malignancy because its characteristics may be difficult to distinguish from metastasis. Nuclear medicine scans using labeled red blood cells that are attracted to the highly vascular tumor are virtually diagnositic in assessing the presence of a hemangioma. These scans demonstrate the tumor as a defect in early phases and display prolonged and persistent uptake on delayed scans. A CT of the liver following an injection of IV contrast demonstrates the hemangioma with peripheral enhancement. MRI demonstrates marked hyperintensity on T2-weighted images, which corresponds with fibrosis within the tumor. Following an IV injection of a gadolinium contrast agent, peripheral enhancement of the hemangioma occurs in early scans, followed by filling in of the tumor (Fig. 5-20), similar to the appearance on an enhanced CT examination.

Hepatocellular Carcinoma (Hepatoma)

Hepatocellular carcinoma, a primary neoplasm of the liver, is uncommon in the United States, accounting for fewer than 2% of all cancers. An association between cirrhosis and hepatocellular carcinoma exists, with chronic hepatitis B or C and alcoholism associated with each. Most primary hepatomas originate in liver parenchyma, creating a large central mass with smaller satellite nodules. Although vascular invasion is common, death occurs from liver failure, often without extension of the cancer outside the liver.

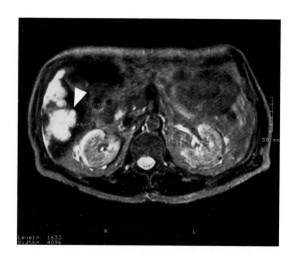

FIG. 5-20 An axial MRI slice through the liver reveals a hemangioma.

Patients with cirrhosis who experience an unexpected deterioration, patients with increased jaundice, abdominal pain, weight loss, a right upper quadrant mass, ascites, or a rapid increase in liver size are suspect for hepatocellular carcinoma. Plain abdominal radiographs may demonstrate hepatomegaly. Ultrasound and CT are often used to reveal the extent of the tumor (Fig. 5-21). Arteriography may demonstrate the increased vascularity associated with a carcinoma. A definitive diagnosis requires a liver biopsy, generally under sonographic guidance.

Surgical resection of the hepatocellular carcinoma represents the only possibility for cure. Those hepatomas that are diffuse or have multiple nodules generally preclude surgery. The general lack of radiosensitivity of these tumors makes radiotherapy ineffective. Patients treated with chemotherapy demonstrate tumor shrinkage and an addition of a few months to their lives. The disease, however, is generally fatal except for those who have had successful resection of a single liver mass.

Metastatic Liver Disease

Metastatic liver lesions are much more common than primary carcinoma because of the liver's

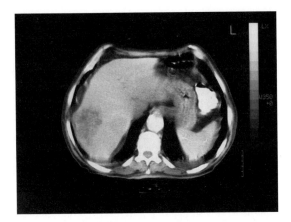

FIG. 5-21 Large, heterogeneous lesion in the liver consistent with hepatoma.

role in filtering blood. The liver is a common site for metastasis from other primary sites such as the colon, pancreas, stomach, lung, and breast (Fig. 5-22). Primary cancers located in the abdomen, especially those drained by the portal venous system, often metastasize to the liver (Fig. 5-23). Ultrasound is most commonly used to screen patients for **metastatic liver disease;** however, CT and MR also offer an accurate diagnosis. Again, liver biopsy, often under sonographic guidance, provides the definitive diagnosis.

Carcinoma of the Gallbladder

Carcinoma of the gallbladder occurs infrequently, but most neoplasms within the gallbladder are malignant. Most primary carcinomas of the gallbladder, approximately 85%, are adenocarcinomas, with the remaining 15% being anaplastic or squamous cell cancers. Carcinoma of the gallbladder is more common in women and the elderly, with gallstones present in about 75% of all cases. The symptoms are nonspecific, right-upper quadrant including pain, jaundice, and weight loss. Another risk factor associated with the development of gallbladder carcinoma is a "porcelain" gallbladder, which results from chronic cholecystitis (Fig. 5-24). Approximately 22% of

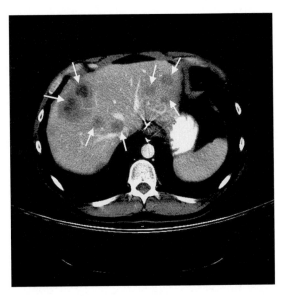

FIG. 5-22 CT of the liver demonstrating metastatic spread from bronchogenic carcinoma *(arrows).*

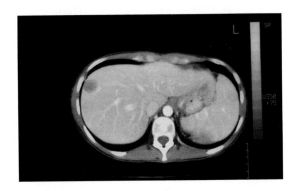

FIG. 5-23 CT scan after duodenal cancer resection in a 21-year-old woman demonstrates local recurrence and metastases to the liver on its lateral border in this slice.

patients with porcelain gallbladders develop carcinoma.

The best methods of imaging gallbladder carcinoma include CT and ultrasound. Radiographically, the appearance of the carcinoma may vary. It may appear as a mass replacing the gallbladder or as a polypoid mass within the gallbladder, or the appearance may be as subtle

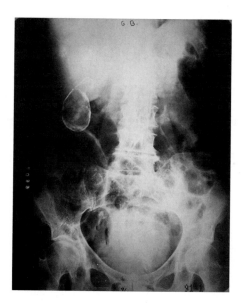

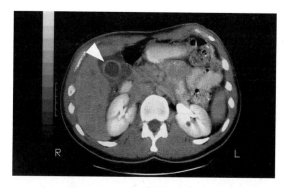

FIG. 5-25 Gallbladder carcinoma, resulting in metastasis to surrounding structures, as seen on this CT of a 23-year-old man. The gallbladder *(arrow)* is surrounded by metastasis, with significant metastasis into the pancreas area and right kidney.

FIG. 5-24 A "porcelain" gallbladder in a 70-year-old man with a history of recurrent indigestion.

as focal thickening of the gallbladder wall. Clinically and radiographically, this cancer may be difficult to differentiate from cholecystitis with pericholecystic fluid accumulation or an abscess. Unfortunately, the prognosis with gallbladder carcinoma is often poor because metastases to the liver usually occur before the primary disease is diagnosed (Fig. 5-25). It may spread via direct invasion of the liver, via intraductal tumor extension, or via the lymphatic system to regional lymph nodes. Approximately 88% of these patients die within 1 year of diagnosis, and only 4% survive 5 years following diagnosis.

Carcinoma of the Pancreas

Pancreatic cancer is usually rapidly fatal and is the fifth most common cause of cancer death within the United States. Its diagnosis is difficult because of the location of the pancreas and lack of symptoms before extensive local spread. Even with advances in CT and ultrasound, the prognosis is poor. In most cases, the tumor is well advanced before the diagnosis is made. Its incidence is greater in men than in women and in blacks than in whites. A clear-cut association with cigarette smoking has been demonstrated, and other risk factors include alcoholism, chronic pancreatitis, diabetes mellitus, and a family history of adenocarcinoma. Most tumors (approximately 90%) arise as epithelial tumors of the duct (adenocarcinoma) and cause pancreatic obstruction (Fig. 5-26). In addition, the majority (60% to 70%) of these neoplasms arise in the head of the pancreas, followed by the body (10% to 15%), and then the tail (5% to 10%). The rich supply of nerves to the pancreas results in pain as a prominent feature of this carcinoma. The tumor infiltrates and replaces normal tissue without significant hemorrhage, necrosis, or calcification. Symptoms are nonspecific, including pain, weight loss, jaundice, fatigue, nausea, vomiting, and diabetes.

Carcinomas of the pancreatic head may be visible on barium studies of the stomach and small bowel because the head of the pancreas lies within the duodenal C-loop. Carcinomas of the body and tail may affect the duodenojejunal junction and cause distortion on a barium-filled small-bowel study. When ultrasound is used to evaluate the biliary tree, the sequence of images begins with the right and left branches of the

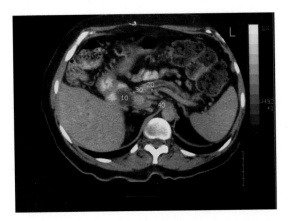

FIG. 5-26 Pancreatic carcinoma in the head of the pancreas, as indicated by atrophy of the pancreatic body and tail. Numbers shown are for density sampling, with 10, 20, and 30 in the pancreas.

common hepatic duct within the liver and concludes by scanning the common bile duct to its termination at the ampulla of Vater. Tumors of the pancreatic head cause enlargement and can result in compression of the duodenum. With the compression of the duodenum, the ampulla of Vater is also compressed, causing a dilation of the distal common bile duct. Sonographic images of a common bile duct that begins coursing normally but increases in size distally to more than 1.0 cm in diameter should suggest the possibility of a pancreatic head mass. CT is the best method of imaging the pancreas, with the most common finding a mass deforming the pancreas. However, in most cases, the tumor is not resectable because of its size by the time the mass is visible on the CT image. If the lesion is not resectable, a percutaneous needle aspiration under CT guidance is performed to biopsy the tissue. In cases where the tumor is resectable, CT offers information regarding the staging of the disease. Radical surgery as a treatment mode is about the only hope for cure, but it carries a high mortality rate. Radiation therapy is difficult because of the proximity to very radiosensitive structures such as the spinal cord, and chemotherapy also produces poor results. The prognosis with pancreatic carcinoma is very poor, demonstrating only a 2% survival rate for 5 years.

PATHOLOGY SUMMARY: THE HEPATOBILIARY SYSTEM

Pathology	Imaging Modalities of Choice	Additive or Subtractive Pathology
Cirrhosis	CT	Both
Ascites	CT and ultrasound	Additive
Hepatitis	CT, nuclear medicine, and ultrasound	None
Cholecystitis	Ultrasound and CT	None
Cholelithiasis	Ultrasound and CT	Calcified stones, additive
Pancreatitis	CT, ERCP, and ultrasound	None
Hemangioma	CT, nuclear medicine, angiography, and ultrasound	None
Hepatoma	CT and nuclear medicine	Additive
Hepatocellular adenoma	CT and ultrasound	Additive
Hepatocellular carcinoma	CT and ultrasound	Subtractive
Metastatic disease of the liver	CT and ultrasound	Subtractive
Carcinoma of the gallbladder	CT and ultrasound	None
Carcinoma of the pancreas	CT and ultrasound	Subtractive

QUESTIONS

1. Bile drains from the liver's right and left hepatic ducts directly into the:
   a. common bile duct
   b. common hepatic
   c. cystic duct
   d. duodenum

2. The noninvasive modality of choice for visualization of gallbladder disease, which does not employ ionizing radiation, is:
   a. CT
   b. diagnostic medical sonography
   c. MRI
   d. nuclear medicine

3. Impairment of normal liver function might result in:
   a. cirrhosis
   b. jaundice
   c. milk of calcium
   d. viral hepatitis

4. Patients with liver cirrhosis have a tendency to develop:
   1. ascites
   2. esophageal varices
   3. jaundice
   a. 1 and 2   c. 2 and 3
   b. 1 and 3   d. 1, 2, and 3

5. Which types of viral hepatitis may be transmitted via blood or blood products?
   a. A   c. C   e. both a and d
   b. B   d. E   f. both b and c

6. The radiographic appearance of a porcelain gallbladder may be an indication of:
   a. biliary obstruction
   b. carcinoma of the gallbladder
   c. cirrhosis
   d. cholelithiasis

7. The yellowish discoloration of the skin associated with jaundice is caused by:
   a. an accumulation of milk of calcium
   b. infected fecal material transmission
   c. paralysis of the small-bowel wall
   d. presence of bilirubin in the blood
   e. none of the above

8. Gallstone ileus refers to impaction of a gallstone in the:
   a. biliary tree   c. liver
   b. gallbladder   d. small bowel

9. The diagnostic imaging modalities of choice for following the progress of a liver malignancy are:
   1. CT   2. radiography   3. ultrasonography
   a. 1,2   c. 2,3
   b. 1,3   d. 1,2,3

10. A malignant liver tumor is a(n):
    a. hepatitis
    b. hemangioma
    c. hepatocellular carcinoma
    d. jaundice

11. Compare and contrast medical versus surgical jaundice.

12. Explain why cholelithiasis in a nonfunctioning gallbladder can be imaged with sonography and an oral cholangiogram would be ineffective in assisting a diagnosis.

13. What are the advantages of imaging the biliary ductal system antegrade with a PTC versus retrograde with an ERCP? What are the disadvantages with PTC?

14. Explain why cancers of the gallbladder and pancreas carry a poor prognosis.

15. Describe the physiologic cause of esophageal varices in conjunction with cirrhosis of the liver.

The Urinary System

UPON COMPLETION OF CHAPTER 6, THE READER SHOULD BE ABLE TO:

- Describe the anatomic components of the urinary system and their functions.
- Discuss the role of other modalities in imaging the urinary system, particularly ultrasound and computed tomography.
- Discuss common congenital anomalies of the urinary system.
- Characterize a given condition as inflammatory, metabolic, or neoplastic.
- Identify the pathogenesis of the pathologies cited and the typical treatments for them.
- Describe, in general, the radiographic appearance of each of the given pathologies.

KEY TERMS

Acute glomerulonephritis	Hypoplasia	Renal calculi
Adenocarcinoma	Malrotation	Renal colic
Bladder carcinoma	Medullary sponge kidney	Renal cyst
Bladder diverticula	Nephroblastoma	Renal failure
Bladder trabeculae	Nephrocalcinosis	Staghorn calculus
Bright's disease	Nephroptosis	Supernumerary kidney
Crossed ectopy	Nephrosclerosis	Uremia
Cystitis	Nephrostomy tube	Ureteral diverticula
Ectopic kidney	Neurogenic bladder	Ureteral stent
Foley catheter	Polycystic kidney disease	Ureterocele
Horseshoe kidney	Pyelonephritis	Urethral valve
Hydronephrosis	Pyuria	Urinary tract infection
Hyperplasia	Renal agenesis	Vesicoureteral reflux

ANATOMY AND PHYSIOLOGY

The urinary system consists of two kidneys, two ureters, a urinary bladder, and a urethra (Fig. 6-1). The urinary system forms urine to remove waste from the bloodstream for excretion. The kidneys are the site where urine is formed and excreted through remarkable processes of filtration and reabsorption, involving up to 180 liters (L) of blood per day. Urine formed in this process amounts to about 1 to 1.5 L per day and passes from the kidneys to the bladder through the ureters. Stored in the bladder, it is eventually excreted through the urethra.

The kidneys are retroperitoneal, normally located between the twelfth thoracic vertebra and the third lumbar vertebra. The right kidney lies slightly lower because of the presence of the liver superiorly. The notch located on the medial surface of each kidney is the hilus, the area where structures enter and leave the kidney. These structures include the renal artery and vein, lymphatics, and a nerve plexus. Microscopically, the nephron is the functional unit of the kidney responsible for forming and excreting urine (Fig. 6-2). The nephron unit terminates into a collecting tubule, which helps to form a tube opening at the renal papilla into a minor calyx. Minor calyces terminate in the major calyces, which, in turn, terminate at the renal pelvis (Fig. 6-3).

The ureters extend from the kidneys to the urinary bladder and are approximately 10 inches

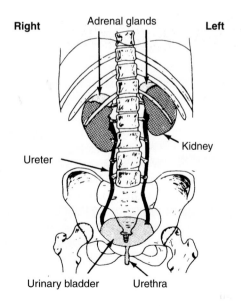

FIG. 6-1 The urinary system.

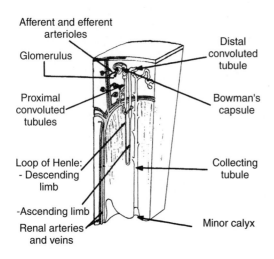

FIG. 6-2 The microscopic structure of a nephron.

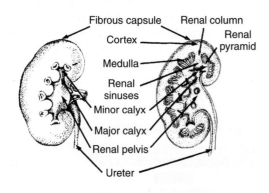

FIG. 6-3 The structure of a kidney.

in length (Fig. 6-4). They normally enter the bladder obliquely in the posterolateral portion of the bladder, equidistant from the urethral orifice in a triangular fashion. A number of variations of this can exist. The function of the ureters is to drain the urine from the kidneys to the bladder.

The bladder is located posterior to the symphysis pubis. It serves as a reservoir for urine

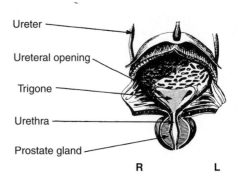

FIG. 6-4 An anterior cutaway view of the bladder.

before it is expelled from the body. The bladder is very muscular and capable of distension. Valves located at the junction of the ureters and bladder prevent the backflow of urine.

The urethra is a tube leading from the urinary bladder to the exterior of the body. In men, it also serves as a part of the reproductive system by receiving watery fluid via prostatic ducts that open into the urethra from the prostate.

IMAGING CONSIDERATIONS

Urinary disorders may be suggested by abnormal laboratory or clinical findings. Clinical findings include frequent urination, polyuria, oliguria, dysuria, or obstructive symptoms. The urine may also present with an abnormal color, resulting from a variety of factors. Kidney pain is generally located in the flank or back around the level of the twelfth thoracic vertebra, whereas bladder pain resulting from cystitis is usually limited to the urinary bladder. Renal function laboratory tests, which should be performed and checked before administering intravenous contrast agents in radiology, include serum creatinine and blood urea nitrogen (BUN). In a normal adult, the serum creatinine production and excretion are constant. Creatinine is a waste product derived from a breakdown of a compound normally found in muscle tissue. BUN levels are influenced by urine flow and the production and metabolism of urea. The BUN designates the urinary system's ability to break down nitrogenous compounds to produce urea nitrogen. Individuals with significant kidney function impairment often have raised blood levels of creatinine and/or urea nitrogen because the glomerulus cannot adequately filter the substances and/or the tubular system is not functioning properly. Intravenous contrast agents should not be used in patients with a BUN greater than 50 mg/dl or a serum creatinine greater than 3 mg/dl.

KUB

A KUB (kidney, ureter, bladder) radiograph is useful in demonstrating the size and location of the kidneys. They may be visible, radiographically, because of the perirenal fat capsule that surrounds them. The kidneys are generally well fixed to the abdominal wall and are seen to move with respiratory effort. As mentioned earlier, the right kidney is usually located inferior to the left kidney because of the presence of the liver. Men's kidneys are generally larger than those of women. The kidneys lie in an oblique plane within the abdomen and tend to parallel the borders of the psoas muscle shadows. Evaluation of the kidneys using only a KUB image is limited because the kidney shadows may often be obscured by bowel content and are difficult to visualize because of the inherent low subject contrast in the abdomen. However, a KUB is the usual beginning for most intravenous urograms (IVU), sometimes referred to as intravenous pyelograms (IVP) (Fig. 6-5). In this case, its primary purposes are to determine if adequate bowel preparation has been accomplished and to visualize radiopaque calculi of the kidneys, ureters, and bladder that may otherwise be hidden by the presence of contrast media. The radiologist also examines areas unrelated to the urinary tract because they may hold clues to the diagnosis and may also assist in differentiating between gastrointestinal and genitourinary disorders.

Intravenous Urography

One common procedure used to assess the urinary system is the intravenous urogram (IVU) or intravenous pyelogram (IVP). It is often the starting point for the diagnosis of urinary tract dysfunction. The indications for performing an IVU include suspected urinary tract obstruction, abnormal urinary sediment (especially hematuria), systemic hypertension, or, frequently in men, symptoms of prostatism. Although few or no serious adverse effects typically accompany the injection of urographic contrast agents, about 1 of 40,000 patients dies as a result of an allergic reaction to the contrast agents. The use of nonionic, low-osmolar contrast agents significantly reduces minor and moderate reactions. These contrast agents still contain iodine, but the molecular makeup prevents them from disassociating into ions (nonionic) in the bloodstream, thus reducing the chances for an anaphylactic reaction. Visualization of the urinary system depends on the concentration of contrast material filtered by the kidneys and present in the collecting system; therefore, the patient must have fairly normal physiologic function for diagnostic images to be obtained. Other imaging techniques such as sonography and CT should be considered in patients with compromised renal function.

Many IVU routines allow for an image to be taken within 30 seconds to 1 minute after contrast medium injection. Because the contrast agents for most IVU examinations are injected by hand, the timing generally begins on completion of the bolus injection and will vary from institution to institution. This is termed the nephrogram phase and may be used to demonstrate the contrast agent in the nephrons before it reaches the renal calyces. Ready visualization of the renal parenchyma allows for an inspection of the renal outline. Indentations or bulges may indicate the presence of disease. The

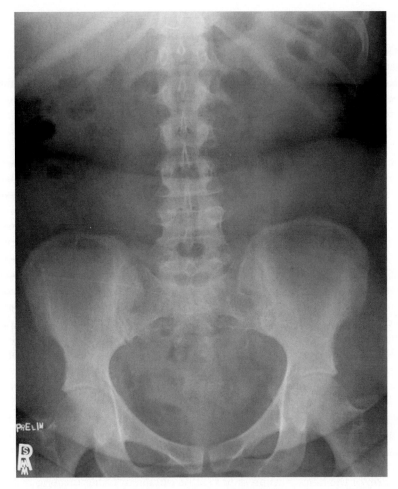

FIG. 6-5 A preliminary or scout image before injecting intravenous contrast for an intravenous urogram. The image demonstrates the renal and psoas major muscle shadows.

nephrogram image is also used to check for normal kidney position, which may be altered by congenital malposition, ptosis, or the presence of a retroperitoneal mass.

Although the number and type of images obtained may vary from one institution to another, a series of collecting system sequence images are the final part of an IVU (Fig. 6-6). The renal pelvis, calyces, ureters, and bladder are examined for any abnormalities. The calyces should be evenly distributed and reasonably symmetrical. Usually, they present as buttercup-shaped projections surrounding the renal papillae. Calyceal dilatation may be demonstrated as a result of acute or chronic urinary tract obstruction, after obstructive uropathy, or reflux. Dilatation secondary to destruction of the renal pyramids is less common.

Because of the peristaltic activity of ureters, only part of their length in a collecting system sequence may be demonstrated (Fig. 6-7). Sometimes nonopaque ureteral calculi cause

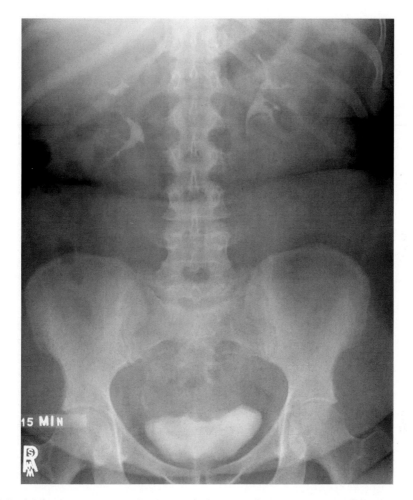

FIG. 6-6 A 15-minute postinjection image during an intravenous urogram demonstrating the normal collecting system.

filling defects and an obstructive dilatation of the ureter. The majority of all urinary tract calculi are found at the vesicoureteral junction. Any pronounced deviation of the ureter suggests the presence of a retroperitoneal mass. Various filling defects may be demonstrated in the contrast agent–filled ureter during an IVU, including tumors, blood clots, and nonopaque calculi. Common bladder defects visualized during an IVU include urinary catheter balloons, normal uterus and colon, and extrinsic deformities such as uterine or sigmoid colon tumors. A "postvoid" image usually completes an IVU procedure and allows assessment of the bladder function (Fig. 6-8).

The physician may also request one of several additional radiographic examinations designed to look at select aspects of the urinary tract. Nephrotomography, for example, may be used as a primary study in lieu of the standard IVU or as an adjunct study, using tomograms of the kidneys taken at suitable intervals

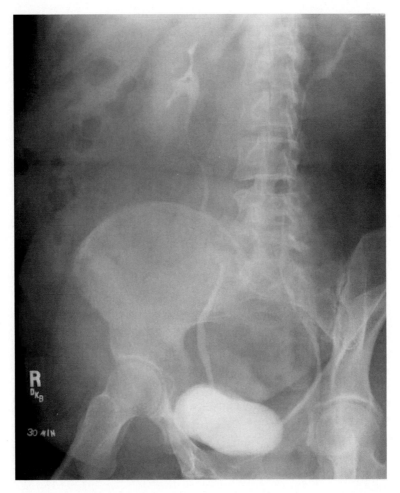

FIG. 6-7 An RPO projection following contrast injection for an intravenous urogram demonstrating the correct entrance of the ureters into the posterior bladder wall.

(Fig. 6-9). Tomographic images obtained before intravenous contrast are used to look for calculi, whereas those after contrast administration are used for closer examination of the renal parenchyma and collecting systems.

Cystogram

The most common examination for studying the lower urinary tract is the cystogram. This involves insertion of a urinary catheter into the urethra and retrograde filling of the bladder with iodinated water-soluble contrast material (Fig. 6-10). A frequent indication for this procedure is to identify vesicoureteral reflux. In the normal bladder, increased pressure as the bladder fills effectively shuts down any chance of reflux. Bladder infection, however, can render the ureteral "valve" incompetent, refluxing infection into the kidney. Cystography is also used to study congenital bladder anomalies, tumors, diverticula (Fig. 6-11), calculi, bladder rupture, or neurogenic bladder. Voiding (mic-

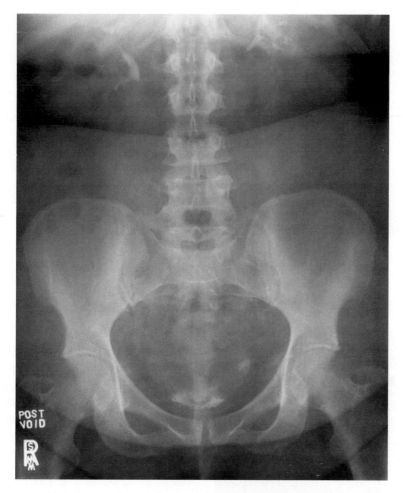

FIG. 6-8 A postvoid image following an intravenous urogram examination.

turition) cystography is sometimes used in conjunction with a retrograde cystogram to allow study of the urethra on voiding. Urethrography may be accomplished antegrade, as with a voiding cystourethrogram, or retrograde when a cystogram is not necessary. The antegrade approach is used to study the posterior urethra, especially in the male patient, and the retrograde approach is helpful in studying the anterior urethra (Fig. 6-12). The usual intent of voiding cystography is to allow study of a urethral stricture (Fig. 6-13).

Retrograde Pyelogram

With retrograde pyelography, a catheter is placed into the ureteric orifice, usually by a urologist, at cystoscopy to allow injection of contrast medium directly into the urinary tract to outline the renal collecting system. It is termed retrograde because the contrast agent is injected through the ureter into the affected kidney, opposite the normal direction of urine flow. Indications for this study may include hematuria of unknown cause, hydronephrosis, and, in cases of a nonfunctioning kidney, where

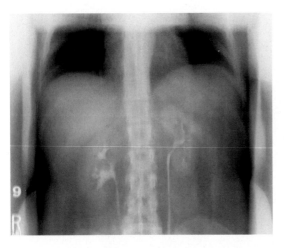

FIG. 6-9 A normal nephrotomogram obtained immediately post injection of an intravenous contrast agent.

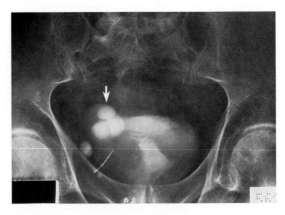

FIG. 6-11 Bladder diverticula in an 88-year-old man demonstrate the presence of numerous calculi within them.

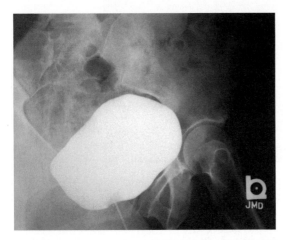

FIG. 6-10 Normal cystogram without reflux as seen in this oblique projection of the bladder in a 56-year-old woman.

further information about possible obstruction is desired.

Ultrasound

Ultrasound (sonography) is a noninvasive method of imaging both functioning and nonfunctioning kidneys. Because sonography can clearly demonstrate the parenchymal structure of the kidney and the renal pelvis without the use of contrast agents, it is often the imaging modality of choice in the evaluation of most renal disorders. It is useful in evaluating kidney stones (Fig. 6-14), calcifications, hydronephrosis (Fig. 6-15), abscesses, renal masses, and renal cysts and to assess renal size and/or atrophy. Ultrasound is the modality of choice for evaluating individuals following kidney transplantation. Doppler techniques are helpful in assessing blood flow in the renal arteries and veins for both transplantation recipients and individuals with suspected renal artery stenosis. Sonography can also be utilized to visualize abnormalities of the urinary system present in the fetus before birth.

Computed Tomography

Computed tomography (CT) is an excellent modality for imaging the kidneys because it can detect small differences in tissue densities within the body. Kidneys can be visualized on CT with or without the use of a contrast agent. Abdominal CT is particularly important in determining the nature of renal masses, either solid or cystic, which may not be visible on a KUB because of the presence of gas in the

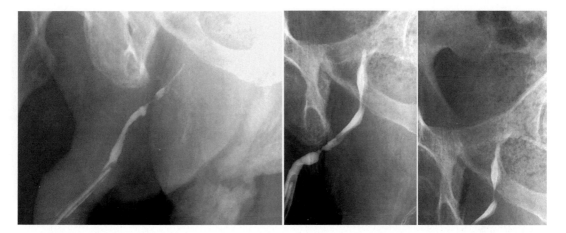

FIG. 6-12 Retrograde urethrogram procedure demonstrating a urethral stricture on a male patient. The location of the stricture is confirmed by its consistent appearance on all three images.

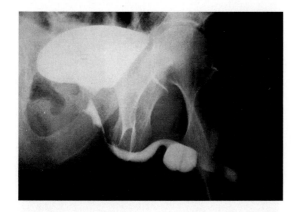

FIG. 6-13 A voiding cystourethrogram demonstrates a urethral diverticula. The mucosal margin of the prostatic urethra is ragged as a result of scarring after transurethral resection.

bowel. CT evaluation of the urinary system generally requires the use of an IV contrast agent to help differentiate renal cysts from solid masses and to evaluate the extent of the lesion (Fig. 6-16). Thin-slice (3–5 mm) images are obtained through the kidneys with thicker slices (10 mm) obtained from the bottom of the kidneys to the iliac crest. Because most institu-

tions use an automatic injector in CT, scanning generally begins at the time the bolus of contrast medium is injected, and a delay is programmed into the scanner to allow the contrast medium to reach the bladder before the pelvis is imaged.

CT is also useful in looking for sites of obstruction caused by **renal calculi** or retroperitoneal masses, which may distort the urinary tract, assessing renal infection or trauma, and staging tumors of the lymph nodes. A CT renal stone study is now often performed instead of an IVU in many medical facilities because the CT stone study is conducted without the use of a contrast agent. Thin slices (5 mm) are obtained from the top of the kidneys through the symphysis pubis. Because CT displays excellent contrast resolution, stones are identified more easily than with conventional radiography (Fig. 6-17). In addition, pelvic CT is the imaging modality of choice for the evaluation of bladder tumors or masses.

Renal Angiography

Renal angiography is one of the most invasive imaging procedures performed on the urinary

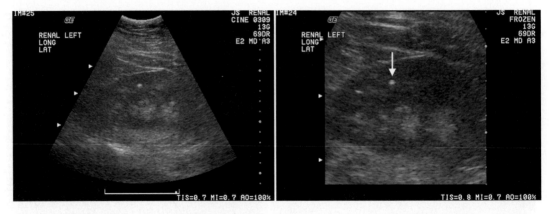

FIG. 6-14 A sonogram demonstrating a renal stone in the cortex of the kidney.

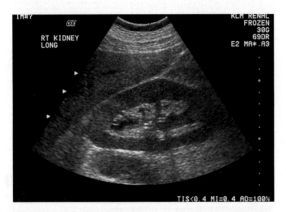

FIG. 6-15 A sonogram confirming hydronephrosis of the kidney and proper placement of a ureteral stent to assist in allowing the kidney to drain properly into the urinary bladder.

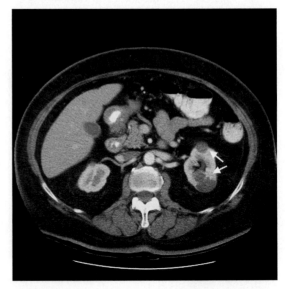

FIG. 6-16 CT of a complex cystic structure of the left kidney post contrast injection during the nephrogram phase.

system. It is usually indicated to further evaluate a renal mass suspected of being malignant; to embolize blood flow to a renal mass; to assess renal artery stenosis that may cause hypertension; as well as to assess other vascular disorders such as aneurysms or congenital anomalies. It is also performed on kidney donors before surgical removal of the kidney to serve as a "road map" of vascular anatomy for the surgeon. In renal angiography, a catheter is introduced peripherally, most commonly into the femoral artery. The catheter tip may be placed into the specific renal artery of interest or the abdominal aorta just superior to the renal arteries. The contrast agent is injected via the catheter to image the vasculature of the kidney or kidneys.

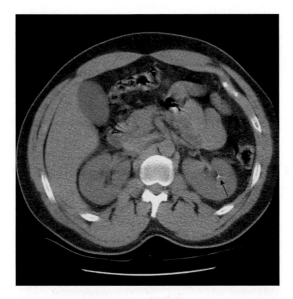

FIG. 6-17 CT demonstrating a calcification in the left kidney indicative of a renal stone without the use of a contrast agent.

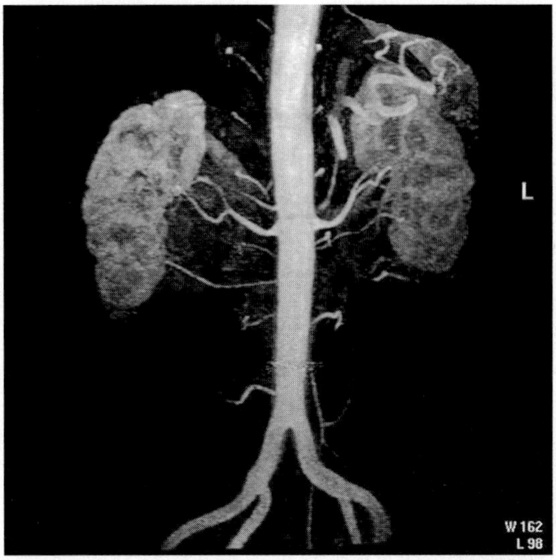

FIG. 6-18 A contrast-enhanced three-dimensional magnetic resonance angiography (MRA) of the renal arteries demonstrating normal renal artery patency.

Magnetic Resonance Imaging

The role of magnetic resonance imaging (MRI) has greatly improved as a result of breath-hold imaging sequences and bolus injections of gadolinium contrast agents. Abdominal MRI is now being used to evaluate for renal artery stenosis (Fig. 6-18) as well as renal carcinoma. Contrast- enhanced three-dimensional magnetic resonance angiography obtains coronal images of the renal arteries in as little as 20 seconds. The images can then be rotated for better visualization. MR is also an excellent modality for demonstrating other vascular anomalies such as thrombosis, aneurysms, and AV malformations. Because it allows for imaging of the urinary system in all three planes, it is also used in conjunction with CT for the evaluation of renal masses and their extension. In cases of renal cyst evaluation, MR is capable of differentiating between fluid accumulation from hemorrhage versus infection. Pelvic MR is utilized to readily demonstrate the seminal vesicles and prostate gland in men as well as masses within the urinary bladder. Because of its ability to clearly image soft tissue, pelvic MR allows thorough evaluation of invasive cancers within the urinary bladder.

Interventional Procedures/Techniques

A percutaneous nephrostogram is an antegrade study in which the contrast medium is injected directly into the renal pelvis. It involves posterolateral insertion of a needle or catheter into the renal pelvis using medical sonography, fluoroscopy, or sometimes a combination of both modalities (Fig. 6-19). The nephrostomy tube may be left in place to provide drainage of an obstructed kidney or to allow retrieval of the calculus with a basket catheter. Sometimes the procedure is used to relieve obstruction in patients for whom immediate surgery is not possible.

Extracorporeal (SWL) is a method used to locate and treat renal calculi. After location of the stone is attained radiographically, fluoroscopy or sonography aids in alignment of a

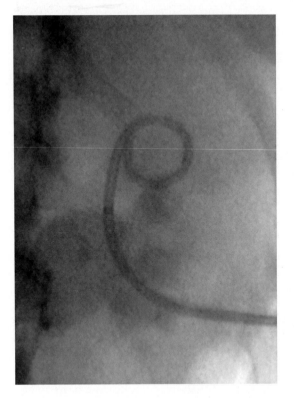

FIG. 6-19 Placement of a right percutaneous renal drainage tube under fluoroscopic guidance.

high-frequency shock wave directed at the stone of a patient. If the treatment is successful, the stone disintegrates into fragments that can be voided by the patient, often sparing a surgical procedure and a much lengthier recovery period (Fig. 6-20).

Percutaneous renal biopsies or drainages may be performed under fluoroscopic, ultrasonic, or computed tomographic guidance. Biopsies help in the evaluation of the histologic origin of renal masses. Percutaneous drainage may be used to aspirate renal cysts or abscesses.

Urinary Tubes and Catheters

When certain types of pathology, such as tumors or stone formation, inhibit the normal flow of urine through the urinary system, several types of tubes may be used to allow drainage of the urine. A **nephrostomy tube** connects the renal pelvis to the outside of the body (see Fig. 6-19). It is inserted percutaneously through the renal cortex and medulla into the renal pelvis to allow the urine to drain outside of the body directly from the renal pelvis. Special care must be taken when dealing with these patients, who are readily prone to infections because of the direct opening into the urinary system.

Ureteral stents may also be placed in cases of ureteral obstruction. Unlike nephrostomy tubes, ureteral stents do not connect the urinary system to the outside of the patient's body (Fig. 6-21). **Ureteral stents** are placed surgically or via cystoscopy, with the upper portion of the stent in the renal pelvis and the lower portion within the urinary bladder. The stent maintains patency of the diseased ureter and enables the urine to flow normally. These stents are radiographically visible on plain abdominal radiographs and on CT examination of the abdomen (Fig. 6-22).

Urinary catheterization is performed to obtain urine specimens, relieve urinary retention, monitor renal function, and manage urinary incontinence. A **Foley catheter** is the most common indwelling urinary catheter. It is placed within the urinary bladder using sterile technique. Once the catheter is placed through the urethra and urinary sphincter, a small balloon is inflated to help the catheter remain in place within the urinary bladder. This catheter is generally connected to a bag that collects the urine as it flows through the catheter to the outside of the body. Care must be taken to ensure that the catheter is not displaced during a radiographic procedure, and the urine collection bag must remain lower than the patient's bladder at all times to prevent the reflux of urine back into the bladder, which could result in a urinary tract infection (UTI). A Foley catheter must be placed in an individual before cystography or cystourethrography is performed to allow the installation of contrast material into the bladder. Again, the impor-

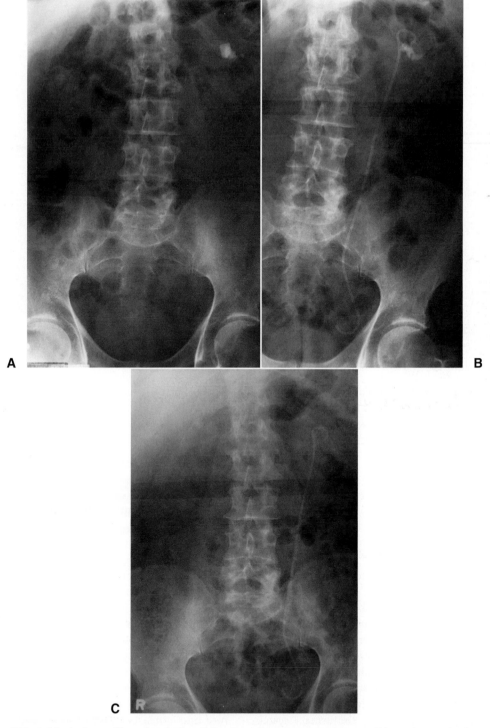

FIG. 6-20 A, Scout film taken before lithotripsy demonstrates a large, solid renal stone in the right kidney. **B,** Two months after lithotripsy, the stone is clearly seen to be fragmented and beginning to descend the right ureter. A stent has been placed in the right ureter to aid in draining urine. **C,** A film taken 2 months later demonstrates further movement of stone fragments down the ureter. The stent is still in place.

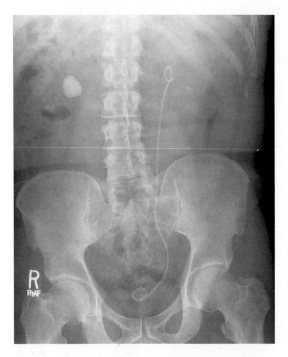

FIG. 6-21 An abdominal radiograph demonstrating bilateral renal calculi with a left ureteral stent properly placed to allow drainage of urine into the urinary bladder.

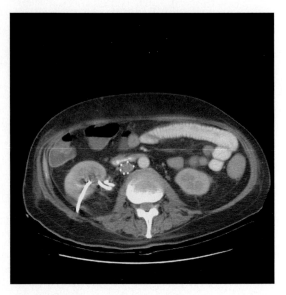

FIG. 6-22 Abdominal CT demonstrating a right percutaneous nephrostomy placement and ureteral stent.

tance of proper sterile technique cannot be overemphasized.

CONGENITAL AND HEREDITARY DISEASES

Anomalies of the kidneys and ureters are caused by errors in development. They can be classified as anomalies of number, size and form, fusion, and position. About 10% of all persons have some sort of congenital malformation of the urinary system, and these congenital anomalies often result in impaired renal function leading to infection and stone formation. At least half of those with kidney anomalies have malformations elsewhere in the urinary system or in other systems, most commonly the reproductive system, which may result in sexual dysfunction or infertility. Surgical correction may

be required for complications associated with the anomaly.

Number and Size Anomalies of the Kidney

Renal agenesis is a relatively rare anomaly that generally demonstrates as the absence of the kidney on one side and an unusually large kidney on the other side (Fig. 6-23), a condition known as compensatory hypertrophy. The left kidney is more frequently missing, and the condition is more common in men than in women. A single kidney occurs in approximately 1 in 1000 individuals. It is more subject to trauma because of its enlarged size. Protection against disease in an individual with only one kidney is very important. The absence of both kidneys, termed Potter's syndrome or bilateral agenesis, is incompatible with life.

A **supernumerary kidney** is also relatively rare and consists of the presence of a third, small, rudimentary kidney. It has no parenchymal attachment to a kidney, with about half of occurrences draining from an independent

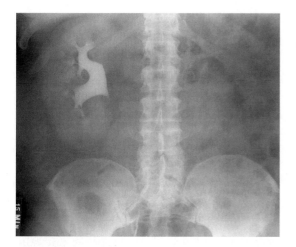

FIG. 6-23 An intravenous urogram demonstrating agenesis of the left kidney accompanied by a large, functioning right kidney.

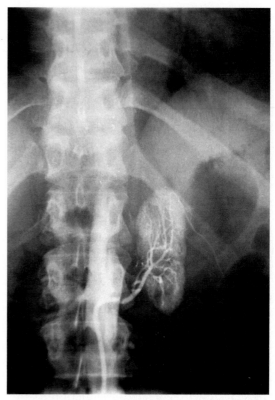

FIG. 6-24 Normal vasculature of this small kidney demonstrates renal hypoplasia.

renal pelvis into the ureter on that side. It often becomes symptomatic as a result of infection.

Hypoplasia is a rare anomaly of size involving a kidney that is developed less than normal in size but contains normal nephrons (Fig. 6-24). Usually hypoplasia is associated with hyperplasia of the other kidney. It requires renal arteriography to differentiate congenital hypertrophic changes from a kidney that is atrophic because of acquired vascular disease (Fig. 6-25). The clinical significance of hypoplasia depends on the volume of functioning kidney; however, hypertension often accompanies this anomaly. **Hyperplasia** is the opposite condition; it involves an overdeveloped kidney. Again, this is often associated with renal agenesis or hypoplasia of the other kidney.

Fusion Anomalies of the Kidney

Fusion anomalies of the kidneys are often distinguishable on plain radiographs. **Horseshoe kidney,** the most common fusion anomaly, describes a condition affecting about 0.25% of the population, with men affected twice as frequently as women. With it, the lower poles of the kidneys are joined across the midline by a band of soft tissues, causing a rotation anomaly on one or both sides. The ureters exit the kidneys anteriorly instead of medially, and the lower pole calyces point medially rather than laterally with this condition (Figs. 6-26 and 6-27). Kidney function is generally unimpaired with this condition; however, if obstruction is present, because of the abnormal location of the ureters, pyeloplastic surgery may be required. The lower bridge frequently lies on a sacral promontory, where it is susceptible to trauma and may be palpated as an abdominal mass.

Crossed ectopy exists when one kidney lies across the midline and is fused to the other kidney (Fig. 6-28). This is the second most common fusion anomaly. Both kidneys demon-

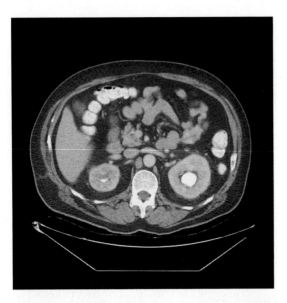

FIG. 6-25 Abdominal CT of an atrophic right kidney.

strate various anomalies of position, shape, fusion, and rotation with crossed ectopy. The crossed kidney generally lies inferior to the uncrossed one, and its ureter crosses the midline to enter the bladder on the proper side. Its

drainage may be impaired by malposition of its ureter within the renal pelvis, which may require surgical pyeloplasty repair.

Position Anomalies of the Kidney

Anomalies of position are relatively common. **Malrotation** consists of incomplete or excessive rotation of the kidneys as they ascend from the pelvis in utero. This is generally of little clinical significance unless an obstruction is created. An **ectopic kidney** is one that is out of its normal position, a condition found in approximately 1 in 800 urologic examinations. Most are asymptomatic throughout life; however, there is an increased incidence of ureteropelvic junction obstruction or vesicoureteral reflux. Ectopic kidneys are usually lower than normal, often in a pelvic (Fig. 6-29) or sacral location. In rare cases, the ectopic kidney may be intrathoracic. In severe cases of ectopy, surgical intervention may be necessary. In some lean and athletic persons, the kidney is mobile and may drop toward the pelvis in an erect position. This is termed kidney prolapse or **nephroptosis.** Nephroptosis can be distinguished from a pelvic kidney by the length of the ureter; if the ureter is short, it is a congenital pelvic kidney.

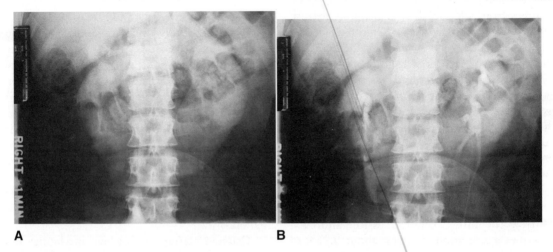

A   **B**

FIG. 6-26 A, Nephrogram phase of an intravenous urogram demonstrates fusing of the lower poles, as consistent with horseshoe kidney. **B,** Further excretion in the intravenous urogram demonstrates emptying of the malrotated kidneys via separate ureters.

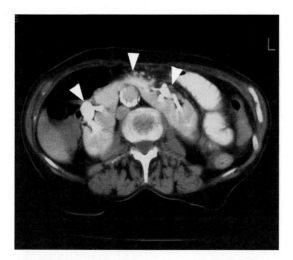

FIG. 6-27 Horseshoe kidney with apparent obstruction as seen on this CT of a 72-year-old woman.

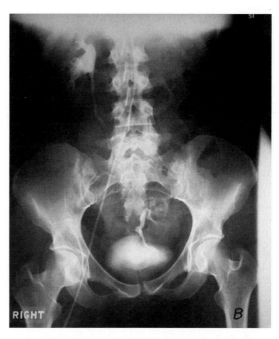

FIG. 6-29 An ectopic kidney, indicated by a urogram film taken at the end of an angiogram, demonstrates the left kidney with a shortened ureter in the left pelvis.

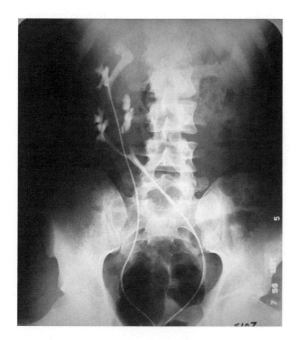

FIG. 6-28 Retrograde pyelogram demonstrates the left ureter crossing midline to connect with the lower pelvis of an anomalous right kidney, as consistent with crossed fused renal ectopy.

Renal Pelvis and Ureter Anomalies

Renal pelvis and ureter anomalies are frequent. They may be unilateral or bilateral, and they have a tendency to be asymmetric. Such anomalies may occur as a double renal pelvis, either isolated or in combination with a double ureter (Figs. 6-30 and 6-31). The problem with these and other upper tract anomalies is that they may impair renal drainage, predisposing the patient to infection and calculi formation.

Lower Tract Anomalies

A simple **ureterocele** is a cystlike dilatation of a ureter near its opening into the bladder. These usually result from congenital stenosis of the ureteral orifice. Radiographically, a ureterocele presents as a filling defect in the bladder with a characteristic "cobra head" appearance. A ureterocele that appears with ureteral

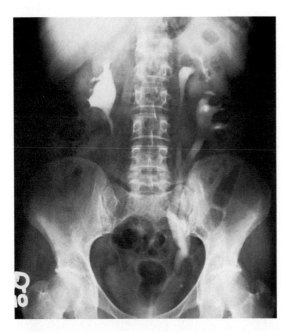

FIG. 6-30 Congenital double ureter is clearly seen on the left side.

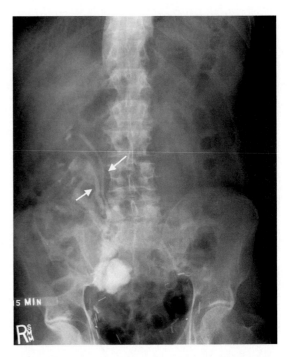

FIG. 6-31 A duplicated right collecting system emptying into a loop of bowel. The urinary bladder has been surgically removed because of bladder carcinoma and replaced with a loop of small intestines.

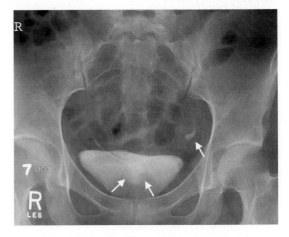

FIG. 6-32 Left ureteric diverticula visible as double densities superimposed on the posterior bladder as seen on this intravenous urogram on a female with recurrent urinary tract infections.

duplication is an "ectopic" ureterocele; it often causes substantial obstruction, primarily of the upper pole, kidney infection, and potentially can lead to **renal failure.** Treatment in this situation involves endoscopic or open surgical repair to allow for increased flow of urine into the bladder.

Ureteral diverticula are probably a congenital anomaly and may actually represent a dilated, branched ureteric remnant. The appearance of these is the same as that of any other diverticula and is best demonstrated by retrograde urography (Fig. 6-32). **Bladder diverticula** (Fig. 6-33) may occur as a congenital anomaly or be caused by chronic bladder obstruction and resultant infection. They usually occur in middle-aged men and may be diagnosed via cystography or cystoscopy. In severe cases the bladder may have to be surgically reconstructed. **Urethral valves** are mucosal folds that protrude into the posterior (prostatic) urethra as a congenital condition. These

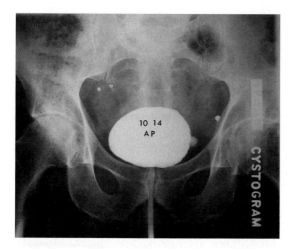

FIG. 6-33 Bladder diverticula visible on the bladder's left margin in this cystogram.

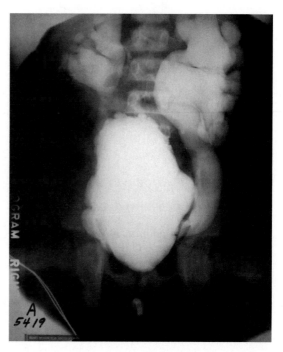

FIG. 6-34 Large, trabeculated bladder and large tortuous ureters and renal pelves seen on this cystogram of a 15-year-old boy, consistent with bladder outflow obstruction secondary to congenital posterior urethral valves.

can cause significant obstruction to urine flow (Fig. 6-34). Such "valves" occur in men and are usually discovered during infancy or early childhood and are commonly diagnosed by voiding cystourethrography. The condition is corrected by endoscopic surgery at an early age to prevent renal damage.

Polycystic Kidney Disease

Polycystic kidney disease is a congenital, familial kidney disorder that may be classified as either autosomal recessive or autosomal dominant. Innumerable tiny cysts within the nephron unit are present at birth and may be discovered by ultrasound in utero. Autosomal recessive polycystic kidney disease is a rare condition causing childhood cystic disease and ultimately resulting in childhood renal failure. Without a family history of autosomal recessive polycystic kidney disease, diagnosis is often difficult. Sonography plays an important role in demonstrating the renal and hepatic cysts and is also utilized for obtaining a tissue sample via percutaneous biopsy.

Autosomal dominant polycystic kidney disease is often asymptomatic in childhood, although it may be visible sonographically. The cysts gradu-

ally enlarge as the patient ages, and clinical symptoms become apparent in adulthood. It is the cause of approximately 10% of end-stage renal disease in adults. This enlargement compresses and eventually destroys normal tissues. The late presentation of the condition occurs because the cysts are initially very small and do not cause problems until tissue destruction becomes significant. Symptoms include lower back pain, UTIs, and stone formation. In addition, approximately 30% to 35% of these individuals have cysts occurring within the liver that do not affect liver function, and 50% are diagnosed with renal hypertension.

Intravenous urographic indications of polycystic kidney disease show bilateral enlargement of the kidneys with poorly visualized outlines (from the presence of cysts) and calyceal

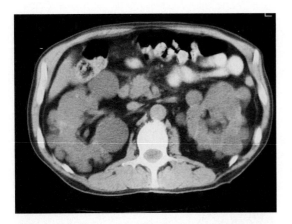

FIG. 6-35 Polycystic kidney disease visible as multiple masses in the kidneys in this CT of a 64-year-old man.

disease in its early stages, before it may be visible on conventional radiographs. Over half of those individuals affected with polycystic kidney disease eventually develop uremia in their mid- to late 50s and require dialysis or kidney transplantation. Therapy for this condition consists of good management of UTIs, basic fluid and electrolyte management, hypertension management, avoidance of physical activities that could cause trauma to the abdomen, and management of pain caused by the occasional rupture of a cyst.

Medullary Sponge Kidney

Medullary sponge kidney is a congenital dilatation of the renal tubules leading to urinary stasis and increased levels of calcium phosphate (nephrocalcinosis). The diagnosis is not usually made until the fourth or fifth decade of life, when infective complications emerge. The only visible abnormality is the dilatation of the medullary and papillary portions of the collecting ducts, usually bilaterally (Fig. 6-36). Calculi are contained in about 60% of symptomatic patients, with infection and

stretching and distortion (Fig. 6-35). The diagnosis of multiple cysts is readily confirmed by ultrasound, which reveals multiple echo-free areas in both kidneys, or by CT evaluation demonstrating a moth-eaten appearance of the functional renal tissue. Both ultrasound and CT have the advantage of demonstrating the

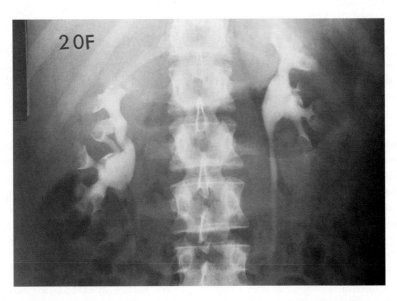

FIG. 6-36 Medullary sponge kidney demonstrated by large bilateral papillae and dilated tubules visible within the papillae in this 20-year-old woman with recurrent cystitis.

intrarenal obstruction common. Intravenous urography reveals linear markings in the papillae or cystic collections of contrast medium in the enlarged collecting ducts. However, this anomaly is often difficult to differentiate from renal cystic disease, tuberculosis, or other disorders resulting in nephrocalcinosis (deposits of calcium phosphates in the renal tubules). Diagnostic sonography is generally unable to demonstrate the cysts because they are very small and generally lie deep within the medulla of the kidney. Therapy for this condition consists of treatment of infection and, if possible, resolution of nephrolithiasis with lithotripsy.

INFLAMMATORY DISEASES

Urinary Tract Infection

Urinary tract infections (UTIs) are the most common of all bacterial infections. They can occur in individuals of all ages and both genders. They are more common in boys in infancy, generally resulting from a congenital anomaly. The incidence increases in girls around the age of 10 years, and by the age of 20, women are twice as likely to develop a UTI as men. Up to 35% of all women experience a UTI at least once in their lifetime. A quantitative urine culture is essential in approaching UTI because its causes are broad. In most cases of UTI, the infecting organism is a gram-negative bacillus that invades the urinary system by an ascending route through the urethra to the bladder to the kidney. Some believe that the offending bacteria ascend during micturition, possibly related to a turbulent stream or reflux on completion of voiding. Research also suggests that sexually active women tend to experience UTIs more frequently than women who are not sexually active, especially when they use a diaphragm and spermicide as forms of birth control. It is believed that the spermicide inhibits the normal flora of the vagina and allows an overgrowth of *E. coli*. The only clearly demonstrated mechanism, however, is by instrumentation of the urethra and bladder by cystoscopy, urologic surgery, or Foley catheter placement. Antibiotics are used to clear the infectious bacteria.

Pyelonephritis

Acute **pyelonephritis** is a bacterial infection of the calyces and renal pelvis and is thought to represent the most common renal disease. Any stagnation or obstruction to urine flow in any part of the urinary tract predisposes the patient to kidney infection. The bacteria involved likely reach the kidney via the bloodstream. Acute pyelonephritis is rare in men with a normal urinary tract but is common in women, especially pregnant women following urinary catheterization or as the increased size of the uterus acts to compress the ureter (Fig. 6-37) and decrease urine clearance of bacteria.

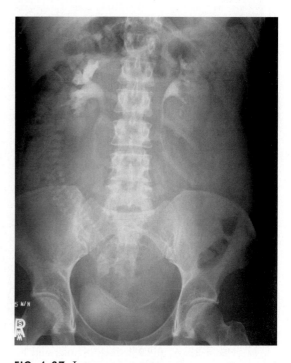

FIG. 6-37 Intravenous urogram on a pregnant female demonstrating hydronephrosis of the right kidney caused by the position of a 31-week-old fetus.

Patients presenting with acute pyelonephritis have fever, flank pain, and general malaise. Urinalysis demonstrates **pyuria,** the presence of pus (white cells) created by the body's reaction to the infection. Abscesses may form in the kidneys and create a flow of pus into the collecting tubules. Diagnosis of the condition is usually made by laboratory results, as radiographic findings are often nonspecific. In most cases, an IVU is normal even during an acute attack. The calyces may be blunted, and collecting structures may be less well visualized because of interstitial edema. Treatment consists of administering antibiotics to eliminate the infectious bacteria.

Recurrent or persistent infection of the kidneys, such as that caused by chronic reflux of infected urine from the bladder into the renal pelvis, can result in chronic pyelonephritis. It generally has no relation to acute pyelonephritis and is sometimes seen in patients with a major anatomic abnormality (e.g., an obstruction) or, most commonly, in vesicoureteral reflux in children. Chronic pyelonephritis is often bilateral and leads to destruction and scarring of the renal tissue, with marked dilatation of the calyces. The eventual result is an overall reduction in kidney size, readily seen on intravenous urography (Fig. 6-38 *A*). The renal pyramids atrophy, giving the calyces a clubbed appearance. Scars may also be seen and appear as indentations of the renal cortex on the kidney outline in the nephrogram phase (Fig. 6-38 *B*). Chronic pyelonephritis may be caused by a congenital duplication of ureters that allows a chronic reflux of urine, by an obstruction of the urinary tract, or by a neurogenic bladder. Hypertension may result from chronic pyelo-

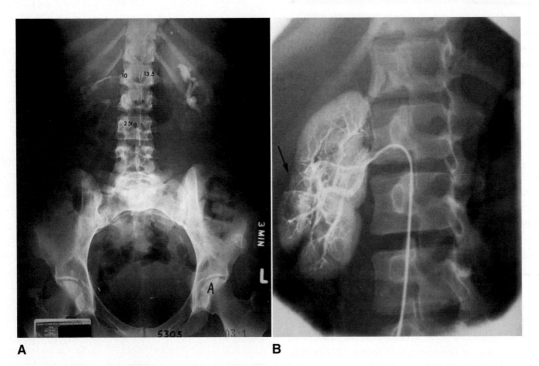

A   **B**

FIG. 6-38 A, Right kidney is small and has a scarred surface, as seen on this intravenous urogram on a 25-year-old woman with recurrent urinary tract infections. **B,** Selective renal angiography demonstrates a thinned cortex caused by scarring and bunching of the renal vessels, as consistent with chronic pyelonephritis.

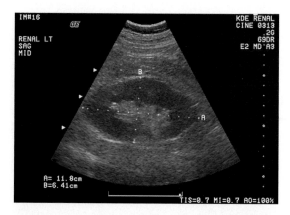

FIG. 6-39 A diagnostic medical sonogram demonstrating the echogenic texture of a normal kidney.

nephritis. Sonography is useful in assessing and grading medical renal disease, including pyelonephritis and renal hypertension. One of the subjective sonographic techniques includes comparing the echogenicity of the kidney to that of the liver because the liver has a homogeneous sonographic texture. For a normal grading, the cortical area of the kidney should be less echogenic than the liver (Fig. 6-39). As the disease breaks down the cortical tissue, the echogenicity becomes equal to that of the liver. In the final phases of renal disease, the kidney exhibits greater echogenicity than the liver. Treatment of pyelonephritis in a chronic stage centers on control of hypertension, removal of any cause for obstruction, and use of antibiotics to control infection.

Acute Glomerulonephritis

An antigen-antibody reaction in the glomeruli causes an inflammatory reaction of the renal parenchyma known as **acute glomerulonephritis** or **Bright's disease.** Often this immunologic reaction occurs following streptococcal infection of the upper respiratory tract or the middle ear. It differs from acute pyelonephritis, which primarily affects the interstitial tissue rather than the nephrons. The condition occurs mainly in children following streptococcal

infection, with most patients recovering completely. The diagnosis is again best made with laboratory results. Radiographically, the kidneys appear larger, particularly during the nephrogram phase of an IVU, because of edematous accumulation. Treatment may include diuretic therapy to lessen edema and its resultant pressure on the glomeruli, as well as anti-inflammatory medications and steroid therapy. Renal dialysis may be used for severe, chronic cases.

Cystitis

Cystitis, inflammation of the bladder, is a fairly common infection, generally caused by bacteria, which may be either acute or chronic. Cystitis is more prevalent in women than in men because their short urethra allows bacteria easier access into the bladder. The bladder lining's natural resistance to inflammation, however, serves as a protective mechanism. Inflammation and congestion of the bladder mucosa cause the patient to experience burning pain on urination or the desire to urinate frequently. Although cystitis is not serious, the infection can cause further problems by spreading into the upper urinary passages, including the renal pelvis and kidney.

Vesicoureteral reflux (VUR), the backward flow of urine out of the bladder and into the ureters, may be seen in cases of cystitis. In the normal urinary tract, vesicoureteral reflux is prevented by compression of the bladder musculature on the ureters during micturition. Failure of this valve mechanism usually results from a shortening of the intravesical portion of the ureter caused by abnormal embryologic development, leading to ureteric orifices that are displaced laterally. As this portion of the ureter lengthens with growth, this type of vesicoureteral reflux may disappear completely with age. Congenital VUR is also seen in duplication of collecting systems and ureters with reflux into an ectopically placed ureter serving the upper pole of the kidney. Vesicoureteral reflux can also result from a **neurogenic bladder,** a bladder dysfunction caused by interference with

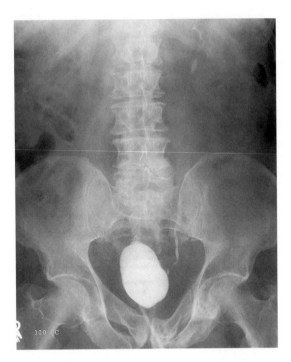

FIG. 6-40 Left ureteral reflux visualized during an intravenous urogram. The patient has suffered a pelvic fracture.

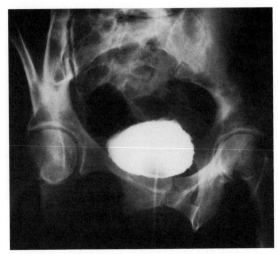

FIG. 6-41 Mildly trabeculated bladder as seen in this 34-year-old woman with a small-capacity bladder.

the nerve impulses concerned with urination. Cystography may demonstrate the presence of reflux (Fig. 6-40) and grade its severity. It may show a roughening of the normally smooth bladder wall, a radiographic appearance referred to as **bladder trabeculae** (Fig. 6-41). Treatment of cystitis includes antibiotic therapy and an abundance of fluids. Prevention of pyelonephritis is paramount.

DEGENERATIVE AND METABOLIC DISEASE

Nephrosclerosis

Nephrosclerosis is intimal thickening of predominantly the small vessels of the kidney. It may occur as part of the normal aging process as well as in younger patients in association with hypertension and diabetes. Reduced blood flow caused by arteriosclerosis of the renal vasculature causes atrophy of the renal paren-

chyma. Local infarction may occur, demonstrating as an irregularity of the cortical margin, usually an indentation. The collecting system of the affected kidney is usually normal, but the kidney itself is decreased in size. Laboratory tests will also demonstrate a gradual increase in BUN and creatinine levels. Other conditions that cause the kidneys to appear smaller than normal include hypoplasia, atrophy following obstruction, and ischemia from large vessel obstruction. Treatment of nephrosclerosis consists of managing the associated hypertension and administration of diuretic agents and proper dietary restrictions (e.g., low-sodium diet).

Nephrocalcinosis

Disturbances of calcium metabolism (e.g., hyperparathyroidism) may result in **nephrocalcinosis,** a condition characterized by tiny deposits of calcium phosphate dispersed throughout the renal parenchyma. These deposits are readily seen on an IVU and even on plain films of the abdomen. Calcium may also be deposited throughout the parenchyma as a result of tissue damaged by some other disease process or injury. In the case of a metabolic cause, treatment of the specific metabolic condition indirectly treats nephrocalcinosis. Treatment designed to lower serum calcium levels is also important.

Renal Failure

Although it can arise acutely, renal failure usually represents the end result of a chronic process such as chronic glomerulonephritis or polycystic kidney disease that gradually results in diminished kidney function. The kidney's normal regulatory and excretory functions become impaired because of loss of glomerular filtration and subsequent deterioration of the renal parenchyma. Uremia, which is characteristic of renal failure, consists of retention of urea in the blood. Although not toxic in itself, urea is normally excreted by the kidneys. Its blood level correlates with retention of other waste products and is thus a measure of the severity of renal failure. Common laboratory findings include a progressive increase in serum creatinine and urea nitrogen. Medical imaging may be requested to locate the cause in cases of acute renal failure. This includes abdominal radiography to rule out urinary calculi and medical sonography or abdominal CT to assess hydronephrosis and kidney size. Renal angiography or radionuclide renal scans may also be indicated when clinical evaluation suggests a vascular anomaly. A renal biopsy may also be necessary if the cause cannot be identified by other, less invasive means.

The gradual deterioration of renal function brings with it a host of changes in other body systems. The affected patient experiences moderate anemia, hypertension, heart arrhythmia, congestive heart failure, and other problems related to the body's severe electrolyte and acid-base imbalances. Treatment consists of dialysis and possible transplantation (Fig. 6-42).

Calcifications

With the exception of the gallbladder, more calculi are found in the urinary tract than anywhere else in the body. Renal calculi are stones

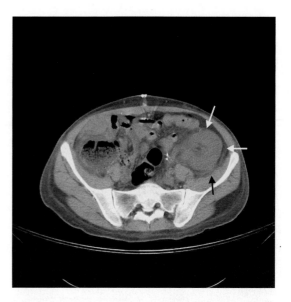

FIG. 6-42 Pelvic CT without contrast enhancement demonstrating the position of a transplanted kidney in the left pelvis.

that develop from urine, which can precipitate crystalline materials, especially calcium and its salts. If the body's normal equilibrium is upset, these products may precipitate out of the solution. Factors that can cause this precipitation include metabolic disorders such as hyperparathyroidism, excessive intake of calcium, and a metabolic rate that causes high urine concentration. Chronic UTIs are also related to stone formation.

Men develop calculi more often than women, especially after age 30. Nearly all urinary tract calculi are calcified to some extent; however, about 5% of stones do not calcify (Fig. 6-43). These are generally made of pure uric acid and present a more difficult diagnosis to the physician because they are one of several filling defects, including blood clots and tumors. Most stones are formed in the calyces or renal pelvis. A staghorn calculus is a large calculus that assumes the shape of the pelvicaliceal junction (Fig. 6-44). Because of the calcium content in renal calculi, most are visible on an

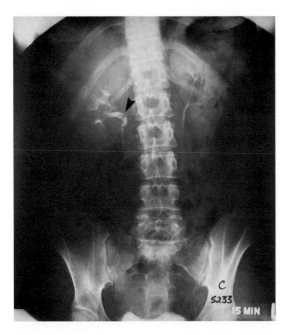

FIG. 6-43 Smooth, oval, noncalcified filling defect is seen in the right renal pelvis, as suggestive of a radiolucent uric acid stone in this 40-year-old woman with hematuria.

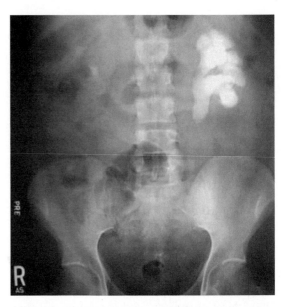

FIG. 6-44 An abdominal radiograph without intravenous contrast demonstrating a large staghorn calculus.

abdominal radiograph, IVU, or retrograde pyelogram. Ultrasound (Fig. 6-45) and noncontrast spiral CT of the abdomen (Fig. 6-46) can be employed to demonstrate stones. In many institutions, a CT "stone study" is the first modality of choice because it does not require contrast administration. It is an excellent method for differentiating abdominal or flank pain caused by renal calculi versus appendicitis or an abdominal aortic aneurysm. In addition, it can detect the location of the stone and the degree of obstruction present.

Stones tend to be asymptomatic until they begin to descend or cause an obstruction. Renal stones generally do not have a smooth texture and often have multiple jagged edges, causing pain as they move through the ureter. The most common site for a calculus to lodge and create an obstruction is the ureterovesical junction (Fig. 6-47). Obstructions can also

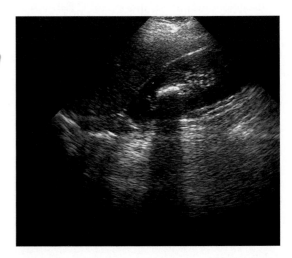

FIG. 6-45 Large calculi seen in the kidney on this ultrasound of a young woman. Note the absence of sound transmission beyond the stone as indicated by the dark pathway beneath it.

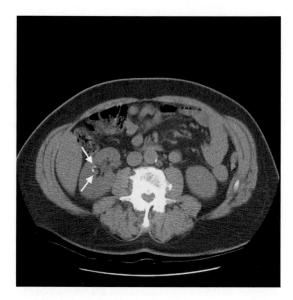

FIG. 6-46 Abdominal CT without contrast enhancement demonstrating a right renal stone without hydronephrosis.

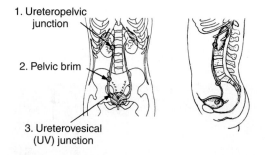

1. Ureteropelvic junction

2. Pelvic brim

3. Ureterovesical (UV) junction

FIG. 6-47 The three usual points where kidney stones become lodged.

occur at the junction of the ureter and bladder and in the ureter at the pelvic brim. Movement of stones or acute obstruction results in severe, intermittent pain known as **renal colic**. So as the stone moves along the course of the ureter toward the flank or genital regions, it is highlighted by sudden, periodic (paroxysmal) attacks,

between which a constant low-grade pain is felt. Renal calculi can also cause bleeding (hematuria), fever, chills, frequent urination, and secondary infection. The physician is generally able to distinguish between biliary and renal colic because biliary colic usually causes referred pain to the subscapular area or epigastrium. The probability for recurrent calculus formation is increased as much as 50% in individuals who develop an initial renal stone, so many patients are placed on a prophylactic regimen such as diuretics, potassium alkali, and increased fluid intake to help reduce their chance of developing further stones.

In most instances, the first treatment is to wait for the stones to pass normally through the urinary system in combination with the administration of antibiotics for the presence of any infection. If the stone is not passed, either lithotripsy of the stone or surgical excision of the cause of obstruction is necessary. SWL is often used to crush calculi less than 2 cm in diameter located in the renal pelvis or ureter. A percutaneous nephrolithotomy may be employed to remove larger renal calculi, and ureteroscopy is necessary to remove larger stones within the ureter. Depending on the size of the stone, it may be removed with a special basket catheter, or it may be crushed into smaller pieces via laser or pneumatic lithotripsy. All of the above methods utilize fluoroscopic guidance.

In addition to the kidneys, other sites of calcification in the urinary tract include the wall of the bladder and the prostate gland in men. Calcification of the bladder wall is very rare and is usually caused by calcium deposition in a tumor extrinsic to the bladder, such as from the ovary or rectum. Rarely, it may also be on the surface of a bladder tumor. Bladder calculi often cause suprapubic pain. Prostatic calcification appears as numerous flecks of calcium of varying size below the bladder. It does not, however, correlate with either prostatic hypertrophy or carcinoma and usually is of no real significance.

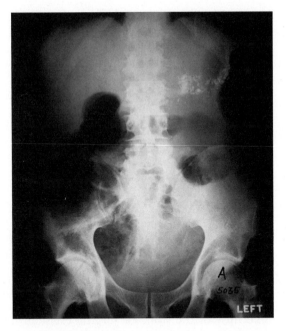

FIG. 6-48 Pancreatic calcification as indicated by the masses of calcium in the left-upper quadrant that conform neatly to the shape of the pancreas.

Urinary tract calcifications are sometimes difficult to distinguish from other abnormal calcifications, such as gallstones, vascular calcifications, and calcified costal cartilages. To be in the kidney, the calcification must remain within the outline of the kidney on both frontal and oblique projections or be confirmed with plain tomography. In the case of gallstones, oblique projections of the abdomen help demonstrate whether the calculus in question is anterior to the kidney. The pancreas may also demonstrate calcification that usually conforms to its shape (Fig. 6-48).

Hydronephrosis

Hydronephrosis is an obstructive disease of the urinary system that causes dilatation of the renal pelvis and calyces with urine. If long-standing, the resultant increase in intrarenal pressure causes ischemia, parenchymal atrophy, and loss of renal function. Although the most

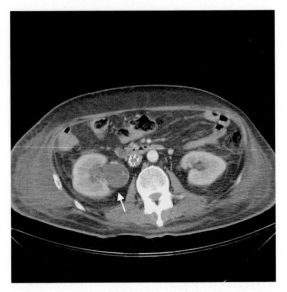

FIG. 6-49 A large hydronephrosis of the right kidney easily identified by CT without the use of a contrast agent.

common cause of hydronephrosis is a calculus (Fig. 6-49), it can also occur as a congenital defect or blockage of the system by a tumor, stricture, blood clot, or inflammation (Fig. 6-50). Patients with hydronephrosis often complain of

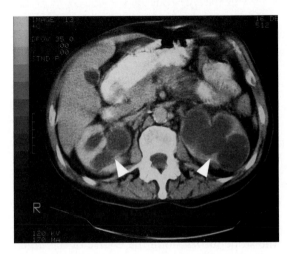

FIG. 6-50 Gross bilateral hydronephrosis as caused by pyelonephritis in this 64-year-old man.

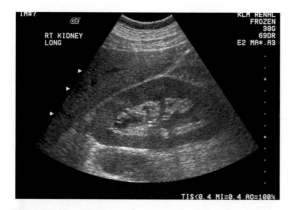

FIG. 6-51 An ultrasound of the kidney demonstrating hydronephrosis.

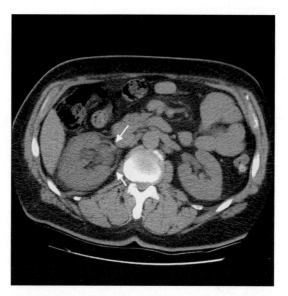

FIG. 6-52 Hydronephrosis of the right kidney demonstrated without contrast enhancement.

pain in their flanks, and their urine may demonstrate blood or pus. The long-term changes of hydronephrosis are reversible if the cause of obstruction is relieved early in the process. As in most urinary system pathologies, abdominal sonography is the initial examination of choice because the kidneys do not have to be functioning properly and intravenous contrast agents are not necessary for the kidneys to be visualized on a sonogram (Fig. 6-51). Additional information regarding increased vascular resistance can be accomplished using Doppler ultrasound. A spiral abdominal CT scan (Fig. 6-52) can diagnose obstruction more than 90% of the time, so CT is quickly replacing the conventional IVU. However, a conventional IVU may be necessary to help differentiate renal cysts or stones from hydronephrosis. In some cases, nuclear medicine renograms may also be indicated.

NEOPLASTIC DISEASES

Masses can cause filling defects in the urinary tract, becoming visible when they stretch and displace the collecting system or form an evident mass. Almost all solitary masses are either malignant tumors or simple cysts.

Profuse hematuria resulting from a blood clot also causes a filling defect. The diagnosis of such depends on the radiologist's awareness of the history of hematuria. The distinction between a blood clot and a tumor is difficult for the physician. However, blood clots tend to have a smooth outline and show change on repeat examinations following treatment.

Renal Cysts

Renal cysts are an acquired abnormality common in adults. It is estimated that more than half of people at age 50 have renal cysts. Simple cysts may be solitary or multiple and bilateral. They are usually asymptomatic and not an impairment to renal function, but they may cause symptoms from rupture, hemorrhage, infection, or obstruction. Their pathogenesis is unknown, but obstruction of nephrons by an acquired disease may have a relationship. They are commonly found in a lower pole of the kidney and are readily demonstrated by CT (Fig. 6-53), MRI (Fig. 6-54), and ultrasound.

Radiographically, cysts have sharply defined margins and show calyceal spreading, but they can be distinguished from tumors by nephroto-

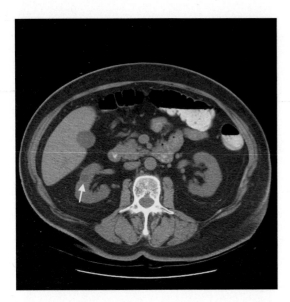

FIG. 6-53 A small, simple cyst on the right kidney demonstrated by an abdominal CT without contrast enhancement.

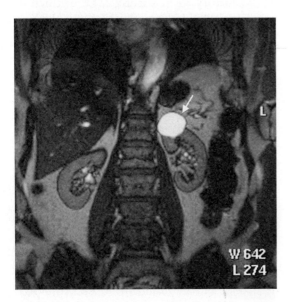

FIG. 6-54 A T2 Tru-Fisp weighted MRI of the abdomen demonstrating a renal cyst of the left kidney.

mography, in which a cyst shows an absence of a nephrogram phase after contrast medium injection. By contrast, tumors, the majority of which have vascularity, may show irregular opacification during the nephrogram phase. Treatment, if needed, consists of aspiration of the cyst contents. Most cysts are asymptomatic, and no treatment is needed.

Renal Carcinoma

The most common malignant tumor of the kidney is **adenocarcinoma** (hypernephroma), arising from the proximal convoluted tubule. It occurs two to three times as frequently in men as in women, with an increased incidence after age 40, and accounts for approximately 2% of adult cancers. Its etiology is unknown, but chronic inflammation as from obstruction, cigarette smoking, and other agents is thought to contribute to the development of renal carcinoma. The affected patient often first presents with hematuria but may also experience flank pain, a fever, or a palpable mass. Renal carcinoma may also be an incidental finding on an abdominal sonogram or abdominal CT examination.

Confirmation of a mass may be accomplished with an IVU, abdominal sonogram, MRI, or CT. Radiographically, the space-occupying lesion may be evident and can distort, stretch, and displace the kidney's collecting system (Fig. 6-55), as visualized on an IVU. CT is useful in demonstrating the density of the renal carcinoma and its degree of metastasis, including extension to adjacent areas and lymph nodes, as well as venous involvement (Fig. 6-56). Abnormal vascularity is also readily visualized during angiography (Fig. 6-57), sometimes surrounding an avascular necrotic center. Magnetic resonance imaging provides information regarding the spread of the renal carcinoma (Fig. 6-58), especially into the renal veins and inferior vena cava.

If the carcinoma is caught early, surgical excision of the kidney provides a good cure

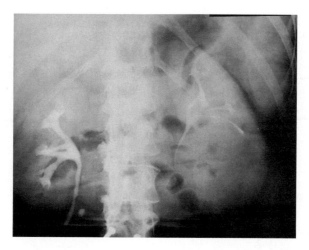

FIG. 6-55 Urography demonstrates displacement of the left lower pole calyces in this 54-year-old woman with hematuria.

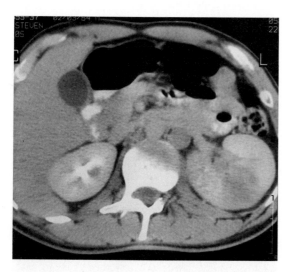

FIG. 6-56 CT demonstration of a large metastatic lesion in the left kidney of this 25-year-old man with renal adenocarcinoma.

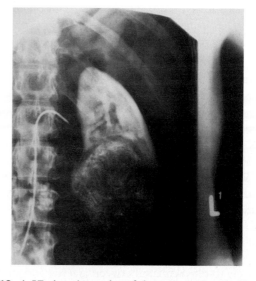

FIG. 6-57 Arteriography of the same patient in Fig. 6-55 demonstrates a large vascularized mass of the left lower pole, with grossly abnormal vasculature, indicative of renal cell carcinoma.

rate, but metastatic renal carcinoma has a very poor prognosis. These tumors are relatively insensitive to chemotherapy and radiation therapy. The tendency of adenocarcinoma to metastasize early from the kidneys, however, poses a serious threat. The most common sites of metastasis are the lungs, brain, liver, and bone. Because pulmonary metastases are common, a chest radiograph should be obtained immediately on discovering a renal carcinoma.

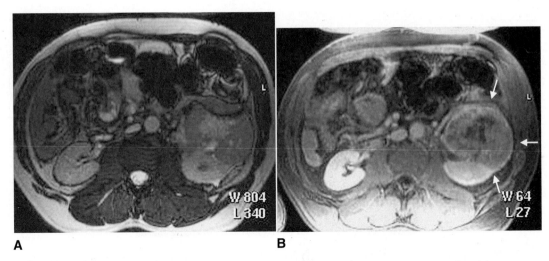

A　　　　　　　　　　　　　　　**B**

FIG. 6-58 A, An axial T2 Tru-Fisp MRI of the abdomen demonstrates a mass involving a large portion of the left kidney. **B,** Axial T1 weighted postcontrast image shows the same mass, consistent with renal cell carcinoma. Notice the internal necrosis *(arrow).*

Nephroblastoma (Wilms' Tumor)

Nephroblastoma is a malignant renal tumor found in approximately 1 child in every 13,500 live births. It almost invariably develops before 5 years of age, with equal incidence between the sexes. Children with nephroblastoma often have no symptoms but may have the tumor discovered by a parent or physician who feels a large, palpable abdominal mass. The relative firmness and immobility help distinguish Wilms' tumor from hydronephrosis and renal cysts. Diagnostic sonography is also used extensively to differentiate between a cystic and solid mass. On urography, the kidneys appear quite enlarged with marked calyceal spreading—an indication nearly diagnostic of the condition when seen in children (Fig. 6-59). Abdominal CT is the modality of choice for assessing the extent and spread of the tumor (Fig. 6-60) and has replaced the IVU in many institutions because CT can demonstrate spread to the lymphatics, liver, and contralateral kidney. Left untreated, the tumor shows widespread metas-

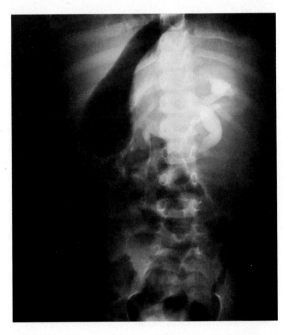

FIG. 6-59 An intravenous urogram on a 4-year-old girl demonstrates an enlarged left kidney with distortion of the collecting system and significant displacement of the stomach by the large mass.

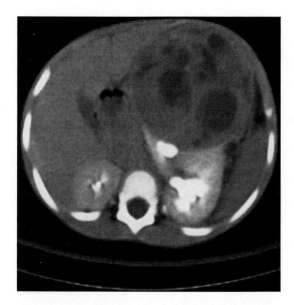

FIG. 6-60 A CT image demonstrates a huge, non-calcified mass arising from the left kidney, as seen in nephroblastoma.

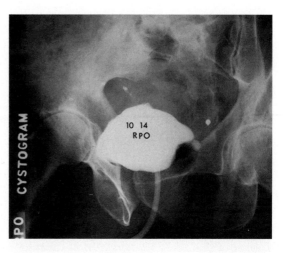

FIG. 6-61 Transitional cell carcinoma of the bladder, seen as a space-occupying lesion on this right posterior oblique view of the bladder on a cystogram of a 67-year-old man.

tases to the lungs, liver, adrenal glands, and bone. Early surgical excision combined with radiation therapy and chemotherapy, results in a cure rate of approximately 80%.

Bladder Carcinoma

Bladder carcinoma is usually seen three times more often in men than in women, particularly after age 50. Its etiology is clearly related to cigarette smoking and certain industrial chemicals, and a link to excessive coffee drinking is being investigated. Bladder carcinoma may be classified as transitional cell carcinoma (most frequent), squamous cell carcinoma (usually resulting from chronic irritation), or adenocarcinoma. Painless hematuria is the chief symptom. Tumors are generally small and located in the area of the trigone. An IVU or cystogram may reveal a filling defect in the bladder (Fig. 6-61), but it is often difficult to distinguish among tumor, stone, and blood

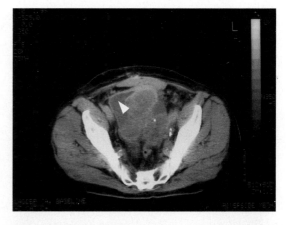

FIG. 6-62 Large bladder carcinoma in this 65-year-old man as seen on CT.

clot. Therefore, cystoscopy is the method of choice for investigation of bladder carcinoma, and diagnosis is made via biopsy or resection. CT (Figs. 6-62 and 6-63), sonography, and MRI are useful in staging the disease once the diagnosis is confirmed.

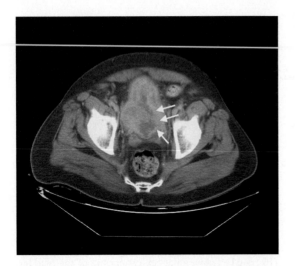

FIG. 6-63 A pelvic CT examination demonstrates an extensive mass in the urinary bladder representing bladder carcinoma.

Treatment consists of resection or a total cystectomy, depending on the amount of involvement and extent of metastasis, if any. Radiation therapy of the region follows. In the case of total cystectomy, the distal ureters are generally attached into a loop of the bowel (Fig. 6-64), most frequently the ileum. Distant metastases are usually late in developing with bladder carcinoma.

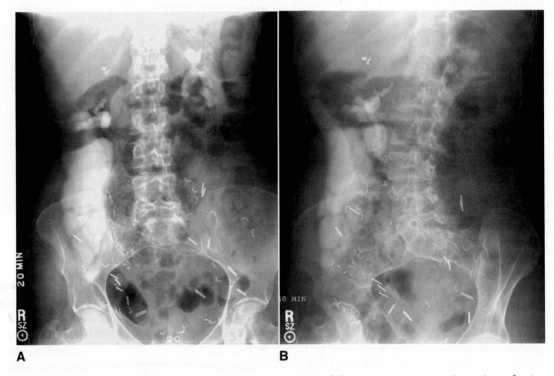

A   **B**

FIG. 6-64 A&B, An intravenous urogram on a patient following a cystectomy. A portion of the cecum has been formed into a pouch to allow the collection of urine.

PATHOLOGY SUMMARY: THE URINARY SYSTEM

Pathology	Imaging Modalities of Choice	Additive or Subtractive Pathology
Congenital anomalies	Ultrasound in the fetus	
Lower tract anomalies	Cystography and ultrasound	
Polycystic kidney disease	Ultrasound and IVU	Subtractive
Medullary sponge kidney	Ultrasound	
Pyelonephritis	Ultrasound	
Cystitis	Cystography and ultrasound	Additive if reflux is present
Nephrosclerosis	Angiography and ultrasound	
Nephrocalcinosis	Ultrasound, CT, and KUB	Additive
Renal failure	Ultrasound, CT, and angiography	
Calcifications	Ultrasound, CT, and IVU	Additive
Hydronephrosis	Ultrasound, CT, and IVU	Additive
Renal cyst	Ultrasound, CT, MRI, and nephrotomography	Subtractive
Renal carcinoma	Ultrasound, CT, MRI, and angiography	
Nephroblastoma	Ultrasound, CT, MRI, and angiography	
Bladder carcinoma	Ultrasound, MRI, CT, and cystography	

QUESTIONS

1. A malignant tumor of the kidney generally occurring in children under 5 years of age is:
   a. adenocarcinoma
   b. hypernephroma
   c. fibroadenoma
   d. nephroblastoma

2. Which of the following statements are true about the anatomy and function of the urinary system?
   1. The amount of urine formed in a typical day is about 1 to 1.5 L.
   2. Urine is formed and excreted in the nephron, the microscopic unit of the kidney.
   3. The left kidney lies lower than the right because of the spleen's presence above it.
   a. 1 and 2
   b. 1 and 3
   c. 2 and 3
   d. 1, 2, and 3

3. Urinary system disorders may be suggested by an abnormal:
   1. BUN blood level
   2. creatinine blood level
   3. coloration of urine
   a. 1 and 2
   b. 1 and 3
   c. 2 and 3
   d. 1, 2, and 3

4. Horseshoe kidney is an anomaly of:
   a. fusion
   b. number
   c. position
   d. size

5. Which of the following statements are true of urinary system anomalies?
   1. Crossed ectopy exists when one kidney lies across midline, fused to the other.
   2. Nephroptosis and a pelvic kidney are identical conditions.
   3. Ureteroceles are ureteral dilatations near the ureter's termination.
   a. 1 and 2
   b. 1 and 3
   c. 2 and 3
   d. 1, 2, and 3

6. Vesicoureteral reflux refers to the backward flow of urine into the:
   a. bladder
   b. major calyx
   c. ureters
   d. urethra
   e. any of the above

7. Arterial and venous renal blood flow for a patient who has received a kidney transplant is best assessed by which of the following imaging modalities?
   a. computed tomography
   b. conventional urography
   c. Doppler sonography
   d. magnetic resonance imaging

8. Which of the following conditions can make the kidneys appear smaller than normal?
   a. atrophy following obstruction
   b. chronic pyelonephritis
   c. hypoplasia
   d. nephrocalcinosis
   e. all of the above
   f. all but one of a through d

9. Medical treatment designed to lower serum calcium levels is important in management of:
   a. cystitis
   b. nephrocalcinosis
   c. nephrosclerosis
   d. polycystic kidney disease

10. Gradual and chronic deterioration of the renal parenchyma eventually results in:
    a. glomerulonephritis
    b. polycystic kidney disease
    c. renal calculi
    d. renal failure

11. Renal failure is characterized by the abnormal retention of what substance in the blood?
    a. bilirubin
    b. calcium
    c. pus
    d. urea

12. Which of the following statements are true of renal calculi?
    1. Precipitation of solutes out of urine is the pathogenesis of renal calculi.
    2. Renal colic causes referred pain into the subscapular area or epigastrium.
    3. Stones tend to be asymptomatic until they move or cause an obstruction.
    a. 1 and 2
    b. 1 and 3
    c. 2 and 3
    d. 1, 2, and 3

13. Significant dilatation of the renal pelvis and calyces as a result of an obstruction from a stone is characteristic of:
    a. hydronephrosis
    b. renal failure
    c. nephroblastoma
    d. vesicoureteral reflux

14. Which of the following statements are true of neoplastic diseases of the urinary system?
    1. Chronic inflammation from obstruction can result in adenocarcinoma.
    2. Wilms' tumor is generally associated with elderly patients in renal failure.
    3. Early excision of nephroblastoma has shown a very high cure rate.
    a. 1 and 2   c. 2 and 3
    b. 1 and 3   d. 1, 2, and 3

15. A patient arrives in the CT department for a contrast-enhanced abdominal examination. What blood lab values must be checked before injecting the patient, and what are the maximum values allowed for contrast administration?

16. A delayed image of the abdomen in an IVU routine demonstrates only a portion of the ureters. Is this cause for concern? Why or why not?

17. How can one distinguish between nephroptosis and a pelvic kidney?

18. Identify at least three mechanisms through which bacteria can enter the urinary tract.

19. A 30-year-old pregnant woman demonstrates fever, flank pain, and general malaise. Although the IVU looks normal, urinalysis demonstrates pyuria. What might you suspect?

20. In renal failure, what causes the kidney to lose its normal regulatory and excretory function?

The Reproductive System

UPON COMPLETION OF CHAPTER 7, THE READER SHOULD BE ABLE TO:

- Discuss the basic anatomic structures associated with the male and female reproductive systems.
- Briefly explain the role of general radiography, mammography, diagnostic medical sonography, computed tomography, and magnetic resonance imaging in the diagnosis and treatment of reproductive system disorders.
- Compare and contrast breast imaging modalities, including diagnostic versus screening mammography, localization techniques, and sonography.
- Differentiate among the major congenital anomalies of the female reproductive system.
- Describe the various neoplastic diseases of both the female and male reproductive systems in terms of etiology, incidence, signs and symptoms, treatment, and prognosis.
- Differentiate among the common disorders during pregnancy and explain the role of diagnostic medical sonography in the management of the gravid female.

KEY TERMS

Adenocarcinoma of the prostate	Follicular ovarian cyst	Polycystic ovaries
Bicornuate uterus	Hydatidiform mole	Polyhydramnios
Breast carcinoma	Hydrocele	Prostatic calculi
Cervical carcinoma	Hysterosalpingogram	Prostatic hyperplasia
Cervical dysplasia	Leiomyoma	Sonohysterography
Corpus luteum ovarian cyst	Mastitis	Spermatocele
Cystadenocarcinoma	Nongravid	Testicular choriocarcinoma
Cystic teratoma	Oligohydramnios	Testicular embryonal carcinoma
Dermoid cysts	Peau d'orange	Testicular seminoma
Ectopic pregnancy	Pelvic inflammatory disease	Testicular teratoma
Endometriosis	Pessary	TURP
Epididymoorchitis	Placental abruption	Unicornuate uterus
Fibroadenoma	Placental accreta	Uterine fibroid
Fibrocystic breasts	Placenta previa	Uterus didelphys

THE FEMALE REPRODUCTIVE SYSTEM

ANATOMY AND PHYSIOLOGY

The female reproductive system comprises one pair of ovaries, which are the primary sex organs, and the secondary sex organs, which include one pair of uterine tubes, the uterus, the vagina, and two breasts (Fig. 7-1). This system functions in the production of the female reproductive cell (the ovum) and hormones and provides a cavity for the development of the zygote.

The external genitalia (the vulva) include the mons pubis, the labia majora and minora, the clitoris, the openings of the urethra and vagina, and the perineum. The vagina connects the external genitalia with the uterus and is the mode of exit of menstrual fluids and conception products.

The uterus is a pear-shaped organ whose purpose is to provide the environment for fetal growth and development. Located within the pelvic cavity, it can be divided into the upper portion, termed the body, and the lower, neck portion, termed the cervix. The cervix connects

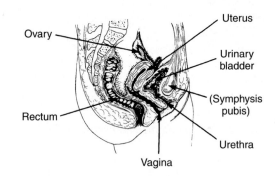

FIG. 7-1 Female pelvic organs.

the uterine cavity with the upper vagina. Anatomically, the uterus is flexed so that the cervix and lower portion of the body lie anterior to the rectum, posterior to the urinary bladder, and with the upper portion of the body normally lying superior to the bladder. The walls of the uterus include an inner, endometrial layer; a middle, muscular, myometrial layer; and an outer layer termed the parietal peritoneum. In actuality, the parietal peritoneum drapes over the upper three fourths of the body but does not enclose the lower fourth of the body or the cervix. The actual cavity within the uterus is fairly small and can be well visualized via hysterosalpingography. It is divided into the internal os leading to the cervical canal and into the external os, which opens into the vagina. The uterus is held in place within the pelvic cavity via eight ligaments. Occasionally, lack of proper uterine support is present, and a device known as a pessary (Fig. 7-2) is inserted into the vagina to provide proper support.

The uterine (fallopian) tubes extend from the upper, outer edges of the uterus and expand distally into the infundibulum located close to, but not attached to, the ovaries. Suspended in place by the broad ligament, they are 8 to 12 cm long and tend to fall behind the uterus. These tubes serve as a passageway for the mature ova and are the normal site of fertilization. In a normal pregnancy, the fertilized ovum continues to travel through the uterine tube and implants into the endometrium of the uterus.

The ovaries are the primary reproductive glands and are responsible for ovulation and for secretion of estrogen and progesterone. Attached to the broad ligament and the posterior uterine wall, each ovary contains numerous graafian follicles enclosing ova. Following puberty, several graafian follicles and ova grow and develop each month. Normally only one follicle matures, migrates to the surface of the ovary, and degenerates, thus expelling a mature ovum. This is termed ovulation.

The breasts, like the uterine tubes, uterus, and vagina, are also secondary sex organs. Breast parenchyma differs according to age and parity. Women in their 20s and 30s, especially nulliparous women, have dense, fibroglandular parenchyma that may hide breast masses on both physical and mammographic examination. However, as age and parity increase, the breast tissue undergoes what is known as involutional change. Involution is the conversion of glandular breast tissue into adipose tissue. As a result of this slow process, the breast changes its architecture and typically becomes fattier. Usually this process begins at the back of the breast and progresses forward to the nipple. Involution aids the radiographer and the interpreting physician because fatty tissue is radiolucent and enhances the radiographic visibility of many breast masses.

Anatomically, the breasts are attached via connective tissue to the pectoral muscles that give the breast its contour and shape. The breast consists of about 12 lobes separated by connective tissue, much like the spokes of a wheel. The lobes are further divided into lobules clustered around small ducts. These small ducts join to form larger ducts, which terminate at the nipple (Fig. 7-3). The breasts function as an accessory reproductive gland to secrete milk for the newborn infant. During

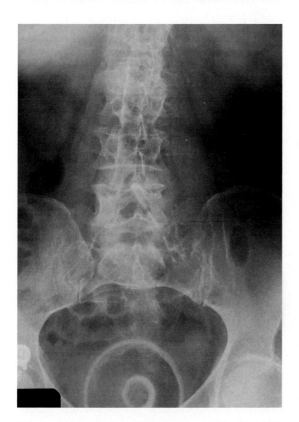

FIG. 7-2 A pessary, inserted into the vagina for uterine support, is readily visible on this abdominal radiograph of an 88-year-old woman.

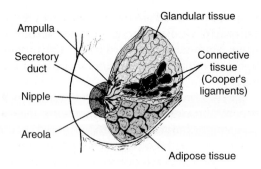

Ampulla

Secretory duct

Nipple

Areola

Glandular tissue

Connective tissue (Cooper's ligaments)

Adipose tissue

FIG. 7-3 Breast, anterior.

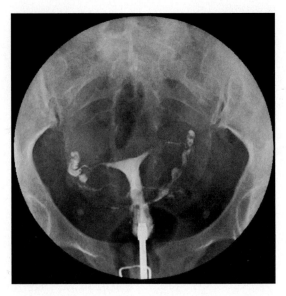

FIG. 7-4 Free spillage of contrast medium bilaterally in this 38-year-old woman indicates uterine tubes are open in this hysterosalpingogram.

pregnancy, changes in the estrogen and progesterone levels prepare the breasts for lactation. Approximately 3 days after delivery, a lactogenic hormone stimulates the secretion of milk.

IMAGING CONSIDERATIONS

Hysterosalpingography

One of the most common radiographic studies of the female reproductive system is the **hysterosalpingogram**. It is an examination performed for screening of the **nongravid** (nonpregnant) woman, especially in cases of suspected infertility. A common finding in cases of infertility is nonpatent fallopian tubes. Additionally, although it does not define the extent of certain conditions such as endometriosis, it is useful in revealing the shape of the uterus and certain characteristics of the fallopian tubes other than their patency. Hysterosalpingography is performed by injecting about 5 to 10 cc of an opaque medium into the uterine cavity. Spillage of the contrast media from the fallopian tubes indicates their patency (Fig. 7-4). Typically, hysterosalpingography is for diagnostic purposes, but it can also be used therapeutically for restoring tubal patency or to dilate or stretch the fallopian tubes.

An adjunct procedure that has potential to replace the conventional hysterosalpingogram is known as **sonohysterography**. This examination is similar to hysterosalpingography in procedural approach; however, with sono-

hysterography, normal saline is injected into the uterine cavity instead of an iodinated contrast agent. Because saline is devoid of complications associated with iodinated contrast agents, the procedure may be better tolerated by the patient. The current application for sonohysterography has been the use of saline to pry apart the layers of the endometrium in order to reveal abnormalities within the uterus. The saline fluid is expelled via the fallopian tubes and can also indicate their patency. This procedure is viewed via the transvaginal ultrasound probe as a physician injects the saline. With real-time images, the dynamics of the reproductive system can be assessed without radiation dose to the patient.

Mammography

The use of mammography as a diagnostic procedure for symptomatic patients is well documented. Mammography provides important information about specific clinical problems such as a breast mass, pain, nipple discharge, and abnormalities of the skin and lymph nodes. With modern mammographic equipment and techniques, radiation exposure is minimal, and there is no evidence to suggest significant risk to women over 35 years of age. If a risk does exist, it is thought to be so minimal that it has never been observed, only inferred, scientifically. The use of mammography for screening purposes is based on its ability to detect nonpalpable breast lesions at an early stage when they are too small to be identified by physical examination. Current literature suggests that mammography can detect some cancers 2 years before they are palpable, and survival depends on tumor size and lymph node involvement. It is generally agreed that women 50 years of age and older should undergo regular mammographic screening because in this age range the breast tissue is less sensitive to radiation, and the incidence of breast cancer increases with age. This also takes advantage of the involutional process making occult lesions easier to identify on a radiograph. The benefits far outweigh associated risks from radiation exposure.

Mammography is also a valuable examination tool in the detection and evaluation of breast disease in individuals with augmentation prostheses. Although experience with augmentation mammoplasty patients is limited, current research indicates that mammography can demonstrate both palpable and nonpalpable breast lesions. In order to provide screening mammography for these patients, it is important to displace the implant so that the native breast tissue can be imaged and assessed for disease. To demonstrate the underlying breast parenchyma in these individuals, technologists are encouraged to use the Eckland maneuver (implant displaced view) to displace the implant from the native breast tissue. The Eckland maneuver is accomplished by having the technologist apply pressure at the area of the nipple and then carefully begin to roll the native breast tissue away from the implant. This maneuver is performed for both the cranio-

caudal and mediolateral projections of the breast. Once the implant is pushed upward away from the native breast tissue, the compression paddle is used to continue to hold the implant so that the native breast tissue can be more fully imaged. Because of the variations in patients' breast tissue and their implants, manual exposure techniques are commonly used.

Needle or guidewire localization is a specialized procedure to identify nonpalpable, mammographically detected abnormalities of the breast. They help direct the surgeon to the lesion in question and allow excision of the suspect tissue for biopsy. Needle guidewire localizations cause minimal morbidity, with complications including hematoma formation, intraoperative wire dislodgement, and wire breakage. The development and refinement of localization techniques have greatly increased the percentage of positive findings on surgical biopsy and allow more accurate diagnosis and treatment of early-stage carcinoma of the breast. Fine-needle and large-core biopsy techniques offer an alternative to surgical biopsy as an initial step in investigation of breast masses. These procedures are performed on an outpatient basis by the mammographer and radiologist or surgeon in the mammography area using a specially designed stereotactic localization unit. Ductal lavage of the breast may also be performed in cases of suspected intraductal disease to obtain a specimen for laboratory analysis. Utilization of ultrasound-guided aspiration and biopsy is also common because ultrasound has the ability to visualize the area in question and note whether the area has been completely removed while the needle or biopsy gun is still in situ. This may prevent additional punctures into the patient's skin during the biopsy procedure.

Ultrasound

Ultrasound is the primary modality for examining the gravid and nongravid female reproductive system because of its excellent accuracy and because it presents no radiation hazards to the fetus or mother. Not only is ultrasound applicable in pregnancy but it is also useful in normal gynecologic examinations to visualize reproductive organs or to follow the progress of a regimen of fertility medication.

The transabdominal pelvic sonography requires a distended urinary bladder to serve as an "acoustic window" for good visualization of the pelvic organs. In addition, the fluid within the urinary bladder helps to displace bowel gas away from the area of interest. Sonography of the uterus and ovaries has been greatly enhanced by the use of a transvaginal transducer, which provides more accurate clinical information as a result of the magnification of images obtained of the internal pelvic structures. The most common indications for sonography in the nongravid female include evaluation of pelvic, uterine, and ovarian masses because ultrasound can give information about mass size, location, internal characteristics, and the effect on surrounding organs. Obstetrically, ultrasound is the method of choice in visualizing the position of the placenta, multiple gestations, and ectopic pregnancies and determining gestational age. It is used to assist and guide the physician during amniocentesis and is invaluable in assessing fetal abnormalities such as anencephaly, hydrocephaly, congenital heart defects, polycystic kidney disease, urinary tract obstructions, and GI tract obstructions as well as determining fetal death.

Ultrasound is an excellent modality for differentiating cystic masses from solid masses within the breast. However, sonography has limitations in the diagnosis of malignant breast disease because of the solid nature of most breast cancers. Recently researchers and clinicians have made great strides in the use of ultrasound to evaluate the dense breast for disease. In order to reduce the radiation dose to these young patients, research continues in order to perfect an accurate and safe screening modality. However, currently, ultrasound is not advocated as a screening modality for breast cancer because it cannot differentiate between a solid benign mass and malignant disease.

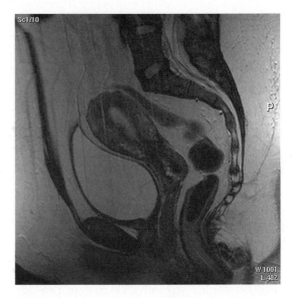

FIG. 7-5 An example of a sagittal T2-weighted MR image of a normal female pelvis demonstrating the bladder and uterus.

Magnetic Resonance Imaging

Magnetic resonance imaging (MRI) is now often used in conjunction with ultrasound in the evaluation of the female pelvis (Fig. 7-5). MRI, like ultrasound, uses no ionizing radiation and is noninvasive. MRI gives detailed information regarding pelvic, uterine, and ovarian masses (Fig. 7-6). In cases of ovarian cancer, MRI accurately demonstrates proliferation into other pelvic structures. In addition, multiple leiomyomas can be detected and localized in a short period of time.

MRI is increasingly being used to assist in differentiating between malignant and benign solid lesions within the breast. Fat suppression imaging is used pre- and postcontrast enhancement. This technique suppresses the normal, fatty tissue of the breast, allowing easier identification of malignant masses through contrast enhancement (Fig. 7-7). MRI is also used to detect faulty or leaking breast implants. Again, fat suppression imaging is utilized to suppress the normal breast tissue and detect the presence of silicone in the surrounding tissues.

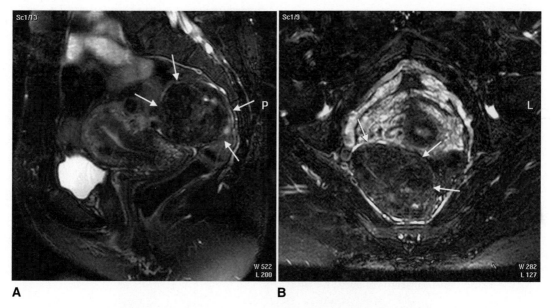

FIG. 7-6 A, A sagittal T2 fat-suppressed MR image demonstrating a large mass, most likely a subserosal fibroid, posterior to the endocervical junction. **B,** An axial T2 fat-suppressed MR image depicting the large subserosal fibroid shown in **A.**

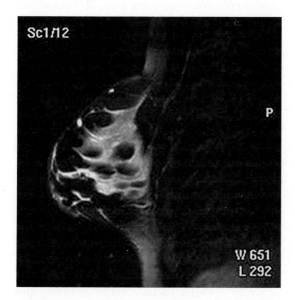

FIG. 7-7 A sagittal T2-weighted fat-suppressed MR image of the left breast.

CONGENITAL ABNORMALITIES

Congenital anomalies of the female reproductive system occur in approximately 1% to 2% of women. The most common anomaly is the **bicornuate uterus,** paired uterine horns that extend to the uterine tubes (Fig. 7-8). A **unicornuate uterus** occurs when the uterine cavity is elongated and has a single uterine tube emerging from it. Often, the kidney on the side of the missing uterine tube is also absent. **Uterus didelphys** is a rare congenital anomaly with complete duplication of the uterus, cervix, and vagina. The most serious complication of these anomalies is problems with reproduction, although various surgical corrections can be employed.

In the normal woman, the fundus of the uterus lies anterior to the cervix as well as away from the rectum. Occasionally, the normal uterus may lie in an abnormal position. If the

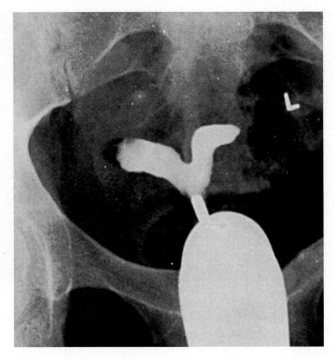

FIG. 7-8 Hysterosalpingogram demonstrates bicornuate uterus.

uterus is more vertical than normal, it is termed retroflexed and lies against the rectosigmoid region of the bowel. A uterus that lies more horizontal is termed anteflexed, and it lies on top of the urinary bladder. Although neither is normal, they are generally of little clinical significance.

INFLAMMATORY DISEASE

Pelvic Inflammatory Disease

Pelvic inflammatory disease (PID) is a bacterial infection of the female genital system, specifically the fallopian tubes, most often caused by gonococcus, *Staphylococcus,* or *Streptococcus* bacteria. It may result from an unsterile abortion or introduction of a pathogen from other sources. This inflammation is generally bilateral, and without treatment the infection spreads to the peritoneum, resulting in bacteremia. Tuboovarian abscess formation may also occur with PID, often resulting in sterility.

Common signs and symptoms of PID include pelvic and abdominal pain, dysmenorrhea, nausea and vomiting, elevated temperature, and leukocytosis. The most common treatment of PID is antibiotic therapy, but healing often results in scarring and obstruction of the fallopian tubes, which predisposes the individual to ectopic pregnancy because of the narrowing of the uterine tubes. It is a common indication for sonographic evaluation in a nongravid woman. Severe cases with abscess formation may also require surgical intervention.

Mastitis

Inflammation of the breast or **mastitis** is most often caused by *Staphylococcus aureus.* This bacterial infection usually occurs in the breasts of lactating women through cracks in the skin surrounding the nipple. Common signs and symptoms of mastitis include pain, redness, and swelling of the affected breast, elevated temperature, and, in severe cases, abscess formation.

Mastitis is treated medically with antibiotic therapy and heat application to the affected breast. Mammography plays a very limited role in the diagnosis and treatment of mastitis.

NEOPLASTIC DISEASES

Ovarian Cystic Masses

Single cystic ovarian masses are fairly common in women within the reproductive age group. They are frequently asymptomatic but can cause abdominal aching and pressure. Acute, sharp abdominal pain may indicate rupture or hemorrhage of the cyst. They include follicular ovarian cysts and corpus luteum ovarian cysts. The formation of follicular and corpus luteum cysts occurs as a part of the normal menstrual cycle. **Follicular cysts** result from faulty resorption of the fluid from incompletely developed follicles (Fig. 7-9). **Corpus luteum cysts** occur when resorption of any blood leaked into the cavity following ovulation leaves behind a small cyst. Changes in the size of follicular and corpus luteum cysts occur quickly and vary with the menstrual cycle. These cysts may occasionally increase in size and cause pelvic discomfort or abnormal pressure on the urinary bladder.

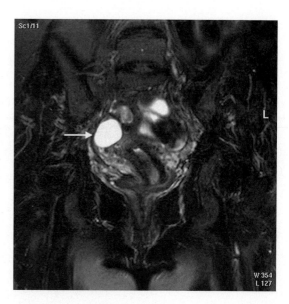

FIG. 7-10 A coronal T2-weighted fat-suppressed MR image of the female pelvis demonstrating a cyst of the right ovary *(arrow)*.

These cysts are readily visible with ultrasound, MRI (Fig. 7-10), and computed tomography (CT) (Fig. 7-11) of the pelvis. Treatment is generally not necessary because they often disappear completely without medical intervention.

Multiple cystic masses may indicate **endometriosis,** a disease caused by the presence of endometrial tissue or glands outside the uterus, in abnormal locations within the pelvis. External endometriosis commonly involves the ovaries, uterine ligaments, the rectovaginal septum, and the pelvic peritoneum; however, it may also attach to the rectal wall, the ureters, or the urinary bladder. The etiology of endometriosis is unknown, but it seems to respond to normal hormonal stimuli and is clinically significant in women between the ages of 20 and 40. The external endometrial tissue contains normal functioning endometrium. Responsive to hormonal changes, it continues to bleed cyclically. These blood-filled cysts are often visible on ultrasonic examination. Long-standing endometriosis results in the development of

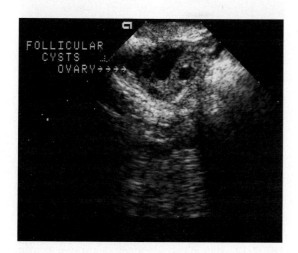

FIG. 7-9 A follicular cyst seen adjacent to the ovary on this transverse ultrasound view.

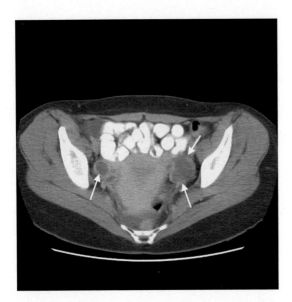

FIG. 7-11 A CT examination of a female pelvis demonstrating bilateral cysts. The patient is currently taking fertility drugs.

fibrosis, adhesions, scarring, and eventually sterility. Common signs and symptoms include pelvic and low back pain, dysmenorrhea, and infertility. Although ultrasound is useful in the diagnosis of endometriosis, a positive diagnosis is generally made via laparoscopy. Mild cases of endometriosis may be treated with hormone therapy; severe cases generally require surgical intervention.

Polycystic ovaries consist of enlarged ovaries containing multiple small cysts. The ovaries are bilaterally enlarged and have a smooth exterior surface, with the multiple cysts lying just below the outer surface. Polycystic ovaries are often associated with Stein-Leventhal syndrome, a fairly rare disease. Women with Stein-Leventhal syndrome rarely ovulate because of an endocrine abnormality that inhibits maturation and release of the ovarian follicle. In addition, these individuals may experience amenorrhea and sterility. The primary treatment is use of drugs to induce ovulation.

Benign **cystic teratomas** of the ovary, often called **dermoid cysts,** account for approximately 20% to 25% of ovarian tumors and are the most common type of germ cell tumor containing mature tissue. These masses arise from an unfertilized ovum that undergoes neoplastic change. Cystic teratomas are composed of tissue derived from the ectoderm, endoderm, and mesoderm, and they often contain hair, thyroid tissue, keratin, sebaceous secretions, and occasionally teeth (Fig. 7-12). A rupture of a cystic teratoma can result in severe peritonitis. The treatment for cystic teratomas is surgical removal of the mass.

Cystadenocarcinoma

Cystadenocarcinoma is a malignant neoplasm of the ovary accounting for more than 75% of all ovarian cancers (Fig. 7-13). It primarily occurs in perimenopausal and postmenopausal women over age 40. Cystadenocarcinoma is the second most commonly diagnosed female genital carcinoma, occurring in 1 out of 70 women in the United States. It is the most

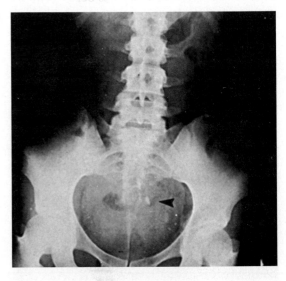

FIG. 7-12 Abdominal radiograph of a young woman demonstrates a radiographically visible tooth within a cystic teratoma.

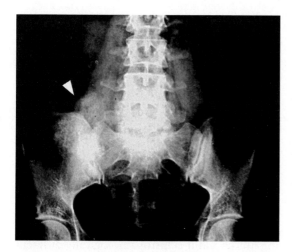

FIG. 7-13 Abdominal radiograph of a 47-year-old woman diagnosed with a cystadenocarcinoma. Note the calcifications within the lesion that make it radiographically visible.

lethal gynecologic malignancy and it is associated with a very poor prognosis.

The etiology of this neoplasm is unknown. However, known risk factors include a diet high in fat, a history of late childbearing or nulliparity, delayed menopause, a family history of cancers of the endometrium, breast, or colon, and the presence of an inherited autosomal dominant gene known as the BRCA gene. Sonographic evaluation demonstrates a rough, irregular ovarian surface with the tumor often containing both cystic and solid areas. Serous tumors are frequently bilateral; mucinous tumors are more likely to be unilateral.

The signs and symptoms of cystadenocarcinoma are very vague, including urinary bladder or rectal pressure, back pain, and bloating. In many cases, the disease is completely asymptomatic and discovered only on routine pelvic examination. This tends to delay diagnosis and treatment, thus reducing the chance for cure. As a woman's age increases, the probability of an enlarged ovary testing positive for ovarian cancer increases proportionately. These tumors often spread to other pelvic organs, the small intestines, the omentum, the stomach, and less

frequently the liver and lungs, presenting with associated ascites and pleural effusions. Common treatment of cystadenocarcinoma includes surgery in combination with chemotherapy or radiation therapy.

Carcinoma of the Cervix

Cervical carcinoma or **dysplasia** is a common malignancy of the female genital system caused by an abnormal growth pattern of epithelial cells around the neck of the uterus. It is the third most common carcinoma of the female genital organs and the eighth most common malignancy in U.S. women. Cervical intraepithelial neoplasias (CIN) are classified or staged as mild (I), moderate (II), or severe (III) and are generally diagnosed by a Pap smear and confirmed by surgical biopsy. Research indicates that cervical cancer is essentially a sexually transmitted disease, as a history of multiple sexual partners or prior sexually transmitted infections predisposes women to this disease. Symptoms commonly associated with cervical dysplasia include abnormal bleeding, especially postcoitally. Additionally, impaired renal function resulting from ureteral obstruction is often seen. If the cancer is invasive, radiography of the chest, urinary system, and skeletal system, in combination with CT or MRI of the abdomen and pelvis, is performed to assist in staging the disease. The treatment of cervical dysplasia varies according to the classification. Pap smears allow early detection of this disease, thus improving the chance of cure and survival. The 5-year survival rate ranges from 90% for stage I dysplasia to less than 15% for advanced disease. The primary treatments are radiation therapy and surgical intervention. Chemotherapy may also be administered in combination with radiation therapy to act as a radiosensitizer.

UTERINE MASSES

Leiomyomas (Uterine Fibroids)

Leiomyomas are benign, solid masses of the uterus that develop from an overgrowth of the uterine smooth muscle tissue. They are present in approximately 25% of all women over age 30 and are the most common benign tumors of the female genital system. Symptoms may include frequent urination if the mass mildly stretches the urinary bladder, affecting its elasticity. The etiology of this neoplasm is unknown; however, they tend to grow under the influence of estrogen, may enlarge during pregnancy, and stop growing at menopause. Following menopause, leiomyomas are replaced largely by fibrous scar tissue, leading to the misnomer **uterine fibroids.** In addition, they often contain radiographically visible calcifications (Fig. 7-14). The tumors vary in size, number (usually occurring in multiples), and location; they are frequently asymptomatic until they grow large enough to place pressure on surrounding structures, and they are usually

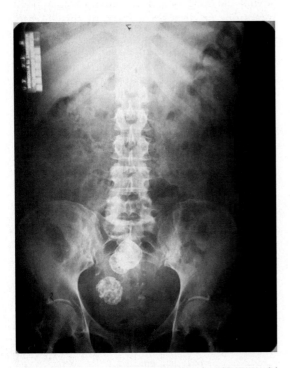

FIG. 7-14 Abdominal radiograph of a 50-year-old woman demonstrates leiomyomas of the uterus with radiographically visible calcifications.

detected on pelvic examination. Ultrasound, CT, and MRI are all useful in confirming the presence of leiomyomas. Sonographically, they appear as sharply circumscribed, encapsulated lesions and may contain cystic areas. Malignant transformation is rare, and treatment depends on patient symptoms, ranging from no treatment to surgical removal of the uterus.

Adenocarcinoma of the Endometrium

Adenocarcinoma of the endometrium is by far the most common malignancy of the uterus, accounting for more than 80% of all endometrial cancers. It is often termed carcinoma of the uterus and it is histopathologically different from cervical carcinoma. Endometrial cancer is one of the most common cancers of the female reproductive system, second only to breast cancer. The incidence of adenocarcinoma of the endometrium has remained fairly static, ranking as the fourth most common malignancy in women, occurring mainly in postmenopausal women, and increasing in incidence with age. The development of this neoplasm has strong ties to hormonal changes within the woman and is more common in nulliparous women. Obesity is also a major risk factor, as well as a family history of breast or ovarian cancer or a history of previous pelvic radiation therapy.

Adenocarcinoma of the endometrium is usually preceded by endometrial hyperplasia. It then passes through an in situ stage before reaching its final invasive stage, often completely filling the uterine cavity. The cancer is graded according to cellular differentiation and staged according to the extent of the disease. The most frequent symptom is irregular or postmenopausal bleeding. Treatment varies with the stage of the disease. Stage 0 is curable via hysterectomy, and stages I and II are usually treated with a combination of surgery and radiation therapy, with a 5-year survival rate ranging from 70% to 95%. Stage III and IV endometrial adenocarcinomas are best treated with chemotherapy, but they have a lower 5-year survival rate of 10% to 60%.

BREAST MASSES

Fibroadenoma

A **fibroadenoma** is a common benign breast tumor. It is usually unilateral and consists of a solid, well-defined mass that does not invade surrounding tissue. The neoplasm is formed by an overgrowth of fibrous and glandular tissue and is commonly located in the upper, outer quadrant of the breast. Fibroadenomas occur most frequently in women between the ages of 15 and 35, appear to be estrogen dependent, and may grow rapidly during pregnancy. These lesions are often painless and can usually be moved about within the breast. Mammography, in conjunction with physical breast examination and ultrasound, plays a vital role in the detection of fibroadenomas (Fig. 7-15) and is useful in distinguishing them from mammary dysplasia (fibrocystic breast disease) and breast carcinoma. Surgical removal of the lesion is curative.

Fibrocystic Breasts

An overgrowth of fibrous tissue or cystic hyperplasia results in **fibrocystic breasts.** This is the most common disorder of the female breast and occurs to some degree in approximately 50% of premenopausal women. This condition may be unilateral; however, it is most frequently bilateral, with variably sized cysts located throughout the breasts (Figs. 7-16 and 7-17). The severity of this disorder varies greatly, and it is believed to result from fluctuations in the hormone levels during the menstrual cycle. The most common sign or symptom associated with fibrocystic breasts is a

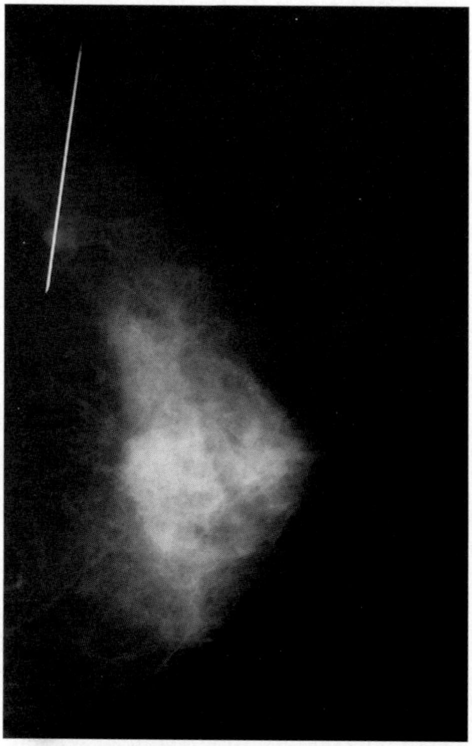

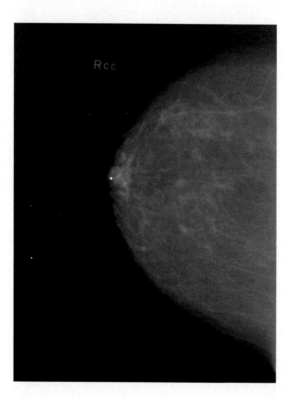

FIG. 7-15 Needle localization of fibroadenoma of the breast pinpoints the location of the mass for surgical biopsy.

FIG. 7-16 Craniocaudad mammographic projection of a moderately fibroglandular breast.

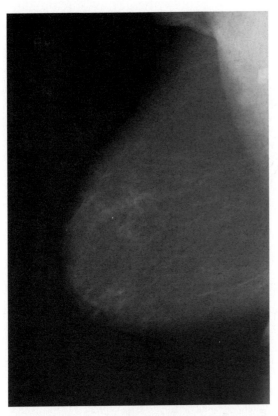

FIG. 7-17 Mediolateral mammographic projection of a moderately fibroglandular breast.

mass or masses that increase in size and tenderness immediately preceding the onset of the menstrual period. Ultrasound is extremely useful as a follow-up to mammography in differentiating solid masses from cystic masses in women with fibrocystic breasts (Fig. 7-18). Large cysts are commonly aspirated for cytologic evaluation of the fluid. If the aspiration is unsuccessful, surgical biopsy is often performed. Although controversy exists about the correlation of fibrocystic breasts and an increased incidence of breast cancer, it is well known that a fibrocystic condition may mask a coexistent cancer. Treatment of the condition is largely symptomatic, including a monthly breast self-examination and proper support.

Carcinoma of the Breast

Breast carcinoma is a very common malignancy among women in the United States and the second leading cause for female cancer deaths, behind only lung cancer. Current literature suggests that one of every eight women in the United States will develop breast cancer during her lifetime, with an increased incidence between the ages of 30 and 50. The incidence continues to rise throughout the postmenopausal years because of changes in estrogen levels, with the mean age for breast cancer at age 60. Approximately 50% of all lesions occur in the upper, outer quadrant of the breast.

Although the exact etiology of breast cancer is unknown, it is believed to be a multifactorial disorder. Heredity, endocrine influence, oncogenic factors (such as viruses), and environmental factors (such as chemical carcinogens) appear to play a role in the development of this disease. The amount of biologically available estrogen and progesterone is a key endocrine factor in the development of breast cancer. Those individuals with an early onset of menstruation (menarche), late menopause, or women with a first pregnancy after the age of 30 are at a higher risk of developing breast cancer. Women using oral contraceptives or estrogen replacement therapy over a 10-year period also have a very small increase in the risk of developing breast cancer. In terms of heredity, a family history including a parent, sibling, or child with breast cancer increases a woman's risk to two to three times that of the normal population. In addition, women who carry BRCA1 or BRCA2, two known breast cancer genes, and men who carry BRCA2 are also at an increased risk of developing breast cancer.

Breast cancers may be classified as in situ carcinoma, ductal carcinoma in situ, lobular carcinoma in situ, invasive ductal or lobular carcinoma, or inflammatory carcinoma. Breast cancers generally are discovered as a lump in the breast by the patient. With the exception of inflammatory breast cancer, which is very virulent with diffuse inflammation and breast

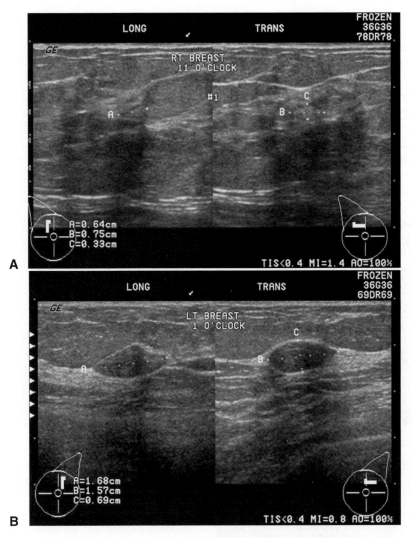

FIG. 7-18 A, Sonogram of the breast demonstrating an enlarged lymph node and cyst in the eleven o'clock axis of the right breast, RUQ. **B,** Sonogram of a hypoechogenic solid breast mass in the left upper quadrant, one o'clock axis.

enlargement, most begin as slow-growing, relatively painless masses, but as they grow, they may infiltrate the suspensory ligaments, causing them to shorten and retract the overlying skin. Physical signs of advanced breast cancer include nipple retraction and distorted breast contour. The neoplasm may infiltrate and block lymphatic vessels, the major route of metastases, especially to the axilla. This infiltration causes edema in the overlying skin and enlargement of the axillary or supraclavicular lymph nodes. As the infiltrating breast carcinoma blocks the lymphatic exchange, the skin's pores open to allow the fluid to escape, therefore causing a rough skin texture from chafing and pore enlargement. The skin edema is known as a **peau**

d'orange appearance. As the tumor progresses, it may attach to surrounding fascia and ulcerate the surrounding skin.

Mammography plays a very important role in the diagnosis and management of breast cancer. In asymptomatic women over 50 years of age, a routine screening mammogram can reduce breast cancer morality up to 35%; therefore, yearly mammograms should be performed on women 50 years of age or older. Annual screening of women between the ages of 40 and 50 years remains controversial. Many breast tumors commonly appear radiographically as dense, irregular, stellate masses that infiltrate surrounding tissue (Fig. 7-19). Many of these

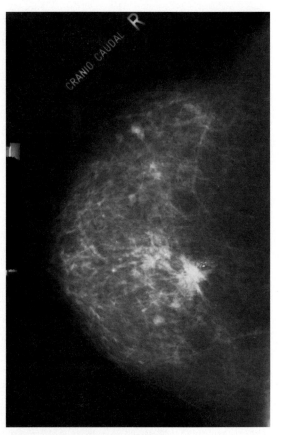

FIG. 7-20 Mammogram of the right breast in an elderly woman demonstrating a stellate mass containing microcalcifications commonly associated with carcinoma of the breast.

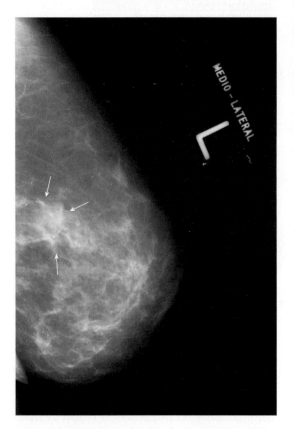

FIG. 7-19 Mammogram of the left breast of a 63-year-old woman demonstrating a stellate mass commonly associated with carcinoma of the breast. Notice the irregular borders of the mass.

neoplasms contain numerous microcalcifications that are radiographically visible (Fig. 7-20). Core needle biopsy is often performed to obtain a specimen of suspect tissue for further evaluation. For patients requiring surgical biopsy, needle localization of mammographically detected, nonpalpable cancerous breast lesions is reliable in directing the surgeon to the lesion in question and allows excision of the suspect tissue. The tissue specimen is radiographed and forwarded to a pathologist for histologic evaluation. Statistics demonstrate that this method of localization causes minimal morbidity, and the development and refinement of mammographic localization has greatly increased the percentage of positive findings on surgical biopsy. This invasive technique allows more accurate diagnosis and treatment of early-stage carcinoma of the breast. If the tumor can be removed before the lesion is palpable, the survival rate is greatly increased.

As discussed earlier in this chapter, MRI may be utilized to detect breast cancer. Research with positron emission tomography (PET) shows promise in terms of predicting the clinical outcome in patients who have been previously treated for breast cancer. Use of 18-fluorodeoxyglucose (FDG) PET may soon be common practice.

Treatment of breast carcinoma depends on the extent of the disease. Once the carcinoma is confirmed by biopsy, an axillary lymph node resection is performed to assist in management of the disease. The 10-year survival rate for patients without node involvement is over 80% but drops to about 40% in patients with one to three positive nodes and about 25% in patients with four or more positive nodes. Much controversy exists in terms of determining the best approach to management and treatment of breast cancers. In the past 40 years, the 5-year survival rate for breast cancer has remained virtually unchanged. Currently, two surgical options are recommended for invasive breast cancers: (1) modified radical mastectomy and (2) breast-conserving surgery followed by radiation therapy. Both methods require axillary lymph node resection, and there is not a significant difference in the survival rate between these two surgical options. Inflammatory cancers are usually treated with a combination of chemotherapy and radiation therapy.

Treatment with an established combination of chemotherapeutic drugs is considered standard care for premenopausal women with lymph node involvement. The chemotherapy may be continued for months or years following the primary therapy, but the adjuvant therapy may decrease the chance of death by 35% in this patient population. Breast carcino-mas are also classified by a hormone receptor test. Many tumors require hormones for continued growth, and these carcinomas may undergo temporary regression if hormonal balances are altered.

DISORDERS DURING PREGNANCY

Diagnostic medical sonography is often used as positive proof of a pregnancy, in addition to aiding in the diagnosis of multiple and ectopic pregnancies. With the use of transvaginal sonography, the sac and early fetal pole can been seen, and a fetal heart detected, as early as 3 weeks of gestation. Sonographic examination may be indicated if the pregnant uterus is too small or too large for the calculated delivery date. Depending on the obstetrician's philosophy, many pregnant women may also receive a sonogram at or between 6 to 8 weeks of gestation to screen for fetal anomalies. Additional laboratory tests such as amniocentesis, chorionic villus sampling, and DNA analysis are performed in cases of suspected congenital anomalies of the fetus. Infant deaths are usually attributed to congenital anomalies or prematurity. Premature delivery may be associated with many anomalies of pregnancy. Examples include multiple pregnancies, placental anomalies, preeclampsia and eclampsia, and congenital anomalies of the uterus, such as bicornuate uterus or cervical incompetence. Cervical incompetence can be demonstrated via sonography of the cervix during the first trimester of pregnancy.

Amniotic Fluid

Amniotic fluid is produced by various physiologic functions within the mother and the fetus. The amount of amniotic fluid present varies with the stage of pregnancy. **Oligohydramnios** occurs when too little amniotic fluid is present, and **polyhydramnios** occurs with an excess of amniotic fluid. The normal fetus swallows several hundred milliliters of fluid per day. This fluid is absorbed by the fetal intestines, with a portion excreted via the fetal urinary system and a portion transferred across the placenta into the mother's circulatory system. The major source of amniotic fluid arises from the fetus urinating fluid once the kidneys are developed. Therefore, oligohydramnios often results from poor fetal kidney function or blockage of the ureters associated with congenital anomalies of the fetal urinary system. If a fetus is unable to swallow because of anencephaly or a high gastrointestinal obstruction, polyhydramnios may occur. It is also an indication of severe growth retardation and fetal death.

Ectopic Pregnancy

Ectopic pregnancy refers to the development of an embryo outside the uterine cavity. It occurs in approximately 1% of all pregnancies. The most common site for an ectopic pregnancy is the uterine tube (Fig. 7-21), but it may also occur in the ovary, cervix, or abdominal cavity. In the case of a tubal pregnancy, the fallopian tube distends to accommodate the growing embryo, causing the blood vessels to

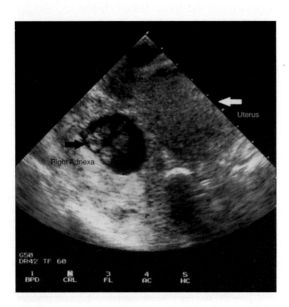

FIG. 7-21 Ectopic pregnancy shown on a sagittal ultrasound image reveals twin fetuses in the uterine tube.

rupture. This may produce serious internal hemorrhage and can be life threatening. If a tubal pregnancy goes untreated, the embryo will develop and survive for only 2 to 6 weeks.

Common signs and symptoms associated with ectopic pregnancy are the same as those of early pregnancy, but distension of the tube causes abdominal pain and tenderness. If internal hemorrhage occurs, loss of blood can cause fainting and shock. Ectopic pregnancies are more common in women who have had PID or have a partial obstruction of the uterine tube. The etiology of tubal pregnancies is obstruction of the normal passageway for the ovum. Although ultrasound is useful in assessing ectopic pregnancies, diagnosis is confirmed via laparoscopy. The treatment is surgical removal of the embryo and the affected uterine tube.

Disorders of the Placenta

The placenta is a temporary organ associated with pregnancy. Its purpose is to exchange nutrients and oxygen from mother to fetus and waste products from fetus to mother for excretion. If a woman begins to bleed during the third trimester of pregnancy, ultrasonography should be performed to evaluate the placenta, because this places both the mother and fetus at high risk. The most common causes of third-trimester bleeding are placenta previa and abruption of the placenta. **Placenta previa** is a condition in which the placenta develops in the lower half of the uterus and encroaches on and partially or completely covers the internal cervical os. In cases of placenta previa (Fig. 7-22), the mother experiences bleeding during the later stages of pregnancy because of the partial separation of the placenta from the uterine wall. Hemorrhage can occur, and this condition can be life threatening to both the mother and fetus. Ultrasound is a good method of determining placenta location in cases of suspected previa and useful in the management of the pregnancy. Normal delivery cannot occur in patients with placenta previa, so a cesarean section is normally performed.

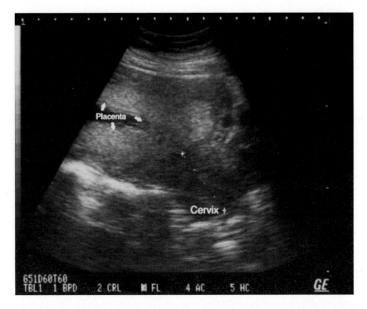

FIG. 7-22 Placenta previa seen on this sagittal ultrasound view reveals the placenta covering the internal os of the cervix.

Occasionally, a normally implanted placenta may prematurely separate from the uterus. This condition is termed **placental abruption** and may be life-threatening to the fetus. **Placental accreta** is an abnormal adhesion of the placenta to the uterine wall. In rare cases, failure of the placenta to separate following birth results in heavy bleeding and the need for an immediate hysterectomy.

Hydatidiform Mole

Hydatidiform mole represents an abnormal conception in which there is usually no fetus. It occurs in about 1 in 2000 pregnancies in North America, although the incidence is much greater in certain other parts of the world for unknown reasons. With this condition, the uterus is filled with cystically dilated chorionic villi that resemble a bunch of grapes (Fig. 7-23). These villi absorb fluid and become swollen, demonstrating a characteristic pattern on ultrasound as well as absence of heart sounds. Usually, these abort spontaneously in the second trimester. If they do not, suction curet-

tage is done, and most patients require no further treatment.

THE MALE REPRODUCTIVE SYSTEM

ANATOMY AND PHYSIOLOGY

The male reproductive system is composed of glands, ducts, and supporting structures. The glands of the male reproductive system include a pair of testes, a pair of seminal vesicles, a pair of bulbourethral glands, and one prostate gland. The testes are enclosed by a white, fibrous covering within the scrotum. They are responsible for the production of sperm and hormone secretion, mainly testosterone. The prostate gland lies just inferior to the bladder, and the urethra actually passes through this gland (Figs. 7-24 and 7-25). The prostate gland is responsible for secreting the majority of the seminal fluid and is normally about the size of a walnut.

The ducts that connect the glands include a pair of epididymides, a pair of vasa deferentia, a

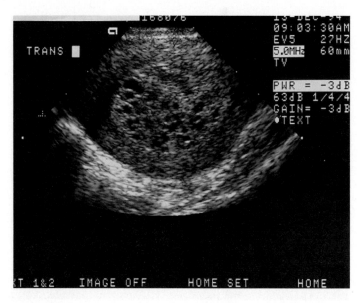

FIG. 7-23 Hydatidiform mole revealed as a grapelike cluster in the uterus on this transverse ultrasound image.

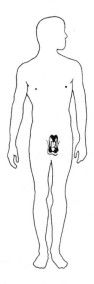

FIG. 7-24 The male reproductive system.

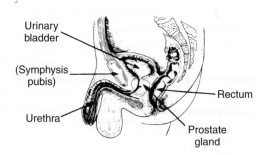

FIG. 7-25 The male urinary bladder, anterior cut away.

pair of ejaculatory ducts, and one urethra. The testes are divided into lobules that contain seminiferous tubules, which converge into larger ducts and emerge at the head of the epididymis. The epididymides lie superior and lateral to the testes and serve as a passageway for sperm. They are also responsible for secreting a portion of the seminal fluid. The vasa deferentia extend from the epididymides and pass through the inguinal canal into the pelvic cavity. They pass superior to the bladder and continue down the posterior surface of the bladder to join the ducts emerging from the seminal vesicles. This junction forms the ejaculatory ducts. These ducts eventually empty into the urethra, which is responsible for delivering the seminal fluid to the exterior of the body.

IMAGING CONSIDERATIONS

Radiographic investigation of the male reproductive system is limited mainly to urethrograms, intravenous urography. However, ultrasound is commonly used to evaluate testicular masses or an enlarged scrotum and to help differentiate between, on one hand, epididymitis and orchiditis and, on the other, testicular torsion. Nuclear medicine is also useful in distinguishing between epididymitis and testicular torsion. Prostatic ultrasound via a rectal probe is used to evaluate nodules and guide the physician during biopsies of the prostate. MRI of the male pelvis is performed to evaluate the seminal vesicles, the prostate gland, and the scrotum (Fig. 7-26). MRI is useful in detecting and staging prostate cancer in men having a positive (+4) prostate-specific antigen (PSA) laboratory test. A specialized rectal coil is used in examining the prostate gland; however, high-

field MRI units may be able to detect pathology without the use of the rectal coil. MRI is also useful in evaluating testicular cancer and can determine if the cancer is present in one or both testicles. This differentiation is especially important for young men who still plan to have children.

CONGENITAL ANOMALIES

Cryptorchidism

As the end of gestation occurs, the male testes normally descend through the inguinal canal into the scrotum. Cryptorchidism is a condition of undescended testes. The rate of malignancy is much greater in men with this condition, so the treatment involves either bringing the testicle down and fixing it surgically or removing it. Ultrasound is often used to locate the testicle.

NEOPLASTIC DISEASES

Prostatic Hyperplasia

Prostatic hyperplasia is a common benign enlargement, palpable through the rectum, of the prostate gland caused by the development of discrete nodules within the organ. Although enlargement may be determined by a digital rectal examination, the results may be misleading, so a laboratory blood test to assess serum PSA should be performed. Results may demonstrate a moderate elevation in PSA, depending on the degree of enlargement and urinary obstruction. The etiology of prostatic hyperplasia is unknown, but it is thought to be caused by hormonal changes associated with aging in that it generally affects men after age 50. The benign nodules most frequently occur in the median lobe and central portions of the lateral lobes of the prostate gland. Because of this location, the nodules often compress the portion of the urethra passing through the prostate gland, thus interfering with urination.

Symptoms associated with this disorder include difficulty in starting, stopping, and maintaining a flow of urine and inability to

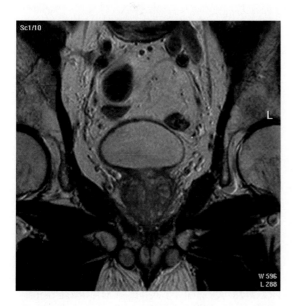

FIG. 7-26 A coronal T2-weighted MR image of the male pelvis depicting the bladder and prostate gland.

completely empty the bladder. Residual urine retained in the bladder tends to become infected, threatening the kidneys with infection. In some cases, urinary tract obstructions may result from an overgrowth of the prostate gland. The most common treatment of prostatic hyperplasia is partial excision of the prostate gland, although nonsurgical treatment is available for some cases. A transurethral resection of the prostate (TURP) is performed by passing an endoscope through the urethra to core out the gland. Prostatic enlargement may be demonstrated on an intravenous urographic examination as a filling defect at the base of the bladder. Hyperplastic changes are also readily visible on MRI and CT examinations of the pelvic area (Fig. 7-27). There is no conclusive evidence to suggest that development of prostatic hyperplasia increases an individual's chance of developing prostatic carcinoma.

Many men over the age of 50 develop small, multiple calcifications within the prostate. These are termed **prostatic calculi** and may be radiographically visible on plain abdominal or pelvic images. The development of these calculi is of no clinical significance.

Carcinoma of the Prostate

Adenocarcinoma of the prostate is a common cancer in men. It most frequently affects elderly men, with the incidence increasing with age. The etiology of prostate cancer is unknown, but it generally affects the outer group of prostate glands and occurs more frequently in the posterior lobe of the prostate. This disease is most often diagnosed by physical examination and an elevation of acid phosphatase levels in the blood. In cases of suspected prostatic disease, MRI or ultrasound may be utilized to determine the location and extent of the disease (Fig. 7-28). Common signs and symptoms associated with prostate cancer include urinary tract obstructions, a hard, enlarged prostate on rectal palpation, and low back pain, often caused by metastatic spread to the pelvis and lumbar spine.

Some types of prostate cancer are fairly dormant, but others are very aggressive and yield a higher mortality rate. If it is diagnosed

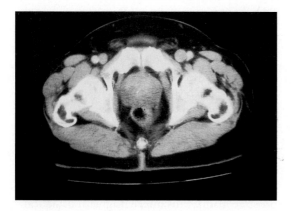

FIG. 7-27 Pelvic CT of a 68-year-old man demonstrating prostatic hyperplasia. Notice the indentation into the urinary bladder.

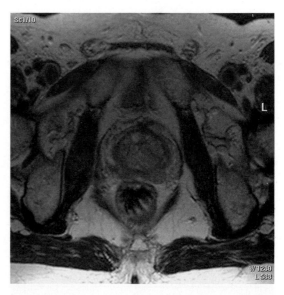

FIG. 7-28 An axial T2-weighted MR image demonstrating enlargement of the posterior left portion of the prostate by prostate carcinoma.

in an early stage, the initial treatment is surgical removal of the tumor. Additionally, this neoplasm is very testosterone dependent, so the testes are often removed along with the prostate. In some instances, female hormones may be administered to control the growth of the tumor by interfering with the testosterone. A new treatment modality involves planting radioactive seeds in the prostate, guided by ultrasound, to destroy the tumor.

Prostate cancer is staged A to D and graded I to III, depending on the extent of the disease. It tends to infiltrate surrounding structures early and extensively, particularly the skeletal system. Skeletal metastases occur in approximately 75% of all cases and manifest on plain radiographs as sclerotic lesions within the bone (Fig. 7-29). Bone pain in an elderly man is particularly suspect for prostate cancer. As the third leading cause of cancer deaths in men, it has a 5-year survival rate of approximately 33%.

Testicular Masses

Testicular torsion occurs if a testicle twists on itself, inducing severe pain and swelling. Failure to correct this surgically in an immediate fashion can result in severe compromise of testicular vascularity. The condition is often evaluated with a nuclear medicine scan, which shows decreased uptake on the affected side (Fig. 7-30). Inflammation of the epididymis, or

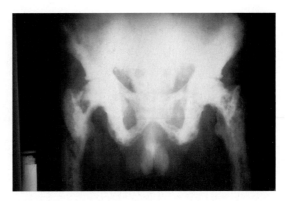

FIG. 7-29 Skeletal metastatic disease of the pelvis and spine secondary to prostate cancer.

epididymitis, can similarly lead to scrotal swelling. This inflammation of the epididymis and testis (**epididymoorchitis**) may result from a bacterial infection such as a urinary tract infection, gonorrhea, or be secondary to the placement of an indwelling urinary catheter. In addition to scrotal edema, signs and symptoms include scrotal pain and erythema. The increased blood flow resulting from it can be detected by ultrasound or a nuclear medicine scan, which demonstrates increased uptake (Fig. 7-31).

Benign masses of the testes may be associated with epididymoorchitis. Other common benign masses include hydroceles and spermatoceles. A **hydrocele** is a common intrinsic

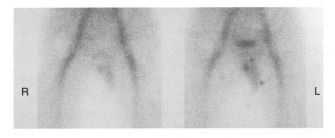

FIG. 7-30 Torsion as seen on a nuclear medicine testicular scan, which reveals a relative absence of blood flow to the right testicle.

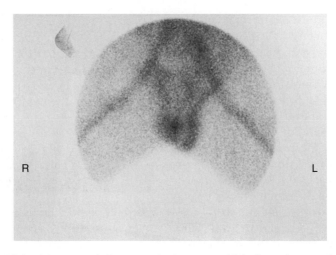

FIG. 7-31 Epididymitis as revealed on a testicular scan, which shows increased uptake in the left testicle.

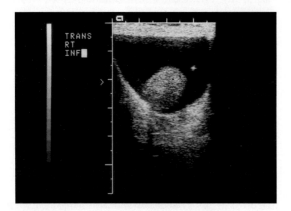

FIG. 7-32 A hydrocele is visualized as the dark collection of fluid surrounding the testicle, as seen on ultrasound of this 52-year-old man.

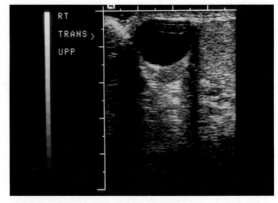

FIG. 7-33 A spermatocele, evidenced by a large fluid collection on the epididymis, as seen on a testicular ultrasound scan of this 33-year-old man.

scrotal mass, sometimes congenital in nature, caused by a collection of fluid in the testis or along the spermatic cord (Fig. 7-32). They may appear as a painless scrotal swelling, or they may demonstrate inflammation in combination with epididymitis and be quite painful. **Spermatoceles** or spermatic cysts are fluid-filled, painless scrotal masses within the testis adjacent to the epididymis (Fig. 7-33). Ultra-

sound may be used to differentiate between benign hydroceles or spermatoceles and solid, malignant neoplasms.

Malignant testicular tumors comprise approximately 1% of all male cancers. It is the most common malignancy among 15- to 34-year-olds and has a peak incidence around age 30 and a second smaller peak around age 75. The etiology of malignant tumors of the testes is unknown, but research has shown a strong hereditary association. The most common signs include enlargement or palpable hardness of the testis. As with other cancers, testicular tumors are staged I to III, depending on the size and extent of the disease. All types of malignant testicular neoplasms are treated with surgical resection. Chemotherapy, radiation therapy, or both may also be used in conjunction with surgery, depending on the type and staging of the disease. There are four types of malignant germ cell tumors: seminomas, embryonal carcinomas, teratomas, and choriocarcinomas.

Seminomas arise from the seminiferous tubules and account for approximately 40% of malignant testicular tumors (Fig. 7-34). Seminomas grow rapidly but tend to remain localized for a fairly long time before metastasizing. These neoplasms have an excellent prognosis because of their extreme radiosensitivity. If treated with radiation therapy, seminomas carry a 10-year survival rate of approximately 90%.

Teratomas arise from primitive germ cells and account for approximately 25% of the malignant testicular masses (Fig. 7-35). These neoplasms are composed of various cell types such as connective tissue, muscle, and thyroid glandular tissue. **Teratomas** are associated with a poorer prognosis than seminomas and carry a 10-year survival rate of approximately 50% to 75%. Like seminomas, teratomas are highly malignant, spreading to the renal hilum via lymphatics and hematogenous spread.

Embryonal carcinomas make up approximately 20% of malignant testicular tumors. They are smaller than seminomas; however, they are very invasive and metastasize fairly quickly. Embryonal carcinomas carry a 10-year survival rate of approximately 35%.

Choriocarcinomas compose the smallest portion of malignant testicular tumors, accounting for only 1% of malignant neoplasms of the testes. However, choriocarcinomas are very small and aggressive neoplasms. They are often nonpalpable and metastasize very early. Choriocarcinomas carry the worst prognosis, with a 10-year survival rate of approximately 10%.

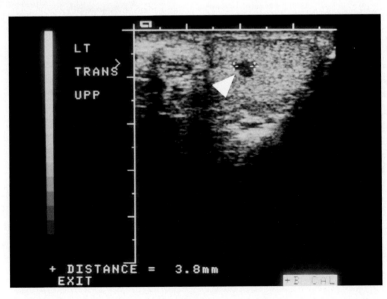

FIG. 7-34 The hypoechoic mass seen in the superior aspect of the testicle on this testicular ultrasound of a 31-year-old man is strongly suggestive of a seminoma.

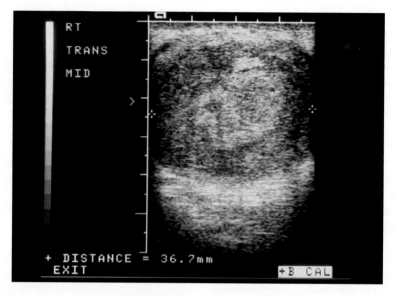

FIG. 7-35 A large, echogenic heterogeneous mass in the right testicle is highly suspicious for a teratoma in the testicular ultrasound scan of this 27-year-old man.

PATHOLOGY SUMMARY: THE REPRODUCTIVE SYSTEM

Pathology	Imaging Modalities of Choice
PID	Ultrasound, hysterosalpingography
Ovarian cysts	Ultrasound, CT, and MRI
Cystadenocarcinoma	Ultrasound , CT, and MRI
Carcinoma of the cervix	Staging: CT and MRI
Leiomyoma of uterus	Ultrasound, CT, and MRI
Adenocarcinoma of endometrium	Staging: CT and MRI
Fibroadenoma of breast	Mammography and ultrasound
Fibrocystic breast	Mammography and ultrasound
Carcinoma of breast	Mammography
Pregnancy status	Ultrasound
Ectopic pregnancy	Ultrasound
Disorders of placenta	Ultrasound
Cryptorchidism	Ultrasound
Prostatic hyperplasia	MRI, CT, and intravenous urography
Carcinoma of the prostate	MRI, CT, and ultrasound
Testicular torsion	Ultrasound, nuclear medicine
Testicular mass	Ultrasound

1. Imaging studies performed on a nongravid woman include:
   a. hysterosalpingography
   b. transvaginal pelvic sonography
   c. transabdominal pelvic sonography
   d. all of the above

2. Regular, yearly mammographic screening should occur in women ___ years of age or older.
   a. 20   c. 40
   b. 30   d. 50

3. The congenital disorder resulting in a complete duplication of the uterus, cervix, and vagina is:
   a. bicornuate uterus
   b. retroflexed uterus
   c. unicornuate uterus
   d. uterus didelphys

4. The formation of which of the following cystic ovarian masses may occur as a part of the normal menstrual cycle?
   1. corpus luteum cysts
   2. cystadenomas
   3. follicular cysts
   a. 1 and 2
   b. 1 and 3
   c. 2 and 3
   d. 1, 2, and 3

5. A malignant neoplasm of the ovary is a:
   a. cystadenocarcinoma
   b. cystadenoma
   c. leiomyoma
   d. fibroadenoma

6. Diagnosis of which type of neoplastic disease is often made via a Pap smear and confirmed by surgical biopsy?
   a. adenocarcinoma of the endometrium
   b. cervical carcinoma
   c. fibroadenoma of the breast
   d. leiomyoma of the uterus

7. The majority of breast masses occur in which anatomic region of the breast?
   a. lower, inner quadrant
   b. lower, outer quadrant
   c. upper, inner quadrant
   d. upper, outer quadrant

8. The presence of excessive amniotic fluid is termed:
   a. abruptio placentae
   b. oligohydramnios
   c. placenta previa
   d. polyhydramnios

9. Prostatic hyperplasia most frequently occurs in men:
   a. under the age of 30
   b. between the ages of 30 and 50
   c. over the age of 50
   d. prostatic hyperplasia is a female condition

10. Benign tumors of the testes include:
   1. hydroceles
   2. seminomas
   3. spermatoceles
   a. 1 and 2   c. 2 and 3
   b. 1 and 3   d. 1, 2, and 3

11. Describe how breast parenchyma changes with age and parity and the effect these changes have on radiographic visibility of potential masses.

12. Identify two purposes for requiring a patient to have a full bladder for female transabdominal sonographic examination.

13. Describe the benefit versus the risk of radiation exposure from routine mammography.

14. What would be the danger of leaving cryptorchidism untreated?

15. A 60-year-old man presents to his physician with complaints of frequent urination, particularly at night. An IVP is ordered. The only visible abnormality is a filling defect at the base of his bladder. What is the likely cause?

The Cardiovascular System

UPON COMPLETION OF CHAPTER 8, THE READER SHOULD BE ABLE TO:

- Describe the anatomic components of the cardiovascular system.
- Explain the appearance of the various portions of the heart on conventional chest radiographs.
- Describe each segment of the cardiac cycle.
- Discuss the role of other imaging modalities in the diagnosis, treatment, and management of cardiovascular disorders.
- Differentiate the major congenital anomalies of the cardiovascular system.
- Identify the pathogenesis of the pathologies cited and typical treatments for them.
- Describe, in general, the radiographic appearance of each of the given pathologies.

KEY TERMS

2-D echocardiography	Foramen ovale	Right and left ventricles
Adventitia	Fusiform aneurysm	Saccular aneurysm
Aneurysm	Gated cardiac blood pool scans	Sinoatrial node
Arteries	Heart	Stent
Atherosclerosis	Infarct	Systole
Atrial septal defect	Intima	Tetralogy of Fallot
Capillaries	Ischemia	Thrombolysis
Cardiomegaly	Lumen	Thrombophlebitis
Coarctation of the aorta	M-mode echocardiography	Thrombus
Congestive heart failure	Media	Transesophageal echocardiography
Cor pulmonale	Murmur	(TEE)
Coronary artery disease (CAD)	Myocardial perfusion scan	Transjugular intrahepatic
Diastole	Myocardium	portosystemic stent (TIPS)
Dissecting aneurysm	Patent ductus arteriosus	Transposition of the great vessels
Doppler echocardiography	Percutaneous transluminal	Valvular stenosis
Ductus arteriosus	angioplasty (PTA)	Veins
Embolization	Permanent catheterization phlebitis	Venous thrombosis
Endocardium	Rheumatic fever	Ventricular septal defect
Epicardium	Right and left atria	

ANATOMY AND PHYSIOLOGY

The cardiovascular system consists of the heart, arteries, capillaries, and veins and may be further divided into two subsystems of circulation. The pulmonary circulation transports blood between the heart and lungs for exchange of blood gases, whereas the systemic circulation transports blood between the heart and the rest of the body.

The Heart

The **heart** acts as a pump to propel the blood throughout the body via the circulatory vessels. It lies in the anterior chest within the mediastinum and is generally readily visible on a chest radiograph. The interior of the heart is divided into two upper chambers, termed the **right and left atria,** and two lower chambers termed the **right and left ventricles** (Fig. 8-1). Note that the heart lies in an oblique plane within the mediastinum; a conventional

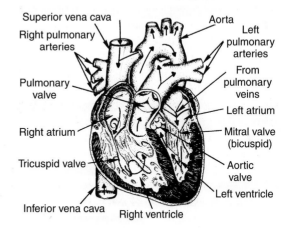

FIG. 8-1 Blood flow through the heart.

posteroanterior (PA) chest radiograph does not clearly demonstrate all chambers of the heart.

A frontal projection of the chest shows a cardiac silhouette, with two thirds of the heart lying to the left of midline; the right side is

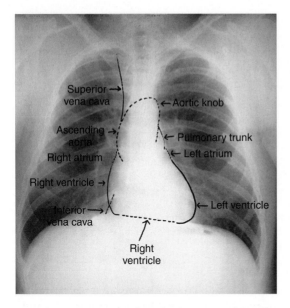

FIG. 8-2 PA chest radiograph with heart chambers and great vessels outlined.

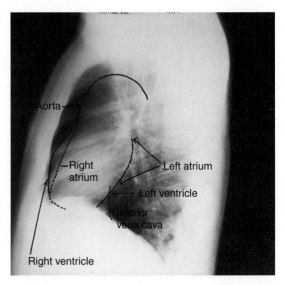

FIG. 8-3 Lateral chest radiograph with heart chambers and great vessels outlined.

composed mainly of the right atrium, and the left side is composed mainly of the left ventricle. The right ventricle lies midline within the cardiac shadow and is located anterior to the right atrium and left ventricle. The left atrium is located midline and is the most posterior aspect of the heart (Fig. 8-2). Therefore, it is necessary to obtain a lateral projection of the chest to best demonstrate the right ventricle and left atrium. On a lateral projection of the chest, the right ventricle constitutes the anterior portion of the cardiac silhouette, and the left atrium and left ventricle constitute the posterior portion of the cardiac shadow (Fig. 8-3).

The heart contains three tissue layers. The innermost layer, termed the **endocardium,** is smooth. The valves located within and between the various chambers are also composed of endocardium. Although the valve tissue is relatively thin, in a normal heart it is able to prevent the backflow and passage of blood when the valve is closed. The middle layer is muscular and is termed the **myocardium.** This is the thickest layer of heart tissue, and the muscle receives blood supply from the right and left coronary arteries that arise directly from the aorta, just superior to the aortic valve. Maximum blood flow through the coronary arteries occurs during diastole, while the heart is relaxed. The outermost layer is a protective covering termed the **epicardium.** The entire heart is enclosed within a pericardial sac, which contains a small amount of fluid to lubricate the heart as it contracts and relaxes, thus reducing friction between the heart and other mediastinal structures.

In the normal heart, the right atrium receives deoxygenated blood from the body via the superior and inferior venae cavae. The deoxygenated blood passes through the right atrioventricular or tricuspid valve into the right ventricle. The right ventricle contracts during systole, thus propelling the blood to the lungs through the pulmonary valve and pulmonary trunk, which bifurcates into the right and left main pulmonary arteries, respectively. Approximately 60% of the deoxygenated blood enters the right lung, and approximately 40% enters the left lung.

The exchange of gases occurs at the capillary-alveolar level within the lungs, and the now oxygenated blood is returned to the left atrium via the four pulmonary veins. The oxygenated blood flows from the left atrium to the left ventricle via the left mitral valve. The left ventricle is responsible for pumping the oxygenated blood throughout the systemic circulatory system; therefore, the left ventricle has a thicker layer of myocardium and contracts with greater force than does the right ventricle. The oxygenated blood flows through the aortic valve into the aorta when the left ventricle contracts.

The Cardiac Cycle

The contraction of the myocardium is termed **systole,** and the subsequent relaxation is termed **diastole.** The pacemaker of the heart is the **sinoatrial (SA) node,** which is located in the upper portion of the right atrium near the superior vena cava. An electrical current is transmitted through the myocardium, resulting in a heartbeat.

Electrocardiography (ECG) graphically displays this electrical activity. The elements of an ECG include the P wave, PR interval, QRS complex, T wave, and QT duration (Fig. 8-4). The P wave is the graphic display of the spread of the electrical impulse from the atria. The PR interval shows the amount of time required for the electrical impulse to travel from the SA node to the ventricular muscle fibers. The spread of the electrical impulse through the ventricles is displayed by the QRS complex, and the period in which the ventricles recover from the spent electrical impulse is graphically displayed by the T wave. The QT duration represents the total time from ventricular depolarization (QRS) to ventricular repolarization (T).

Circulatory Vessels

Arteries are blood vessels that carry blood away from the heart and are generally named for their location or the organ they supply (e.g., splenic artery). They are composed of three layers. The outermost layer is termed the **adventitia,** the middle layer is the **media,** and the innermost layer is the **intima.** The internal, tubular structure of the vessel is termed the **lumen. Veins** are blood vessels that carry blood

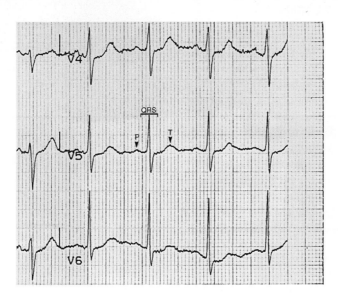

FIG. 8-4 Electrocardiograph demonstrating the P wave, QRS wave, and T wave.

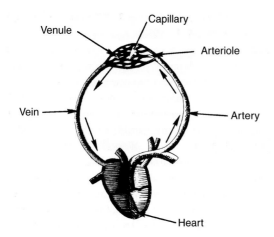

FIG. 8-5 General systemic circulation.

to the heart. They are composed of the same three layers; however, venous walls are thinner than arterial walls, and veins contain valves at set intervals to help with blood return to the heart. **Capillaries** are microscopic vessels that connect the arteries and veins (Fig. 8-5). They are responsible for the exchange of substances necessary for nutrient and waste transport.

IMAGING CONSIDERATIONS

Radiography

Although a number of imaging modalities play an important role in evaluation of the cardiovascular system, conventional radiography continues to play a very important role in the diagnosis and management of cardiovascular disease. Chest radiographs provide information concerning heart shape and size, and radiographers must be aware that many factors may affect the cardiac image. Heart size is best assessed on serial radiographs of the chest because severe coronary artery disease (CAD) may often be present in a normal-sized heart, making it difficult to identify heart disease based on one chest image. Because the atria and ventricles overlap and may be obscured by other structures, estimating exact heart chamber size is also difficult with conventional radiography.

However, chest radiography is excellent in demonstrating the great vessels and vascular changes within the lung fields, which offer critical information regarding cardiac function.

Factors that the technologist can control include patient posture, degree of inspiration, correct positioning, geometric factors, and exposure technique selection. Whenever possible, chest radiographs should be taken with the patient in an erect position. If a patient is semi-recumbent or recumbent, the heart appears to be enlarged because the abdominal organs push the diaphragm and heart up into the thoracic cavity. It is important to identify cases in which the patient is not erect to aid the physician in diagnosis and interpretation.

Chest radiographs obtained without a good inspiration also distort heart shape and size (Figs. 8-6 and 8-7). Remember, at least 10 pos-

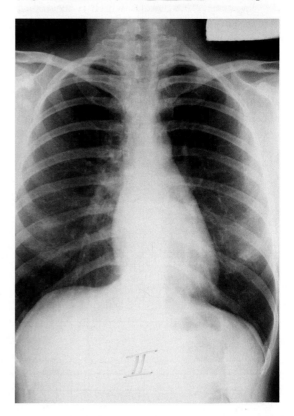

FIG. 8-6 PA chest radiograph with good inspiration.

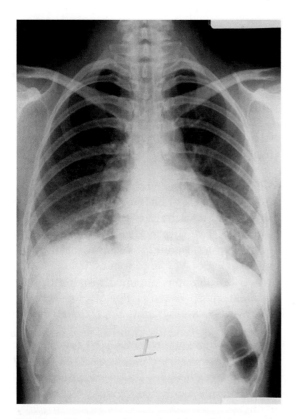

FIG. 8-7 PA chest radiograph with expiration on the same patient as in Fig. 8-6; notice the enlargement of the cardiac shadow on this radiograph.

terior ribs should be visible within the lung fields on a good inspiratory chest radiograph. The sternoclavicular joints should be an equal distance from the spine, and the scapulae should be rolled forward out of the lung fields on a well-positioned PA chest radiograph. To position a patient for a lateral chest, the arms and shoulders should be placed above the patient's head to ensure that they are above the apices.

Geometric factors affecting heart shape and size include source-to-image receptor distance (SID) and object-to-image receptor distance (OID). Conventional chest radiographs are generally obtained using a 72-inch SID to decrease magnification of the heart to an approximate factor of 10%. Again, it is impor-

tant to document variations in SID to aid in the proper diagnosis of heart disorders. Because the heart is fairly anterior in the mediastinum, it is preferable to obtain PA chest images whenever possible. This places the heart closest to the image receptor, allowing for the smallest OID. Positioning the patient for a PA projection also helps decrease magnification of the cardiac silhouette. A third geometric factor that is frequently overlooked is the anode-heel effect. Radiographers can use this phenomenon to their advantage by placing the anode over the apical region and the cathode toward the base of the lungs, when possible, thus distributing the radiographic density more evenly throughout the chest radiograph.

Adequate penetration of the mediastinal structure is also critical in chest radiography and requires the use of a relatively high kilovoltage. A minimum of 100 kilovolts peak (kVp) should be used. Compensating filters, such as trough filters, may also be used to ensure adequate penetration of the mediastinum while maintaining optimum visualization of the vascular markings within the lung fields. Vascular markings within the chest help the physician assess ventricular function. The pulmonary vessels also provide information about pulmonary artery pressure. Dilatation of these vessels often indicates problems with the right ventricle. Exposure times of one tenth of a second or less should be used whenever possible to decrease involuntary cardiac motion. It has been documented that heart motion may increase the size of the cardiac shadow. The heart may look larger if the radiograph is exposed during diastole.

In most institutions, chest radiography is the most commonly performed procedure, and radiographers all too often underestimate the importance of these basic radiographic principles. Well-positioned diagnostic chest radiographs are crucial in the diagnosis and treatment of cardiovascular disorders. In a normal adult, the transverse diameter of the cardiac shadow should be less than half the transverse diameter

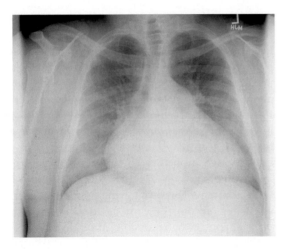

FIG. 8-8 PA chest radiograph demonstrates cardiomegaly secondary to congestive heart failure.

of the thorax on a PA erect chest radiograph. An enlarged heart is termed **cardiomegaly** (Fig. 8-8), which is indicative of many cardiovascular disorders and is a nonspecific finding.

Factors affecting cardiac shape and size that are not under the technologist's control include patient body habitus, bony thorax abnormalities, and pathologic conditions, such as a pneumo-thorax or pulmonary emphysema. Bony abnormalities of special concern include scoliosis and pectus excavatum. Individuals with pectus excavatum present a funnel-shaped depression of the sternum. The abnormal placement of the xiphoid causes displacement of the heart to the left and distortion of the cardiac shadow. Vascular lines and tubes are discussed in Chapter 3 of this text.

Echocardiography

Echocardiography encompasses a group of noninvasive sonographic (ultrasound) procedures that can provide detailed information about heart anatomy, function, and vessel patency (Fig. 8-9). Sonographic imaging may be performed using M-mode, two-dimensional (2-D) imaging, spectral Doppler, color Doppler, or stress echocardiography.

M-mode echocardiography uses a stationary ultrasound beam to provide an examination of the atria, ventricles, heart valves, and aortic root allowing evaluation of left ventricular function. M-mode cardiac sonography is also used to measure the thickness of the ventricular walls; however, it has largely been replaced by

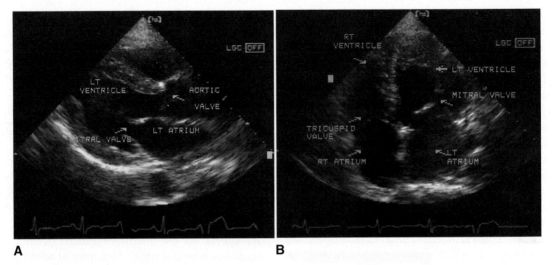

A   **B**

FIG. 8-9 A, Echocardiographic visualization of heart anatomy of a 47-year-old man as seen in a parasternal, sagittal view. **B,** A coronal view of the same heart via echocardiography.

2-D echocardiography. 2-D imaging allows for spatially correct, real-time imaging of the heart. It provides multiple tomographic projections of the heart and great vessels in a cine-like (dynamic imaging) presentation. In addition, it is an excellent modality for visualizing the ascending and abdominal aorta in cases of suspected aneurysm. Both M-mode and 2-D images are obtained by placing the transducer over the thorax at the sternal borders, cardiac apex, between the ribs, or at the suprasternal notch. Smaller transducers have been developed to allow for **transesophageal echocardiography (TEE),** in which the patient swallows a mobile, flexible probe containing the transducer. With TEE, the heart's structure can be readily visualized without interference from structures such as the skin, rib cage, and chest muscles. It is especially helpful in imaging the aortic arch and aortic root. Smaller transducers can also be placed on intravascular catheters to assess vessel anatomy and blood flow.

Stress echocardiography combines an exercise test with an echocardiogram to check the heart's contraction ability and its pumping efficiency. If exercise is not possible, a drug, dobutamine, can be used to increase the cardiac output to assess how well the heart pumps during infusion.

Doppler sonography is an adjunct, noninvasive procedure used to study peripheral vasculature. It has been a mainstay of vascular imaging since the 1970s and is used to determine the direction and velocity, as well as the presence or absence, of blood flow in both arteries and veins. Using ultrasound, the Doppler effect is the principle that sound coming toward you has a higher pitch than sound going away. The return of pulsed ultrasound allows calculation of the shift in the direction of blood flow and creates a spectral display from which velocity is calculated (Fig. 8-10). The spectral signal is displayed on a strip chart or videotape. With Doppler sonography, the flow of blood is not affected until any obstruction present is at least 60% complete. The

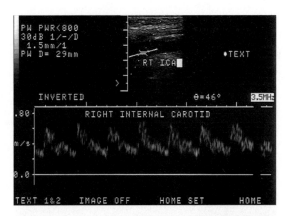

FIG. 8-10 Illustration of the Doppler effect with normal arterial flow in the internal carotid artery depicted above a graph of the arterial flow.

percentage of stenosis present dictates the treatment of vascular disease, and usually this consists of surgery (e.g., endarterectomy). Such vascular imaging is said to be duplex in that it helps reveal physiologic characteristics, and the imaging component defines anatomy (e.g., plaque morphology). The most common conditions imaged by 2-D Doppler sonography are carotid stenosis (significantly reducing carotid angiography) (Figs. 8-11 and 8-12), lower

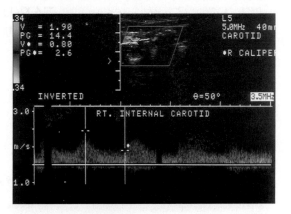

FIG. 8-11 A Doppler sonogram of an abnormal internal carotid artery spectrum caused by heterogeneous calcified plaque. Note the difference of appearance of the graphic representation as compared to Fig. 8-10.

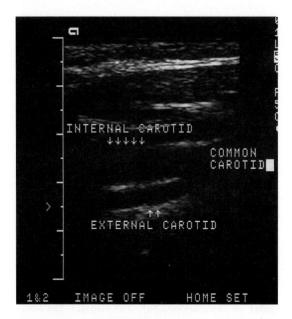

FIG. 8-12 A Doppler sonogram of a normal carotid bifurcation from the common carotid into the internal and external carotid arteries.

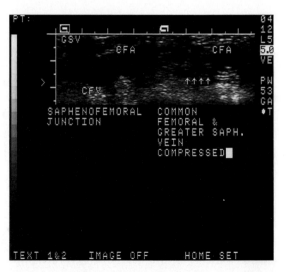

FIG. 8-13 Doppler sonographic portrayal of normal flow on the left of the image through the greater saphenous vein (GSV), common femoral vein (CFV), and common femoral artery (CFA). Compression on the right side of the image depicts normal closure of the common femoral vein and greater saphenous vein, as expected.

extremity arterial stenosis, and deep venous thrombosis (Figs. 8-13 and 8-14), largely supplanting traditional venography. The blood flow may be encoded with color to differentiate blood flowing toward the transducer (red) from blood flowing away from the transducer (blue); this is termed "color Doppler echocardiography."

Nuclear Cardiology

Nuclear medicine procedures used in the assessment of cardiovascular disease include myocardial perfusion scans, gated cardiac blood pool scans, and positron emission tomography (PET). They are useful in assessing CAD, congenital heart disease, and cardiomyopathy.

A **myocardial perfusion scan** is the most widely used procedure in nuclear cardiology. It may be performed on patients with chest pain of an unknown origin, to evaluate coronary artery stenosis, and as a follow-up to bypass surgery, angioplasty, or thrombolysis. It is especially useful in detecting regions of myocardial

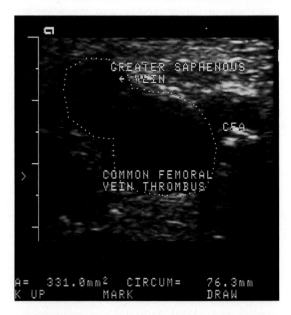

FIG. 8-14 This transverse view of the greater saphenous vein and common femoral vein indicates their failure to close on compression because of the large venous thrombus contained within.

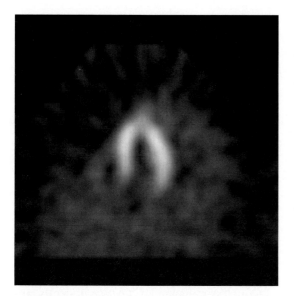

FIG. 8-15 The appearance of a normal heart on a nuclear medicine perfusion scan with the isotope distribution equal throughout the myocardium at rest.

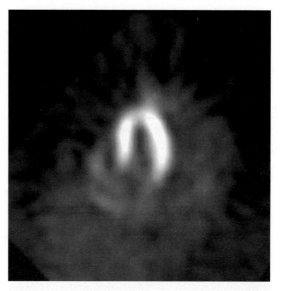

FIG. 8-16 The appearance of a normal heart on a nuclear medicine perfusion scan on the same patient as Fig. 8-15 during exercise. Notice the increased activity in the myocardium.

ischemia and scarring (Figs. 8-15 and 8-16). In this study, a special agent is used to dilate the coronary arteries, and then a radionuclide, usually radioactive technetium sestamibi or thallium, is injected. It concentrates in the areas of the heart that have the best blood flow. Those areas lacking blood flow demonstrate filling defects, visualized between images taken at rest and under stress. Patients may be stressed by exercise using a treadmill or by the use of pharmaceuticals such as dipyridamole. Myocardial perfusion scanning is performed using a single photon emission computed tomographic (SPECT) camera, allowing the camera to rotate around the patient to obtain tomographic images of the heart parallel to the short and long axis of the left ventricle. SPECT myocardial perfusion scans can detect significant CAD in 90% of patients presenting with CAD.

PET may also be used for imaging myocardial perfusion using a variety of positron perfusion and metabolic agents. A PET unit is more sensitive than conventional nuclear medicine cameras, and the spatial resolution is superior to conventional cameras. It is highly accurate for detecting CAD that interferes with blood flow to the heart muscle and can identify injured but viable heart muscle. PET can also provide quantitative data about the distribution of the radionuclide within the body.

Gated cardiac blood pool scans, sometimes called radionuclide ventriculograms, are used to evaluate ventricular function and ventricular wall motion. These images are obtained with the patient at rest and during exercise. They are synchronized with the patient's heart beat using an ECG to image the heart during specific phases of the cardiac cycle with the use of the radionuclide technetium-99. Images are obtained over a 5- to 10-minute time period. The images are displayed in a cine-like format allowing the wall motion of the beating heart to be evaluated. Ventricular function can be assessed by calculating the ejection fraction, ejection and filling rates, and left ventricular volume.

Computed Tomography

Computed tomography (CT) is a relatively noninvasive modality used to assess cardiac and vascular disease. Studies may be performed using conventional, spiral, or electron beam CT (EBCT). Cardiac scoring is performed without the use of a contrast agent. It was introduced in 1990, and a scoring algorithm was developed for evaluating the amount of calcium present in the coronary arteries.

EBCT was introduced in the mid-1980s and is a technique used primarily to examine the heart, particularly as related to coronary artery calcifications. It uses a scanning focused x-ray beam to provide complete cardiac imaging in 50 ms—fast enough to "freeze" heart motion without the need for ECG gating. An electron gun produces an electron stream that is magnetically focused onto four tungsten targets. Each target emits two fan beams of x-rays, which are directed through the patient and registered on detectors arranged in a semicircle above the patient. The net result is that extremely thin slices are readily demonstrated, either as a cine loop or single images. This allows for coronary calcium scoring, which may represent a predictor of atherosclerosis and current heart disease. A low calcium score implies a low risk for obstructing coronary disease. However, cardiac catheterization is still recommended for a final diagnosis. EBCT is not of value in patients with a history of a previous heart attack, angioplasty, or bypass surgery.

Multidetector spiral CT units with specialized cardiac software may also be used to perform calcium scoring and have better reproducibility than EBCT examinations. The software enables ECG gating and fast, multiple-section scans to obtain images without interference from the normal heart motion. Images are generally captured during the R-wave to acquire the image during the diastolic phase of the heart. The gating may occur prospectively or retrospectively. Images of 2.5 mm are obtained, generally at 2.5-mm intervals. Multidetector CT cardiac scoring employs software to analyze the histogram information obtained during the scans and compute image and region scores, similar to EBCT.

ECG-gated CT is also employed to perform noninvasive angiography (CTA) allowing evaluation of the right and left coronary arteries, the circumflex artery, and the anterior descending artery. Currently, CTA can identify a stenotic cardiac vessel in almost 70% of the cases because of its ability to image soft atherosclerotic plaque. Postprocessing software can reproduce three-dimensional images of the heart to assess the coronary arteries, heart chambers, and assess bypass grafts. The contrast-enhanced CT images may also be reviewed in a cine loop to allow evaluation of heart motion and assessment of cardiac function and perfusion.

Contrast-enhanced CTA was recently approved by the FDA. It is less invasive and is more cost-effective than conventional angiography. In combination with 3-D reconstruction, it is used to image vascular structures for organ donors, to diagnose pulmonary embolisms, to evaluate vascular stenosis and peripheral vascular disease, and for imaging abdominal aortic aneurysms (Fig. 8-17). CTA helps the surgeon determine the necessary stent type and size in the presurgical planning of abdominal aortic aneurysms and in the evaluation following surgery to assess the stent's effectiveness.

Magnetic Resonance Imaging

Magnetic resonance imaging (MRI) has recently gained popularity as a modality that cardiologists are using to evaluate many cardiac, mediastinal, and great vessel anomalies (Fig. 8-18). It may be used to evaluate myocardial wall thickness and chamber volumes and is especially helpful in diagnosing right ventricular dysplasia. Most protocols involve obtaining imaging sequences and putting them into motion using a cine loop to evaluate how well valves of the heart are functioning. Like nuclear cardiology, contrast-enhanced MRI can demonstrate myocardial perfusion, and blood flow velocities within the heart can be measured. As with

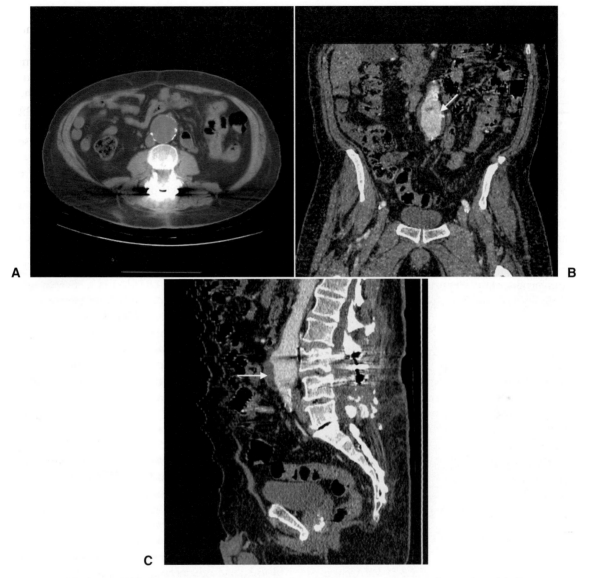

FIG. 8-17 CTA demonstrating an abdominal aortic aneurysm in three planes: **A,** axial; **B,** coronal; **C,** sagittal.

many other imaging modalities, information may be ECG-gated to acquire the images during specific portions of the cardiac cycle.

MRI is also used to evaluate aortic aneurysms, dissections, and aortic stenosis, especially in patients who are unable to have contrast-enhanced CT scans because of renal failure.

Contrast-enhanced magnetic resonance angiography (MRA) is widely used to evaluate the vasculature from the aorta to the brain (Fig. 8-19). This technology takes only about 1 minute to acquire data and is considered non-invasive. The larger coronary arteries may also be assessed using MRA.

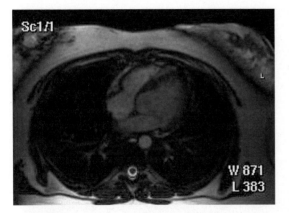

FIG. 8-18 A T2 Tru Fisp image of the heart demonstrating normal heart anatomy.

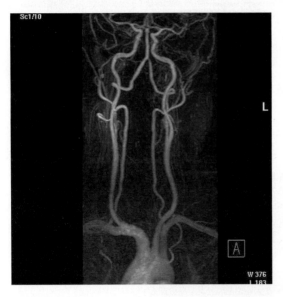

FIG. 8-19 A contrast-enhanced 3-D MRA image of the aortic arch, carotid and vertebral arteries, and Circle of Willis.

Angiography

Angiography is still the most commonly performed procedure for cardiovascular disease. It may be performed for diagnostic purposes or for therapeutic reasons. As discussed above, traditional diagnostic angiography is being challenged by less invasive procedures such as MRA and CTA. Cardiac catheterization is an invasive procedure specific to the heart and great vessels. It is performed on patients with CAD, conduction disturbances, or congenital heart disease and provides information regarding heart and vessel anatomy. Intracardiac and arterial pressures are measured as the catheter passes through the various areas of the heart. This provides information regarding the function of the cardiac valves. Angiocardiography is performed by injecting the contrast material into the heart chambers and obtaining cine images of the heart and great vessels in motion.

Therapeutic angiography continues to steadily increase through expanded use of interventional procedures. Percutaneous transluminal coronary angioplasty (PTCA) is a therapeutic procedure commonly performed to open stenotic coronary vessels, and **stents** may be placed in the vessel to maintain the patency of narrowed vessels. **Thrombolysis** is a procedure in which a high-intensity anticoagulant, such as streptokinase, is dripped over a period of hours directly onto a clot to dissolve it (Fig. 8-20). With **embolization,** devices such as coils are used to clot off vessels (Fig. 8-21). Common examples of the use of embolization include clotting of vessels feeding brain tumors, arteriovenous malformations, or other abnormalities of the brain to prevent excessive bleeding during open cranial surgery. In a **transjugular intrahepatic portosystemic stent** (TIPS) procedure, a catheter is used to connect the jugular vein to the portal vein to reduce the flow of blood through a diseased liver (Fig. 8-22). Arterial stents are devices placed in arteries (Fig. 8-23), typically the iliac, aorta, renal, and coronary, to open occluded vessels. Insertion of a stent is often preceded by **percutaneous transluminal angioplasty** (PTA) with a balloon catheter to open up the vessel's occlusion before stent placement (Fig. 8-24). In **permanent catheterization,** a catheter is placed in the subclavian or jugular vein and tunneled under the skin to allow for improved dialysis access.

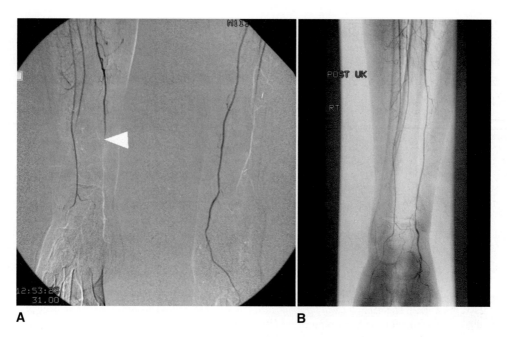

FIG. 8-20 A, An apparent embolus in the right popliteal artery prevents blood flow to the foot in this 91-year-old woman. **B,** In this thrombolysis procedure, urokinase is sprayed onto the embolus and then allowed to drip over a 30-minute period. Patency is restored.

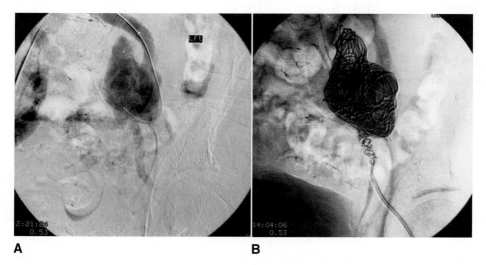

FIG. 8-21 A, A large aneurysm is seen angiographically in the left common iliac artery of this 74-year-old man. **B,** Embolization of this large aneurysm was accomplished by progressive insertion of a variety of coils and guide wire fragments.

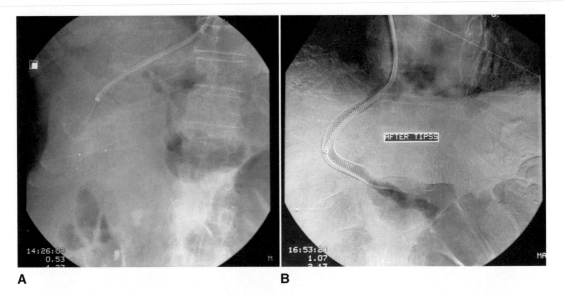

FIG. 8-22 A, A specialized catheter is used to create an opening through a cirrhotic liver of a 69-year-old man for the beginning of a TIPS procedure. **B,** Following dilation of the pathway using standard angioplasty technique, a shunt is installed to connect the right hepatic vein to the right portal vein, restoring blood flow.

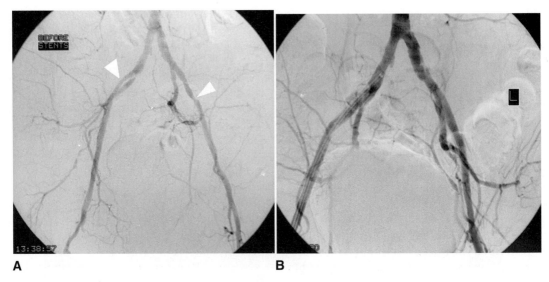

FIG. 8-23 A, A bilateral lower extremity arteriogram reveals stenosis of both external iliac arteries. **B,** Following balloon angioplasty, stent placement in each external iliac artery results in restored flow of blood.

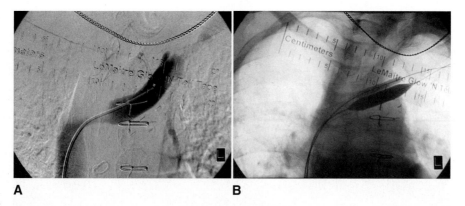

A   **B**

FIG. 8-24 A, Catheterization and angiography of the left brachiocephalic vein of this 56-year-old man reveal significant narrowing. **B,** Balloon angioplasty and a stent are used to open up the stenotic left brachiocephalic vein. Excellent blood flow was restored in subsequent images.

Vena caval filters are basket-like devices placed in the inferior vena cava to catch clots before they enter the heart (Fig. 8-25). Besides typical contrast media, some of these procedures utilize carbon dioxide as the contrast agent for patients who do not tolerate normal agents (Fig. 8-26). The role of interventional angiography will continue to grow and reduce costs and complications from certain surgical procedures it replaces.

CONGENITAL AND HEREDITARY DISEASES

Because fetal circulation and blood-gas exchange occur within the placenta, certain characteristics are present in the fetal circulatory system that should normally disappear at birth. These characteristics include an opening in the septum between the atria, termed the **foramen ovale,** which allows the blood to bypass the pulmonary circulatory system, and a small vessel termed the ductus arteriosus, which connects the pulmonary artery and the descending aorta. If these anatomic structures persist, a variety of congenital anomalies can develop in the newborn. The incidence of congenital cardiovascular anomalies is approximately 1 per 120 live births.

Etiology of congenital heart disease includes inherited genetic disorders, chromosomal aberrations (such as Down syndrome), and environmental factors (such as drugs, alcohol, infection, radiation, and maternal disease). In addition, individuals with congenital anomalies of the heart are at an increased risk of developing endocardial infections. Immediate diagnosis to determine the type and severity of the anomaly and treatment of the cardiac anomaly are vital to survival. The outcome of the disease depends on the pressure differences created between the right and left side of the heart, abnormal ventricular load, and defects that obstruct blood flow. Radiography and diagnostic medical sonography play a critical role in the diagnosis and treatment of congenital anomalies, along with the diagnosis of heart murmurs by physical examination and abnormal heart rates and ventricular hypertrophy demonstrated by ECG. A **murmur** is an abnormal heart sound resulting from disturbed or turbulent flow, often through malformed valves. Common signs of heart failure include tachycardia,

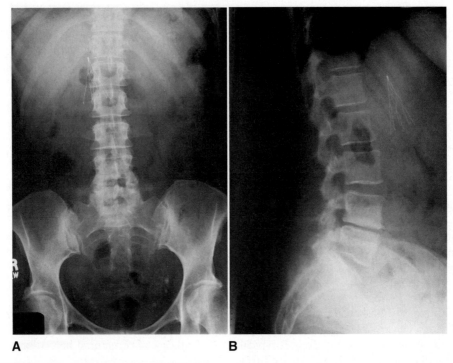

FIG. 8-25 A, Greenfield filter placement in the inferior vena cava, as seen on an AP abdomen radiograph. **B,** Greenfield filter placement in the inferior vena cava, as seen on a lateral abdomen radiograph.

respiratory distress, cyanosis, and a weak or impalpable pulse.

Patent Ductus Arteriosus

The **ductus arteriosus** is a temporary vessel that serves during in utero life. It shunts blood from the pulmonary artery into the systemic circulation because the pulmonary circulation is unneeded during this time. If it does not close at birth, **patent ductus arteriosus** results (Figs. 8-27 and 8-28). This condition is more common in premature infants, occurring in approximately 80% of infants born before 28 weeks of gestation, especially in those who have respiratory distress syndrome.

Because the left ventricle contracts with more force than the right ventricle, the arterial blood within the aorta is shunted into the pul-

monary trunk via the open ductus arteriosus instead of out into the systemic circulation. This increases the volume of blood propelled into the lungs, thus increasing pulmonary vascular congestion and the volume of blood returning to the left atrium. Infants with this condition generally have a heart murmur and display cyanotic features resulting from the shunting. Echocardiography is the imaging method of choice for evaluating the severity of this anomaly usually demonstrating a left atrial diameter larger than the aortic root. Color Doppler technology demonstrates the reverse pulmonary artery flow during diastole and can show the full length of the ductus arteriosis. Chest radiographs of the infant demonstrate cardiomegaly with prominence of the left side of the heart and ascending aorta and increased

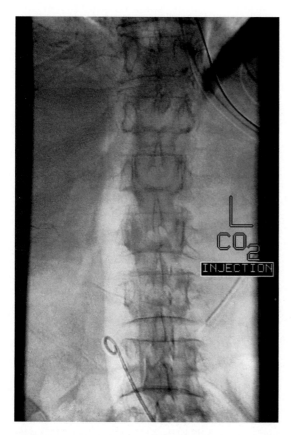

FIG. 8-26 Use of carbon dioxide (CO₂) as a contrast medium is demonstrated in this inferior vena cavagram (appearing white along the right of the spine) on a frail 75-year-old man.

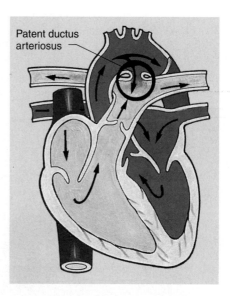

FIG. 8-27 Patent ductus arteriosus.

pulmonary vascular congestion. In premature infants, treatment includes fluid restriction and diuresis, the use of drugs, or surgical intervention. Surgery is used as a last resort on premature infants and generally does not occur until the infant is 1 to 2 years in age. In full-term infants, surgical ligation is necessary in cases of heart failure. In full-term infants without distress, elective surgery is generally performed between the ages of 6 months and 3 years to decrease the chance of the infant developing infective endarteritis.

Coarctation of the Aorta

Although the ductus arteriosus may close normally at birth, a narrowing of the aorta may occur at the junction site. This anomaly is termed **coarctation of the aorta** (Fig. 8-29) and is the cause of 7% to 8% of all congenital cardiac anomalies. It occurs anatomically inferior to the vessels responsible for circulation to the head, neck, and upper extremities, so circulation to these anatomic regions is not affected. However, blood flow to the abdomen and lower extremities is compromised, and the femoral pulse is very weak in most individuals possessing this anomaly. This anomaly may lead to heart failure. Radiographically, two bulges of the aorta are demonstrated in the aortic arch region, one superior to and one inferior to the stenosis. Rib notching, another radiographic indication of coarctation of the aorta, refers to well-defined bony erosions along the lower rib margins as a result of the enlargement of anastomotic vessels. Coarctation of the aorta may be successfully treated surgically by removing the narrowed region of the aorta and reattaching

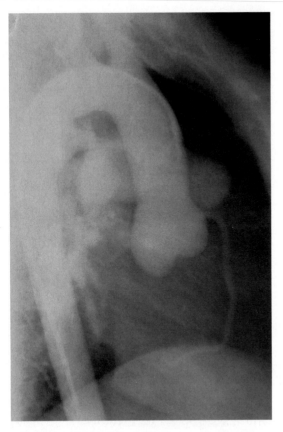

FIG. 8-28 Aortogram demonstrating patent ductus arteriosus. Notice filling of the pulmonary vessels as well as the aorta.

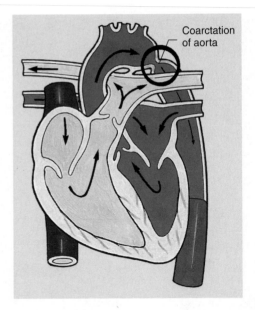

FIG. 8-29 Coarctation of the aorta.

the normal aorta superior and inferior to the coarctation.

Septal Defects

A defect in either the ventricular or atrial septum allows the blood to be shunted between the two chambers (Figs. 8-30 and 8-31), mixing pulmonary and systemic blood. The blood is generally shunted from the left to the right chamber because of increased pressure in the left side of the heart. This shunting of the blood results in an enlargement of the right side of the heart and increased pulmonary vascularity as the lungs overload with blood.

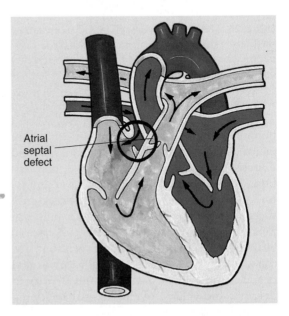

FIG. 8-30 Atrial septal defect.

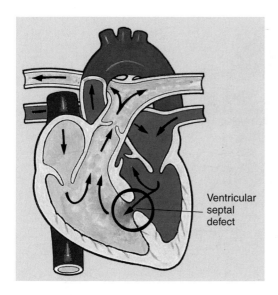

FIG. 8-31 Ventricular septal defect.

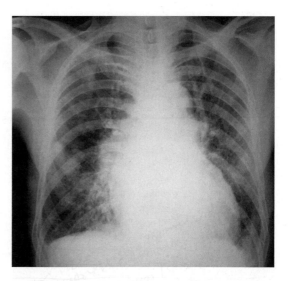

FIG. 8-32 Chest radiograph depicting ventricular septal defect. Notice the enlargement of the right heart border.

If the foramen ovale does not close at birth, an opening remains between the right and left atria. **Atrial septal defects** are the most common congenital heart defect, responsible for about 10% of all cases of congenital heart disease. This defect also occurs twice as frequently in girls as in boys and is generally detected clinically by an audible heart murmur at the upper left sternal border around the age of 1 year as well as by atrial dysrhythmias on ECG evaluation. Doppler and 2-D echocardiography may also be performed to confirm the diagnosis. Radiographically, the right atrium and ventricle are enlarged, resulting in cardiomegaly. There is also evidence of increased pulmonary blood flow within the lung fields. In most cases, this does not require surgical intervention. However, if surgical intervention is necessary, a preoperative cardiac catheterization may be performed to evaluate the size of the defect, left ventricular function, and the vessel anatomy.

Ventricular septal defects involve defects between the two ventricles and are more serious because the pressure difference is greater between the ventricles than between the atria. Clinically, these patients also present an audible heart murmur; however, it is heard a little lower on the left sternal border and at a younger age than the murmur associated with an atrial defect. In significant cases of ventricular septal defect, the murmur may be audible in infants as young as 2 to 3 weeks old. In these cases, intervention is necessary, as signs of heart failure may develop between 6 and 8 weeks of age. In addition, these infants are at an increased risk for developing severe viral or bacterial pneumonia and infective endocarditis. Again, color flow **Doppler echocardiography** is the imaging method of choice. Radiographically, the left atrium and ventricle are enlarged, resulting in cardiomegaly (Fig. 8-32). Increased pulmonary flow is also evident in the lung fields. Surgical intervention depends on the size of the defect and the risk of developing bacterial endocarditis at the site of the defect.

Transposition of Great Vessels

Transposition of great vessels is an anomaly in which the aorta arises from the right

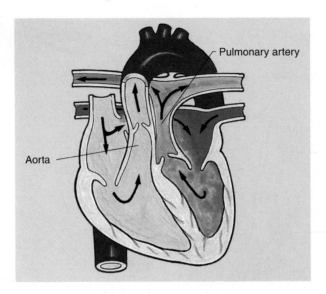

FIG. 8-33 Transposition of great vessels.

ventricle instead of the left ventricle and the pulmonary trunk arises from the left ventricle instead of the right ventricle (Figs. 8-33 and 8-34). This serious congenital defect does not allow the pulmonary and systemic subsystems to communicate and comprises over 5% of all cardiac anomalies. Deoxygenated blood returns to the right atrium, travels through the right ventricle, and is pumped through the aorta back into the systemic subsystem without becoming oxygenated. The oxygenated blood returns to the left atrium, travels through the left ventricle, and is pumped through the pulmonary trunk back to the lungs for gas exchange to occur. A conventional chest radiograph demonstrates a narrow mediastinum because the vessels are superimposed and the main pulmonary trunk is not in the usual location. Pulmonary congestion is also visible in the lung fields. Obviously, this anomaly is incompatible with life. Because immediate recognition and treatment of this defect are imperative, echocardiography is performed to confirm the diagnosis. Emergency cardiac catheterization and balloon septostomy must be performed to enlarge the opening between the atria to

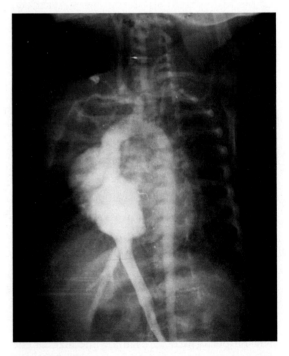

FIG. 8-34 Angiogram demonstrating transposition of great vessels. Notice the "closed" system of the right side of the heart. The blood is returned via the venae cavae and redistributed via the aorta, thus bypassing the lungs.

increase mixing of venous and arterial blood and to decompress the left atrium. Surgical correction of this anomaly is indicated within the first 10 days of life.

Tetralogy of Fallot

Tetralogy of Fallot is a combination of four defects: pulmonary stenosis, ventricular septal defect, overriding aorta, and hypertrophy of the right ventricle (Fig. 8-35). The narrowing of the pulmonary valve prevents passage of a sufficient volume of blood from the right ventricle to the lungs and results in the most common cause of cyanosis in infants with cardiovascular anomalies. Normally, the aorta should arise from the left ventricle, but, in patients with Tetralogy of Fallot, the aorta arises from a ventricular septal defect. In other words, it overrides the right ventricle, which, in turn, results in hypertrophy of the right ventricle. Enlargement of the right ventricle is demonstrated radiographically as a boot-shaped cardiac shadow caused by displacement of the heart apex (Fig. 8-36). Corrective surgery is usually performed after the age of 1 year.

VALVULAR DISEASE

Abnormalities of the heart's valves often cause cardiac symptoms such as dyspnea, fatigue, syncope, or chest pain, and signs such as murmurs. Additionally, lesions of the valves often result in abnormal pulses detectable through palpation. Clinicians are often able to diagnose most valve abnormalities by assimilating historical and physical findings. Noninvasive techniques add to the precision of diagnosis, and invasive studies are reserved for surgical candidates.

The most common cause of chronic valve disease of the heart is **rheumatic fever.** This condition most frequently affects the bicuspid (mitral) and aortic valves and is more common in women than in men. Because of advances in pharmaceuticals, technology, and medical care, the incidence of rheumatic heart disease is on

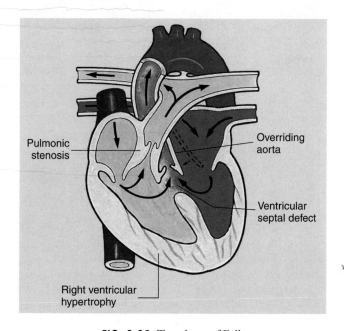

FIG. 8-35 Tetrology of Fallot.

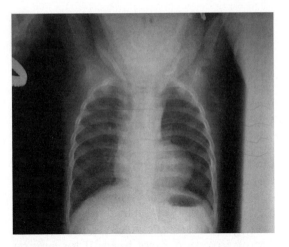

FIG. 8-36 Chest radiograph on an infant with Tetralogy of Fallot. Notice the "boot-shaped" cardiac shadow.

the decline. Rheumatic fever produces inflammatory changes within the connective tissues of the body, thus affecting the valves within the heart. It may result in stenosis, insufficiency, or incompetency. Individuals suffering from rheumatic heart disease present a distinct heart murmur audible on physical examination.

Valvular stenosis (Fig. 8-37) is caused by a scarring of valve cusps that eventually adhere to one another. The results of valvular stenosis become apparent in adult life because it generally takes years for the scarring to affect valve function. Mitral valve stenosis inhibits blood flow from the left atrium into the left ventricle. It slows the blood flow through the lungs and the right side of the heart, resulting in an enlargement of the right side of the heart and the left atrium. Insufficiency and incompetency

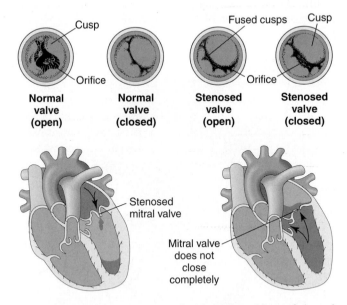

FIG. 8-37 Valvular stenosis and regurgitation. **A,** Normal position of the valve leaflets, or cusps, when the valve is open and closed. **B,** Open position of a stenosed valve *(left)* and open position of a closed regurgitant valve *(right)*. **C,** Hemodynamic effect of mitral stenosis. The stenosed valve is unable to open sufficiently during left atrial systole, inhibiting left ventricular filling. **D,** Hemodynamic effect of mitral regurgitation. The mitral valve does not close completely during left ventricular systole, permitting blood to reenter the left atrium.

occur when the valves do not close properly and allow blood to reflux during systole. This complication often follows endocarditis or is seen in the case of mitral valve prolapse. Mitral valve prolapse is a genetic disease caused by an autosomal dominant inheritance occurring in about 6% of the population and is generally diagnosed by clinical examination. Echocardiography is usually performed to confirm the diagnosis and has approximately a 95% accuracy rate. Patients with mitral valve prolapse are at an increased risk of developing endocarditis, so prophylactic treatment is necessary.

Damaged valves are often replaced surgically, especially in patients experiencing symptoms of heart failure. Patients with a reduced ejection fraction diagnosed by either nuclear medicine studies or echocardiography are also candidates for surgery. These patients must receive prophylactic medication to prevent endocarditis both preoperatively and postoperatively. Cardiac catheterization is performed before surgery to assess the valve function and to evaluate the presence of CAD. Following surgery, patients are generally placed on a variety of medications to help maintain proper cardiac function.

Radiographically, manifestations of mitral stenosis may be subtle. More progressed cases may show the heart silhouette as enlarged with a straightening of the left cardiac border and a prominent main pulmonary artery. The diseased valves may contain small calcifications visible during echocardiographic or CT evaluation. Mitral valve insufficiency appears radiographically as an enlargement of the left atrium and ventricle with right upper lobe pulmonary congestion. Color Doppler echocardiography provides quantification or grading of the severity of regurgitation; however, TEE provides the most information in terms of mitral valve function. In cases of aortic valvular disease, both conventional chest radiographs and echocardiograms may demonstrate calcification of the cusps of the valve and hypertrophy of the septum. Left ventricular enlargement is generally present only when the left ventricular

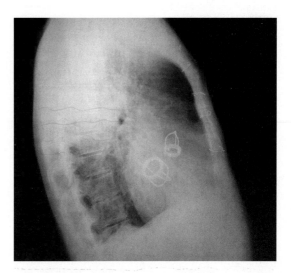

FIG. 8-38 Lateral chest radiograph demonstrating two prosthetic valve replacements clearly visible within the heart.

myocardium is damaged. In cases of tricuspid damage, the right side of the heart is affected, and chest radiographs will reveal enlargement of the superior vena cava, right atrium, and right ventricle. The right ventricular enlargement is best demonstrated on the lateral projection of the chest. Doppler and 2-D echocardiograms confirm the diagnosis by demonstrating increased dimensions in the right side of the heart. Following valve replacement, the prosthetic devices are clearly visible on conventional chest radiographs (Fig. 8-38).

CONGESTIVE HEART FAILURE

Congestive heart failure occurs when the heart is unable to propel blood at a sufficient rate and volume. This results in congestion of the circulatory subsystems and does not allow a sufficient supply of blood to reach the tissues of the body. Congestive heart failure is most commonly caused by hypertension but may result from other disease processes that overburden the heart, such as valvular disease. Congestive heart failure may affect either side of the heart, but both sides are commonly affected together. It may develop gradually or have a quick onset in combination with pulmonary edema. Regardless of the original side affected, prolonged strain on the heart eventually affects the entire organ. Signs and symptoms may vary with the extent and location of the disease. The treatment of congestive failure is usually medical but depends on the cause and severity of the disease and may include surgical intervention, especially in cases of valvular disease.

Left-Sided Failure

When the left ventricle of the heart cannot pump an amount of blood equal to the venous return in the right ventricle, the pulmonary circulatory subsystem becomes overloaded. The fluid that accumulates in the capillaries of the lungs leaks into the interstitial tissues within the lungs. This results in rales and pulmonary edema, which can be a life-threatening condition. Radiographically, the heart is enlarged, and the hilar region of the lungs are congested with increased vascular markings (Fig. 8-39). On physical examination, individuals with left-sided heart failure present an increased heart

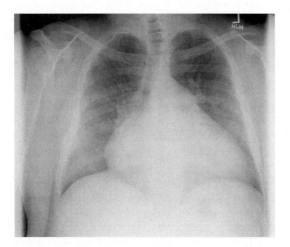

FIG. 8-39 Chest radiograph demonstrating cardiomegaly resulting from congestive heart failure.

rate because the heart tries to compensate for the deficiency. Individuals commonly complain of difficulty in breathing or shortness of breath on exertion and respiratory distress severe enough to awaken them during the night. As the disease progresses, sleeping in a recumbent position becomes impossible. The most common cause of left-side failure is hypertension, but other causes include aortic and mitral valvular disease and CAD.

Right-Sided Failure

Right ventricular failure is not as common as left-sided failure and occurs when the right ventricle cannot pump as much blood as it receives from the right atrium. This causes the venous blood flow to slow down, producing engorgement of the superior and inferior venae cavae and edema of the lower extremities. A common complaint from individuals with right-sided failure is swelling of their ankles. Radiographically, the right atrium and right ventricle appear enlarged. Common causes of true right-sided failure are pulmonary valve stenosis, emphysema, and pulmonary hypertension secondary to pulmonary emboli.

COR PULMONALE

Cor pulmonale results from some type of lung disorder producing hypertension in the pulmonary artery and an enlargement of the right ventricle of the heart. It may be acute, in the case of a pulmonary embolism, or chronic, as a result of chronic obstructive pulmonary disease (COPD). This disease results from alveolar hypoxia, and common symptoms include dyspnea and syncope on exertion. Patients may also experience chest pain. Conventional chest radiographs reveal enlargement of the right ventricle and a proximal pulmonary artery. Echocardiography and nuclear medicine examinations are performed to demonstrate and evaluate right ventricular function. A right heart catheterization may be performed to confirm the diagnosis. These patients are at an increased risk for venous thrombosis and may be placed on long-term anticoagulants.

DEGENERATIVE DISEASES

Atherosclerosis

Atherosclerosis is a degenerative condition affecting the major arteries of the body, often termed hardening of the arteries. It is the most prevalent disease in humans, occurring in epidemic proportions in the United States. It affects sexes equally; however, it tends to affect men at an earlier age than women. Women are not generally affected until after menopause. Atherosclerosis may occur in any artery (Fig. 8-40), but it has a predilection for the

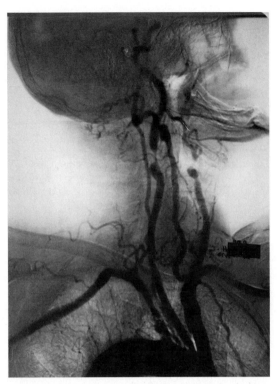

FIG. 8-41 A digital subtraction arteriogram demonstrating atherosclerotic disease of the carotid artery. Notice that the carotid artery is almost completely occluded.

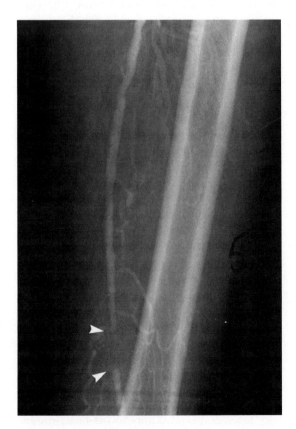

FIG. 8-40 Arteriogram on a 47-year-old man demonstrates how atherosclerosis occludes the femoral artery.

aorta, coronary arteries, and cerebral arteries (Fig. 8-41). Risk factors associated with this disorder that cannot be controlled include increased age and a strong family history of atherosclerosis. Risk factors that can be altered include increased serum low-density lipoproteins (LDL), reduced levels of high-density lipoproteins (HDL), hypertension, cigarette smoking, obesity, and a sedentary life style. In addition, some other disease processes, such as diabetes mellitus, predispose individuals to atherosclerotic disease.

Atheroma formations (fibrofatty plaques) are comprised of intracellular and extracellular lipids, muscle, and connective tissue. They begin as fatty streaks progressing to fibrous

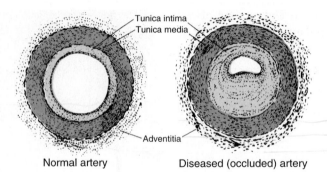

FIG. 8-42 The development of arteriosclerosis.

plaque, which collects within the vessel and reduces its ability to expand during systole (Fig. 8-42). The cause of the development of these formations within the vessel is currently being debated, but two hypotheses, the chronic endothelial injury theory and the lipid theory, are most prominent. The chronic endothelial injury theory suggests that the disease process first affects the intima or inner layer of the artery as a result of injury, resulting in an accumulation of platelets, monocytes, and T-cell lymphocytes at the site of injury. These cells cause a migration of the smooth muscle tissue from the media, forming a fibrous plaque. The lipid theory suggests that an increase in LDL within the blood plasma causes lipid accumulation in smooth muscle cells. The LDL becomes oxidized, and this modification affects the monocytes, creating fat-laden macrophages and foam cells. As these cells enlarge and project into the vessel lumen, platelets aggregate to the site. Oxidized LDL has been found to be toxic to endothelial cells and may be responsible for their dysfunction. The reality may be a combination of the two theories because the oxidized LDL may injure the endothelium, attracting the monocytes and macrophages as described in the endothelial injury hypothesis. As the disease slowly progresses, the vessel becomes stenotic, and the atheroma may calcify (Fig. 8-43), hemorrhage, ulcerate, or include a superimposed thrombosis. These arterial changes often occur

silently, and symptoms may not be present until atheroma formation occludes more than two thirds of the vessel. In some cases, this slow narrowing allows enough time for the formation of collateral vessels to maintain blood supply distal to the stenotic site. If normal blood supply is decreased or stopped completely, **ischemia** occurs. Unfortunately, the most common signs and symptoms associated with atherosclerotic disease result from ischemia of a vital organ, such as the heart or brain, or a weakening of a vital artery resulting in an aneurysm. Atherosclerotic disease is the most common cause of coronary heart disease and cerebrovascular accidents.

Cardiovascular angiography is often used in the diagnosis and treatment of atherosclerosis through the use of PTA. Doppler sonography also plays a major role in diagnosis of atherosclerosis (Fig. 8-44). MRI (Fig. 8-45) and echocardiography are both noninvasive modalities that may also visualize blood flow without the use of contrast agents.

Coronary Artery Disease

CAD results from the deposition of atheromas in the arteries supplying blood to the heart muscle. As the plaques accumulate in the coronary arteries, blood supply to the heart muscle is decreased, resulting in ischemia, a local and temporary impairment of circulation caused by obstruction of circulation, and myocardial

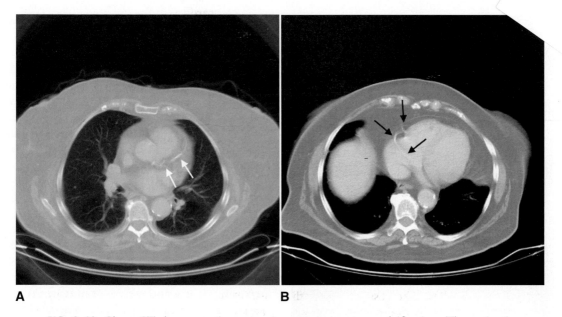

A **B**

FIG. 8-43 Chest CT demonstrating extensive coronary artery calcification. The patient's major complaint was shortness of breath.

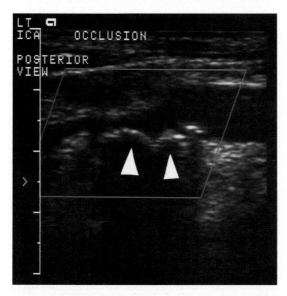

FIG. 8-44 Atherosclerosis as seen in Doppler sonography of the internal carotid artery in a 75-year-old man. Arrows point to the "hilly" plaque deposit on the lower surface of the artery; the lack of echo signal underneath them indicates calcium contained within the plaque.

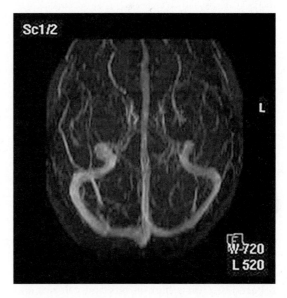

FIG. 8-45 2-D time flight MR image of normal venous blood flow of the brain within the sagittal and transverse sinuses.

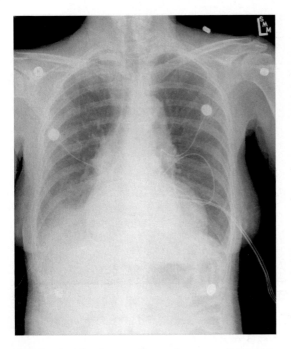

FIG. 8-46 PA chest radiograph on patient with known CAD demonstrates cardiomegaly with left ventricular configuration and mild dilatation of the thoracic aorta.

damage as an **infarct,** an area of ischemic necrosis (Fig. 8-46). Major complications of CAD include angina pectoris (chest pain), myocardial infarction, and subsequent myocardial necrosis, if the patient survives the heart attack. CAD is responsible for over 30% of all annual deaths in the United States and is the single most frequent cause of death in both men and women. Most cases, on autopsy, demonstrate significant widespread atherosclerotic disease of the coronary arteries.

As mentioned earlier, the exact etiology of plaque formation is unknown. However, risk factors for CAD are well known and include tobacco use, diets high in fats and calories and low in phytochemicals and fiber, and poor physical fitness. Recent research has demon-

strated the possibility that a common variant of the platelet fibrinogen receptor may also be a strong predictor of CAD.

Medical treatments of CAD may include antianginal drugs to improve circulation and decrease the amount of oxygen consumed by the myocardium. Other cases may be treated surgically with coronary artery bypass grafts, which involve bypassing the obstruction with a segment of the saphenous vein. A portion of the saphenous vein is removed from the patient's leg, and one end is attached to the aorta above the level of the coronary arteries. The lower end of the graft is attached to the coronary artery, beyond the site of the occlusion.

Nuclear medicine studies such as myocardial perfusion scans and gated examinations are important noninvasive methods of determining the presence and extent of CAD; these studies also assist in the clinical management of post-myocardial patients. In addition, echocardiography may be used to provide needed clinical information in the diagnosis, treatment, and management of CAD. It is also helpful in demonstrating abnormalities in the left ventricular wall motion when the diagnosis of myocardial infarction is uncertain.

Myocardial Infarction

Myocardial infarction is most commonly caused by an acute thrombus of the coronary arteries and primarily affects the left ventricle of the heart. The ability of the heart to continue pumping blood depends on the extent of muscle damage. Clinical signs and symptoms of myocardial infarction include a sudden onset of severe crushing chest pain that may radiate down the left arm or up into the neck. It may be accompanied by profuse sweating, shortness of breath, nausea, or vomiting. In milder cases, it may be passed off as indigestion, and women often experience atypical chest discomfort. Immediate medical attention is critical to the survival of individuals experiencing a myocar-

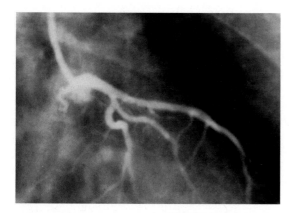

FIG. 8-47 Coronary angiography demonstrates a normal left anterior descending artery as shown in this RAO projection.

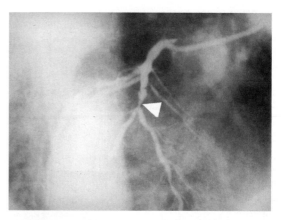

FIG. 8-48 A major stenosis is seen in this coronary arteriogram in an LAO projection, just as the left coronary artery bifurcates into the left anterior descending artery to the right and a major diagonal branch to the left.

dial infarction. Approximately 20% to 25% of these patients die before reaching the hospital, primarily from ventricular fibrillation. Early medical intervention significantly increases survival. Survival rates are approximately 85% for those first attack victims receiving medical attention within the first 30 minutes after the attack. The prognosis of CAD is variable, depending largely on the location of the occlusion, the extent of damage to the heart muscle, and the amount of collateral circulation available.

Cardiac angiography plays a major role in the diagnosis of stenotic or occluded heart vessels (Figs. 8-47 and 8-48). Thrombolytic therapy is a widely accepted treatment, and it is most effective if administered within hours of the onset of a myocardial infarction. If therapy is started within 3 hours, the chances of survival are better. The most common thrombolytic agents include streptokinase, anistreplase, alteplase, and reteplase. In some cases, PCTA may be performed to open these vessels and has been found to be as effective as thrombolytic therapy.

ANEURYSMS

A localized "ballooning" or outpouching of a vessel wall is called an **aneurysm.** It results when the vessel wall has been weakened by atherosclerotic disease, trauma, infection, or congenital defects. Aneurysms are usually classified as saccular, fusiform, or dissecting (Fig. 8-49). A **saccular aneurysm** is a localized bulge involving one side of the arterial wall (Fig. 8-50). Usually, it is located in a cerebral artery. If this bulging includes the entire circumference of the vessel wall, it is termed **fusiform.** This type is often found in the distal abdominal aorta. A **dissecting aneurysm** results when the intima tears and allows blood to flow within the vessel wall, thus forming an intramural hematoma (Fig. 8-51). Symptoms of a dissecting aneurysm often mimic those of a heart attack.

Although an aneurysm may occur anywhere in the aorta, the majority (75%) occur in the abdominal aorta, with 90% of those occurring below the level of the renal arteries. Abdominal aortic aneurysms (AAA) may cause pain, or the patient may remain symptom-free. Conventional

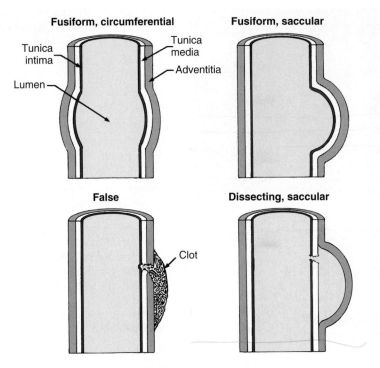

Fusiform, circumferential

Tunica intima

Tunica media

Adventitia

Lumen

Fusiform, saccular

False

Clot

Dissecting, saccular

FIG. 8-49 Types of aneurysms.

abdominal images are of little value; however, a cross-table lateral abdomen radiograph may show enlargement of the aorta with calcification of the vessel wall. Diagnostic medical sonography, MRI, and CT are fairly noninvasive and are of value in determining the size and extent of the aneurysm (Figs. 8-52 and 8-53). Aortography is an invasive procedure that also helps delineate the aneurysm, especially in cases where the aneurysm extends above the renal arteries. Surgical repair is necessary for AAAs larger than 6 cm in diameter. The aneurysm is removed, and the section of the vessel is replaced with a synthetic graft (Fig. 8-54), possibly extending to the iliac arteries.

Thoracic aortic aneurysms most commonly result from congenital anomalies or blunt chest trauma. These are visible on conventional chest radiographs (Fig. 8-55); however, CT, MRI, and transesophageal ultrasound are most helpful in assessing the size and extent of the aneurysm. As in the case of AAAs, thoracic aortic aneurysms are surgically repaired if they are equal to or greater than 6 cm in diameter. Aneurysms may also occur in the extremities, most commonly in the popliteal artery. These often are bilateral and occur in conjunction with an abdominal aortic aneurysm. Popliteal aneurysms are generally confirmed by ultrasonic evaluation or CT. Arteriography may also be performed. Intracranial aneurysms are discussed in Chapter 10 of this text.

VENOUS THROMBOSIS

The formation of blood clots within a vein is called **venous thrombosis.** These clots commonly form in the veins of the lower extremities (Fig. 8-56) and result from a slowing of the blood return to the heart. The contraction of the leg muscles assists with venous blood return; therefore, postoperative or bedfast

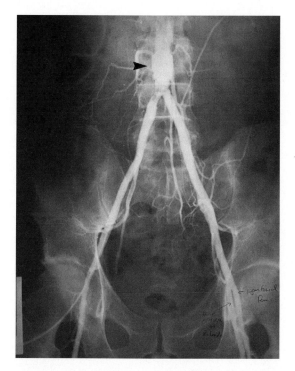

FIG. 8-50 Abdominal aortogram on a 53-year-old man demonstrating a saccular abdominal aneurysm and bilateral areas of stenosis at the bifurcation of the aorta into the common iliac arteries.

patients are especially prone to this disorder. **Phlebitis,** an inflammation of the vein, is often associated with venous thrombosis. The medical term used to specify the combination of these disorders is **thrombophlebitis.** The **thrombus** formation generally begins in the valves of the deep calf veins where thromboplastin traps red blood cells to create the blood clot. Patients may be placed on anticoagulant drugs or receive thrombolytic therapy.

Sonography is performed to determine the location and the extent of this disease, primarily in the lower extremities, and venography may be of use in confirming the diagnosis. One major complication associated with deep vein thrombosis is the development of a pulmonary embolism. Filters may be placed in the patient's inferior vena cava to prevent these clots from reaching the kidneys and chest. These filters may be inserted under fluoroscopic control and are clearly visible on plain radiographs of the abdomen (Fig. 8-57).

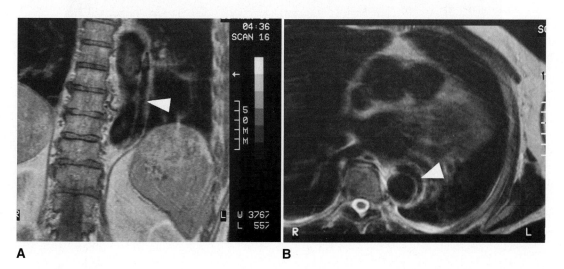

FIG. 8-51 A, A dissecting aneurysm in a 79-year-old man seen in a coronal MRI view, with clear depiction of the extraluminal flow. **B,** A dissecting aneurysm in a 79-year old man, seen as extraluminal flow in this transverse MRI view, which represents a view looking down into the aorta.

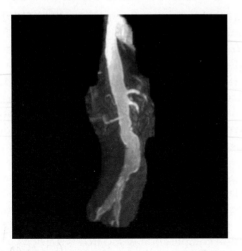

FIG. 8-52 A 3-D reconstruction of an MRA demonstrating an abdominal aortic aneurysm below the level of the renal arteries.

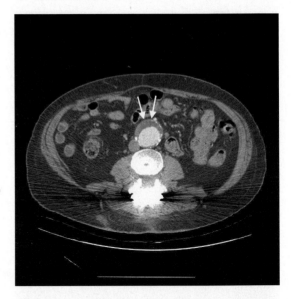

FIG. 8-53 A contrast-enhanced axial CT image showing an infrarenal abdominal aortic aneurysm approximately 4 cm in diameter.

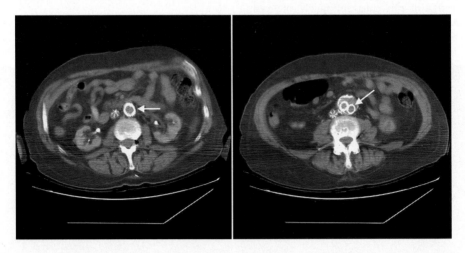

FIG. 8-54 CT examination of a patient after graft placement for AAA.

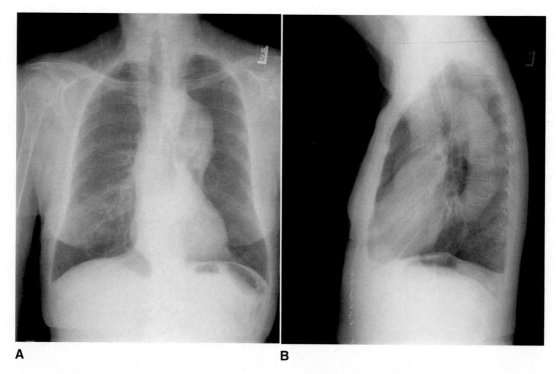

A   **B**

FIG. 8-55 A, PA chest radiograph demonstrating a widened mediastinum as a result of a thoracic aortic aneurysm. **B,** Lateral projection of the chest on the same patient as in **A.**

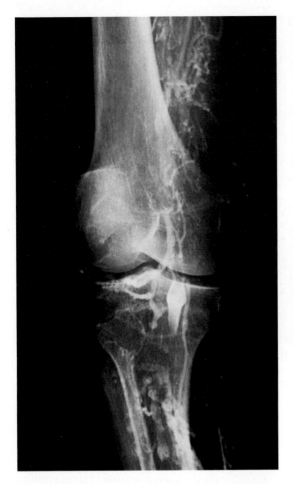

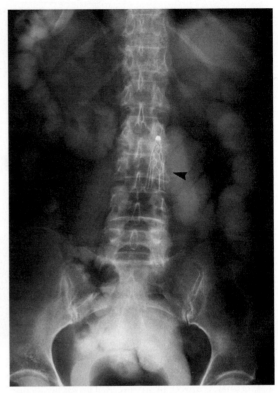

FIG. 8-57 Abdominal radiograph on an elderly woman demonstrating the proper placement of a vena cava filter.

FIG. 8-56 Venogram of the left lower extremity demonstrating deep vein thrombosis.

PATHOLOGY SUMMARY: THE CARDIOVASCULAR SYSTEM

Pathology	Imaging Modalities of Choice	Additive or Subtractive Pathology
Patent ductus arteriosus	Echocardiography	
Coarctation of the aorta	Echocardiography and chest radiography	Additive because of enlarged mediastinum
Septal defects	Echocardiography, chest radiography, and cardiac catheterization	Additive because of enlarged mediastinum
Transposition of great vessels	Echocardiography and cardiac catheterization	
Tetrology of Fallot	Echocardiography, chest radiography	Additive because of enlarged mediastinum
Valvular disease	Echocardiography, cardiac catheterization, and chest radiography	Additive because of enlarged mediastinum
Congestive heart failure	Chest radiography	Additive because of fluid in great vessels and lungs
Cor pulmonale	Echocardiography, nuclear medicine cardiac studies, chest radiography	Additive because of enlarged rt. ventricle and pulmonary a.
Atherosclerosis	Ultrasound and angiography	
Coronary artery disease	Echocardiography, nuclear medicine cardiac studies, CT	
Myocardial infarction	Cardiac catheterization and nuclear medicine cardiac studies	
Aneurysm	Ultrasound, MR, and CT	
Venous thrombosis	Ultrasound	

QUESTIONS

1. The heart chamber located most anteriorly and comprising the anterior border of the cardiac shadow on a lateral chest radiograph is the:
   a. left atrium
   b. left ventricle
   c. right atrium
   d. right ventricle

2. The bicuspid valve is also known as the:
   a. left atrioventricular valve
   b. right atrioventricular valve
   c. aortic valve
   d. pulmonary valve

3. Contraction of the myocardium is termed:
   a. diastole
   b. systole
   c. peristole
   d. myostol

4. How many posterior ribs should be visible on a good inspiration PA chest radiograph?
   a. 12
   b. 10
   c. 8
   d. 6

5. In a fetus, the ductus arteriosus connects which two structures?
   a. aorta and SVC
   b. aorta and pulmonary trunk
   c. right and left atria
   d. right and left ventricles

6. Tetralogy of Fallot includes which of the following defects?
   a. pulmonary stenosis
   b. ventricular septal defect
   c. hypertrophy of right ventricle
   d. a and c
   e. a, b, and c

7. A condition in which the left ventricle cannot pump an amount of blood equal to the venous return of the right ventricle is:
   a. coronary artery disease
   b. left-sided congestive heart failure
   c. right-sided congestive heart failure
   d. patent ductus arteriosus

8. Risk factors associated with atherosclerosis include:
   1. low blood sugar levels
   2. hypertension
   3. cigarette smoking
   a. 1 and 2   c. 2 and 3
   b. 1 and 3   d. 1, 2, and 3

9. A decrease in tissue blood supply is termed:
   a. atheroma   c. ischemia
   b. infarction   d. necrosis

10. The single most frequent cause of deaths in the United States is:
    a. congestive heart failure
    b. coronary artery disease
    c. transposition of great vessels
    d. valvular disease

11. Clinical signs of a myocardial infarction include:
    1. shortness of breath
    2. crushing chest pain
    3. neck pain
    a. 1 and 2   c. 2 and 3
    b. 1 and 3   d. 1, 2, and 3

12. Which type of vessels are used as the graft material for coronary artery bypass grafts?
    a. arteries
    b. capillaries
    c. veins

13. Aortic aneurysms most commonly occur in the:
    a. abdominal aorta above the level of the renal arteries.
    b. abdominal aorta below the level of the renal arteries.
    c. thoracic aorta.

14. Imaging procedures that may be used to demonstrate an abdominal aneurysm include:
    1. angiography
    2. CT
    3. sonography
    a. 1 and 2
    b. 1 and 3
    c. 2 and 3
    d. 1, 2, and 3

15. Venous thrombosis most often affects the:
    a. deep veins of the upper extremities.
    b. deep veins of the lower extremities.
    c. superficial veins of the upper extremities.
    d. superficial veins of the lower extremities.

16. What common imaging procedures provide functional information regarding the heart?

17. Which type of aneurysm results when the intima tears and allows blood to flow within the vessel wall?

18. An elderly patient presents with shortness of breath on exertion and overall respiratory distress. A chest radiograph reveals an enlarged heart and a congested hilar region, with some pulmonary edema. What is a likely cause?

19. Identify at least two common sites for atherosclerosis to occur.

20. What is the cause of ischemia in coronary artery disease?

The Hemopoietic System

UPON COMPLETION OF CHAPTER 9, THE READER SHOULD BE ABLE TO:

- Identify the major constituents of blood and describe the function of each constituent.
- Specify the various blood types.
- Explain the role of the lymphatic system in terms of immunity.
- Describe the pathogenesis, prognosis, and signs and symptoms of the disease processes discussed in this chapter.

ANATOMY AND PHYSIOLOGY

The hemopoietic system consists of blood, lymphatic tissue, bone marrow, and the spleen. The circulating blood contains both plasma and blood cells, with the plasma comprising approximately 55% of the total blood volume. The plasma is about 90% water and 10% solutes such as proteins, glucose, amino acids, and lipids. Three basic types of blood cells—erythrocytes, leukocytes, and thrombocytes (Table 9-1)—make up the remaining 45% of the total blood volume.

The **erythrocytes** or red blood cells are very small in relation to the other blood cells. They do not possess a nucleus and are shaped like biconcave disks. Erythrocytes are responsible for transporting oxygen and carbon dioxide to and from the various organs of the body. This is accomplished via the hemoglobin in the erythrocytes, which allows oxygen or carbon dioxide molecules to attach to the cell for transport. Individuals with a hemoglobin level of less than 12 g per 100 ml of blood have **anemia** and are considered "anemic" because they have less than normal oxygen or carbon dioxide transportation occurring. The total percentage of red blood cells in blood volume is determined by a laboratory test termed **hematocrit.**

Erythrocytes are formed by specialized cells called **hemocytoblasts** that are located in the myeloid tissue found within red bone marrow. These cells live approximately 120 days and are phagocytosed by the **reticuloendothelial system,** which consists of specialized cells in the liver, spleen, and bone marrow. During the phagocytosis, the iron within the hemoglobin is released, and bilirubin is formed. The iron is used again in the development of new erythrocytes, and the bilirubin is excreted in the bile.

Erythrocytes may contain various antigens that determine blood type. This is especially critical for blood transfusions because blood

TABLE 9-1 BLOOD CELL TYPES

Type	Formed by	Function	Life span
Erythrocyte	Myeloid tissue within red bone marrow	Transporting O_2 and CO_2	120 days
Leukocyte			
Granular	Red bone marrow	Body defense	2 weeks
Nongranular	Lymphatic tissue	Immunity	Years
Thrombocyte	Myeloid tissue within red bone marrow	Blood clotting	10 days

type incompatibility can have fatal results. Erythrocytes may contain no antigens, either the A or B antigen, or both the A and B antigens. The resulting blood types are O (no antigen), A, B, and AB. If incompatible blood types are mixed (e.g., a type O patient receives type AB blood), the erythrocytes from the donor clump together in the serum of the recipient. Because the type O recipient does not possess the A or B antigen, antibodies are formed to fight against the foreign red blood cells. This is termed **agglutination.** Eventually, the recipient destroys the donor erythrocytes, with the rejection possibly resulting in immediate shock. In some cases, the reaction may be delayed, resulting in fever, pain, and ultimate renal failure as the kidneys try to excrete the by-products produced from the destruction of the erythrocytes. Cross-matching of blood types to eliminate the chance of a recipient's receiving incompatible blood is essential.

Type O blood is considered the universal donor because it does not contain any antigens and can be given to anyone, regardless of blood type. Type AB is considered the universal recipient because it possesses both antigens and can receive any type of blood (Table 9-2). In addition, the Rh blood factor should also be considered. The **Rh factor** is termed such because it was first discovered in the blood of the rhesus monkey. Approximately 85% of the human population contains this factor and are classified as **Rh-positive.** Individuals not possessing the Rh factor are **Rh-negative.** The Rh factor

becomes a problem if an Rh-positive father transmits the Rh factor to a fetus carried by an Rh-negative mother. The first pregnancy generally progresses normally, but in subsequent pregnancies the mother's anti-Rh antibodies, made during the first pregnancy, attack the Rh-positive fetal blood. This scenario can be avoided by Rh immunization of the mother before pregnancy.

Leukocytes or white blood cells may be classified as granular or nongranular. Granular leukocytes contain cytoplasmic granules and irregular nuclei. They are formed within the red bone marrow and include basophils, neutrophils, and eosinophils. The names of these cells correspond to the manner in which they respond to certain dyes for microscopic inspection. Nongranular leukocytes do not contain cytoplasmic granules, and they possess regular nuclei. They are mainly formed in the lymphatic tissue of the spleen and include lymphocytes and monocytes. Leukocytes play an important role in the body's defense system. They are able to move out of capillaries into tissue to "attack" and phagocytose foreign substances. The life span of leukocytes varies, depending on the type of cell. Granular leukocytes live for only about 2 weeks, whereas lymphocytes may live for years. Normal blood contains between 5000 and 9000 leukocytes per milliliter. Changes in the number of leukocytes often indicate the presence of disease.

The third major type of blood cells are the **thrombocytes** or platelets. These cells are

TABLE 9-2 CROSS-MATCHING OF BLOOD TYPES

Recipient	Acceptable Donor Type			
Blood Type	A	B	AB*	O†
A	yes	no	no	yes
B	no	yes	no	yes
AB*	yes	yes	yes	yes
O†	no	no	no	yes

*AB, Universal recipient
†O, Universal donor

necessary for blood to clot properly and respond within seconds to initiate the coagulation process. The thrombocytes are also formed in the myeloid tissue within the red bone marrow and have a life span of approximately 10 days.

The lymphatic system is a subsystem of the circulatory system. Its major function is in assuring immunity through production of lymphocytes and antibodies, but it is also responsible for absorbing fat from the intestinal tract and for manufacturing blood under certain circumstances. The lymphatic system is comprised of both lymphatic vessels and nodes. Lymphatic vessels contain a milky liquid substance termed **lymph.** The **lymph nodes** are small ovoid bodies attached in a chain-like pattern along the vessels. They filter out particles and foreign materials from the blood. Major areas of lymph node chains include the neck, mediastinum, axillary, retroperitoneal, pelvic, and inguinal regions. These lymph nodes often become enlarged when the body is invaded by an infectious agent and in cases of neoplastic disease.

The spleen, which is also part of the lymphatic system, is an oval organ in the left upper quadrant. Its chief function is production of lymphocytes and plasma cells. Additionally, it stores red blood cells and functions in phagocytosis. It is occasionally ruptured in abdominal trauma and can be removed without detrimental effects.

Mature **lymphocytes** are the most important cells in the development of immunity. T lymphocytes are derived from lymphatic tissue of the thymus gland, and B lymphocytes are derived from the bone marrow. These two types of lymphocytes work together with macrophages to ingest foreign substances and process the specific foreign antigens. Via a complex process, an antibody is formed capable of attacking the foreign antigen. An antibody is an immunoglobulin produced by plasma cells and can be categorized into one of five classifications: IgG, IgM, IgA, IgD, and IgE. This is the systemic response that can have a negative effect on tissue grafts and organ transplants. The human body sees the transplant as foreign; therefore, the lymphocytes and macrophages try to destroy the foreign antigens, resulting in rejection of the graft or organ.

Although the risk of whole-body radiation exposure is of little concern in diagnostic radiology, it is important for the radiographer to remember that exposure to x-rays or γ-rays can have a harmful effect on the blood marrow and lymphoid tissue. It takes a whole-body dose of approximately 0.5 to 0.75 Gy (50 to 75 rad) to cause a detectable change in the blood cells. The most radiosensitive blood cells are the lymphocytes, followed by the leukocytes and thrombocytes.

IMAGING CONSIDERATIONS

Radiography plays a limited role in the diagnosis and treatment of hemopoietic disorders. Skeletal radiography may be used in cases of multiple myeloma and for some types of leukemia. Chest radiographs are helpful in identifying lymphatic changes within the mediastinum and various opportunistic infections associated with acquired immune deficiency syndrome (AIDS). Abdominal computed tomography (CT) is also of great value in the assessment of lymph node enlargement (Fig. 9-1) and may be followed by lymphography to further determine the location and extent of neoplastic diseases of the lymphatic system. CT and magnetic resonance (MR) evaluation of the brain may also assist in the diagnosis and treatment of central nervous system (CNS) complications associated with HIV.

Magnetic resonance imaging (MRI) is quite useful in imaging bone marrow and the diseases that affect the marrow. Although MRI produces a signal void in areas of compact bone, changes in the marrow pattern are quite visible and useful in the diagnosis of many disorders (Fig. 9-2).

Many bloodborne pathogens may be transmitted to the health care worker. Therefore, it

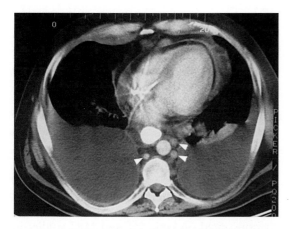

FIG. 9-1 CT of the lower chest and upper abdomen demonstrating enlargement of lymph nodes on a 27-year-old man with lymphoma.

is of utmost importance that radiographers always practice standard precautions in terms of blood and body fluids. Gloves should be worn when performing venipuncture or whenever the possibility of contamination with blood or other body fluids exists. Additional protective apparel may be necessary if large amounts of body fluids may be encountered. Needles should not be recapped; they should be placed in puncture-proof containers for hazardous waste disposal. Handwashing cannot be over-emphasized because it plays an important role in good infection control practices. It is the single most significant factor in infection control.

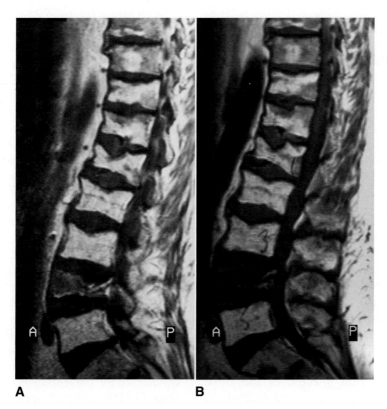

A   **B**

FIG. 9-2 A, A T2-weighted sagittal MRI view without gadolinium demonstrates an obvious L4 lesion. **B,** A T2-weighted sagittal MRI view with gadolinium demonstrates L4 destruction consistent with multiple myeloma in this 55-year-old man.

ACQUIRED IMMUNE DEFICIENCY SYNDROME

Acquired immune deficiency syndrome (AIDS) was first recognized in 1981. It is caused by one of two related human immunodeficiency retroviruses, HIV-1 and HIV-2, and results in a wide range of clinical manifestations. HIV-1, identified in 1984, paralyzes the normal immune mechanisms within the human body, resulting in severe immunosuppression or AIDS. It is responsible for most cases of AIDS in the Western Hemisphere. Less virulent than HIV-1, HIV-2 is the principal agent of AIDS in West Africa. Retroviruses contain reverse transcriptase, an enzyme that converts viral RNA into a DNA copy that becomes integrated into the host cell DNA. Each time the cell divides, the retroviral DNA is duplicated. Both types of HIV also contain HIV protease, an enzyme that converts immature, noninfectious HIV to its infectious state within the cell. The HIV infects a part of the T lymphocytes termed *T4* or *CD4* as well as nonlymphoid cells such as macrophages. Infected individuals experience a brief antibody-negative period immediately following infection, during which time the virus rapidly reproduces until the immune system begins to react to the infectious agent.

Because HIV inhibits the body's response to the presence of a variety of diseases, one major sign of AIDS is the presence of unusual opportunistic infections such as *Pneumocystis carinii,* *Toxoplasma gondii,* cryptococci, *Mycobacterium avium,* and herpes. AIDS is also directly linked to an increased incidence of malignancies such as Kaposi's sarcoma, non-Hodgkin's lymphoma (NHL), Hodgkin's disease, and primary CNS lymphoma. It is the most common disease associated with lymphocytopenia or the depletion of lymphocytes. This occurs through the destruction of CD4+ T cells infected by the virus. Anemia, thrombocytopenia, and leukopenia also commonly occur in HIV-infected patients.

Signs and symptoms associated with HIV and AIDS are broad and may mimic other diseases. They include generalized lymphadenopathy, malaise, fever, and joint pain within 1 to 4 weeks following infection. Weight loss may occur as a result of nausea, vomiting, and diarrhea. As mentioned earlier, leukopenia, anemia, and thrombocytopenia also occur. AIDS can affect the CNS, resulting in apathy, memory loss, inability to concentrate, and dementia. Headaches, fever, or photophobia associated with acute aseptic meningitis; encephalopathy with seizures; or motor, sensory, or gait deficits may be the first manifestations of the disease. Atrophy of the brain cortex is commonly demonstrated on brain CT and MRI studies in patients with subacute encephalitis related to AIDS. In cases of toxoplasmic encephalitis, CT and MRI will demonstrate contrast-enhanced lesions within the basal ganglia.

With no known cure, AIDS remains a major health crisis and places a burden on the health care system in the United States. As a result of advances in the production and use of highly active antiretroviral therapy (HAART) in the United States, the number of individuals diagnosed with AIDS and the number of deaths associated with AIDS have declined since 1996 and leveled off since 1999. In addition, the number of individuals living with AIDS has steadily increased since 1996.

HAART has reduced the incidence of opportunistic infections and extended the lives of individuals infected with AIDS. However, the use of antiviral drugs in the treatment of HIV is continually being reevaluated, and recommendations regarding specific drug regimens are in flux. The use of only one drug results in mutation of the virus as well as resistance to the drug and loss of efficacy of the therapy. Currently, the most common therapy calls for a three-drug regimen to include reverse transcriptase inhibitors and protease inhibitors. Guidelines for preventing opportunistic infections for HIV-affected persons were updated for a fourth time in 2001 by the U.S. Public Health Service and the Infectious Diseases Society of America. Additional information can be accessed at the Centers for Disease Control and Prevention (CDC) web site. Bone marrow evaluation is common in HIV-positive individuals. This diagnostic tool is used to evaluate decreased blood cell counts, to stage malignancies, and to obtain cultures for associated infections.

Although it can affect anyone, regardless of age or sexual orientation, HIV most frequently affects homosexual and bisexual men and intravenous (IV) drug users. The virus is transmitted through sexual contact and exposure to infected blood and body fluids.

One of the most common lung infections associated with HIV is tuberculosis (TB). TB may be the first indication of HIV infection in areas of the world where TB is prevalent. In developed countries, such as the United States, HIV has caused increased rates of TB. The lungs are also a common site for opportunistic infections associated with AIDS such as *Pneumocystis carinii* pneumonia, often in combination with a cytomegalovirus. This fungal infection occurs in over half of all AIDS patients; however, in developed countries the risk of these infections has been reduced through the use of effective prophylactic treatment. Bacterial pneumonias are also common in IV drug users infected with HIV. Chest radiographs demonstrating localized consolidation usually indicate a bacterial infection (Fig. 9-3). *Pneumocystis carinii* infections (Fig. 9-4) generally reveal bilateral perihilar reticular-interstitial infiltrates that rapidly progress within 3 to 5 days to diffuse consolidation.

Kaposi's sarcoma is the most common malignancy in AIDS patients, especially in homosexual or bisexual men who are often coinfected with herpes virus 8. It is present in approximately 25% to 30% of AIDS patients

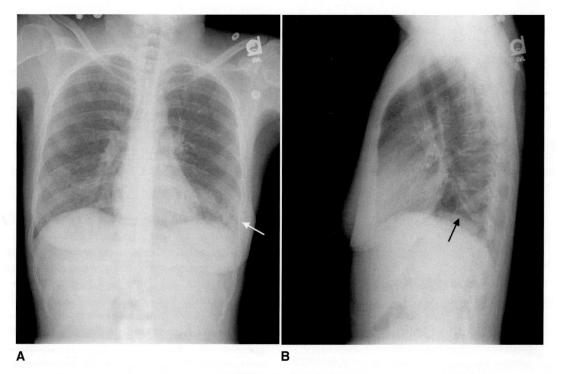

A   **B**

FIG. 9-3 PA (**A**) and left lateral (**B**) chest radiographs of a patient with known AIDS demonstrating a left lower lobe infiltrate.

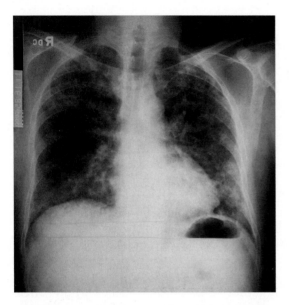

FIG. 9-4 Chest radiograph of a 53-year-old man diagnosed with AIDS. The radiograph demonstrates *Pneumocystis carinii* pneumonia with diffuse bilateral airspace parenchymal infiltrative densities.

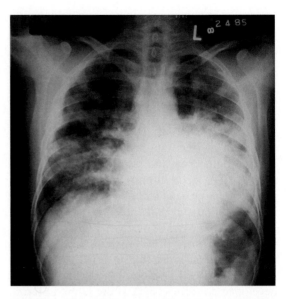

FIG. 9-5 Chest radiograph of a 27-year-old man with Kaposi's sarcoma of the skin and pulmonary involvement showing nodular diffuse patchy parenchymal infiltration with nodular densities in the upper lobes.

and may affect the connective tissue in various sites within the body. It most often affects the skin, lymph nodes, and gastrointestinal system. About 20% of patients with Kaposi's sarcoma also demonstrate pulmonary involvement. Radiographically, the patients present hilar adenopathy, nodular pulmonary infiltrates, and pleural effusion (Fig. 9-5). Endobronchial Kaposi's sarcoma is frequent and may result in atelectasis or postobstruction pneumonia.

NEOPLASTIC DISEASE

Multiple Myeloma

Multiple myeloma is a neoplastic disease of the plasma cells that results in cell proliferation. It is usually confined to the bone marrow and forms discrete tumors that weaken the affected bone.

Multiple myeloma most frequently affects the pelvis, spine, ribs, and skull, resulting in multiple osteolytic lesions and hypercalcemia. The abnormal plasma cells produce large amounts of protein, specifically the immuno-

globulins, which create a variety of problems in addition to skeletal involvement. This protein is excreted via the urine and disrupts normal renal function. The protein can be detected in both blood and urine. The etiology of multiple myeloma is not known, however, researchers suggest a relationship to the type of herpes virus associated with Kaposi's sarcoma, which promotes myeloma growth and stimulates bone resorption.

Multiple myeloma is typically seen in persons over the age of 40, and its signs and symptoms include progressive bone pain, anemia, fatigue, bleeding disorders, renal insufficiency or failure, hypercalcemia, and recurrent bacterial infections, especially pneumococcal pneumonia. It is slightly more common in men than women and in blacks than whites. Radiography plays a vital role in the diagnosis and treatment of multiple myeloma because about 90% of these patients have bony involvement. Skeletal survey radiographs demonstrate diffuse osteoporosis with discrete punched-out, osteolytic regions

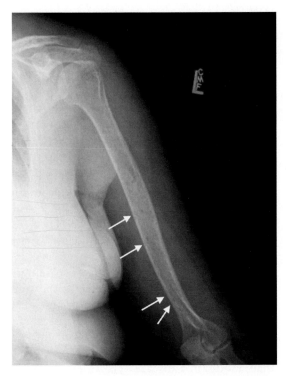

FIG. 9-6 Humerus radiograph of a patient with multiple myeloma demonstrating the presence of discrete, lytic, well-circumscribed skeletal defects.

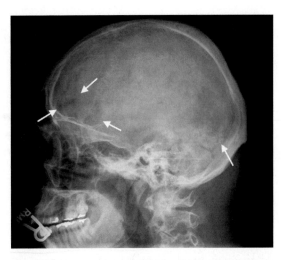

FIG. 9-7 Lateral skull radiograph of a patient with multiple myeloma demonstrating the presence of discrete, lytic, well-circumscribed skeletal defects.

(Figs. 9-6 and 9-7). These patients are at risk for pathologic fractures and vertebral compression fractures because multiple myeloma primarily affects the axial skeleton. A 30% bone loss is necessary before the disease can be visualized with conventional radiography, but MRI is useful in the diagnosis and management of early-stage multiple myeloma. Chemotherapy and palliative radiation therapy may be prescribed, but the prognosis is poor because as the disease progresses it leads to multiple bone lesions, renal failure, and infections. The median survival of patients with multiple myeloma is approximately 2 to 3 years.

Leukemia

Leukemia is a term associated with neoplastic disease of leukocytes that results in an overproduction of white blood cells. This increase in leukocytes interferes with normal blood cell production and may lead to anemia, bleeding, and infection. Leukemias can infiltrate lymphatic tissue and organs such as the liver and spleen. The cause of leukemia is unknown, but exposure to irradiation and certain chemicals (especially benzene), as well as genetic defects such as Down syndrome, seem to predispose individuals to developing this disorder. Current research also indicates an association between leukemia and two viruses: the Epstein-Barr virus and the human T-cell leukemia/lymphoma virus.

Leukemias are classified according to cell type and cell maturity. Granulocytic or myelocytic leukemias develop from primitive or stem cells. Monocytic leukemias develop from precursor cells (the cells from which leukocytes are derived) and are the least common type of leukemia. Lymphocytic leukemias arise from lymphoid cells. Additionally, leukemias are classified as either acute or chronic. Acute leukemias have an abrupt onset and may present as a hemorrhagic episode. They generally are associated with primitive or poorly differentiated cells. Chronic leukemias progress at a relatively slow pace with nonspecific signs such as fatigue and weakness. They are associated with mature or well-differentiated cells. These terms are used in combination to describe the specific type of leukemia.

Acute lymphocytic leukemia (ALL) predominantly affects children. Chronic lymphocytic leukemia (CLL) predominantly affects individuals over age 60. Chronic myelocytic leukemia (CML), also called chronic granulocytic leukemia (CGL), most often affects adults between the ages of 20 and 50. Acute myelocytic leukemia (AML) and acute monoblastic leukemia (AMOL) can affect anyone at any age. Leukemias, in general, account for approximately 33% of all cancer deaths in children under the age of 15 years.

In many cases, proper therapy can stop the pathologic process. Regardless of the type of leukemia, all forms require the destruction of cells by either radiation or antileukemic drug therapy that renders the patient severely immunosuppressed. In some cases, bone marrow transplants may be attempted. Most patients with acute leukemias die within 6 months without treatment. More than 90% of ALLs carry a 5-year remission rate of 50% or better following treatment. Acute myelocytic and AMOLs result in 70% to 85% remission following treatment. In all cases, survival depends on complete remission. CGL, however, is progressive, with an average survival of about 3 to 4 years after the onset of the disease and a 5-year survival rate of approximately 20%. Radiography plays a limited role in the diagnosis and treatment of most leukemias.

Non-Hodgkin's Lymphoma

NHL is a malignancy of the lymphoid cells found in the lymph nodes, bone marrow, spleen, liver, and gastrointestinal system. It is the most common type of lymphoma, and its incidence increases with age. Some patients tolerate NHL very well, and others die very quickly from the disease. Although its etiology is unknown, research indicates that a virus may cause this disease because there is an increased incidence of NHL in HIV patients. Most cases arise from B cells (80% to 85%), and approximately 15% arise from T cells. There are currently two ways to classify lymphomas: Working Formulation, which deals with the prognosis or grade of the disease; and a newer pathologic classification system termed the Revised European-American Lymphoma (REAL) classification.

The signs and symptoms of NHL are varied. In a few cases, the patient presents general lymphadenopathy before developing lymphoma. Many patients also present anemia. Diagnosis is made from a histologic examination of the diseased tissue to differentiate NHL from Hodgkin's disease, leukemia, and metastatic disease. CT of the abdomen and pelvis is commonly employed to stage the disease and demonstrates the extent of disease in the lymphatic system around the aorta and mesentery (Figs. 9-8 and 9-9). A bone biopsy may also be performed, as bone marrow involvement and organ infiltration are more common with NHL than Hodgkin's disease. Treatment of NHL depends on the stage of the disease. It consists

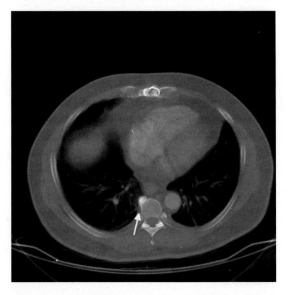

FIG. 9-8 Chest CT of a patient with non-Hodgkin's lymphoma (NHL) demonstrating a necrotic lymph node in the cardiophrenic angle.

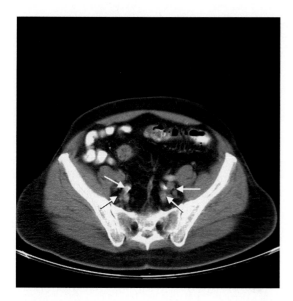

FIG. 9-9 Pelvic CT of a patient with non-Hodgkin's lymphoma (NHL) demonstrating enlarged inguinal lymph nodes.

of chemotherapy and radiation therapy, either in conjunction with one another or independently. In some advanced cases, radiolabeled antibody therapy may also be used.

Hodgkin's Disease

Hodgkin's disease is another neoplastic disease affecting the lymphoid tissue and is also a type of lymphoma. Hodgkin's and NHL generally have a different nodal distribution as seen on CT, as Hodgkin's disease is generally retroperitoneal with less mesenteric involvement than NHL.

Hodgkin's disease has an unknown etiology, commonly affects individuals between the ages of 20 and 40 and those over 60 years of age. It tends to affect men slightly more often than women. Common signs and symptoms associated with Hodgkin's disease are general malaise, fever, anorexia, and enlarged lymph nodes. Mediastinal lymph nodes are often visible on a chest radiograph, and definitive diagnosis is made via biopsy of the lymphatic tissue. **Reed-Sternberg cells** differentiate Hodgkin's lymphomas from other types of lymphatic disease. As with other neoplastic disorders, Hodgkin's disease is staged according to the extent of the disease, most commonly using the Ann Arbor staging system.

CT examinations of the chest, abdomen, and pelvis are used to assist in staging the disease and commonly demonstrate enlarged retroperitoneal nodes. Nuclear medicine gallium scans and MRI of the abdomen may also be useful in staging Hodgkin's disease. In some cases, a laparotomy, including splenectomy, may also be indicated. Stage I denotes one anatomic node location, and stage IV denotes extranodal spread to the bone marrow, the lungs, or the liver.

Hodgkin's disease is most commonly treated and cured with a combination of radiation and chemotherapy. Stage I and IIA Hodgkin's lymphoma can be treated with radiation therapy alone and are associated with a 5-year survival rate of 85% to 90%. Stage IV Hodgkin's disease has approximately a 70% to 80% complete remission rate with more than 50% remaining disease-free for up to 15 years.

PATHOLOGY SUMMARY: THE HEMOPOIETIC SYSTEM

Pathology	Imaging Modalities of Choice
AIDS	CT and MRI
Multiple myeloma	MRI and radiography
Non-Hodgkin's lymphoma	CT
Hodgkin's disease	CT

QUESTIONS

1. The majority of blood volume is comprised of:
   a. erythrocytes
   b. leukocytes
   c. plasma
   d. thrombocytes

2. Bilirubin is formed during the destruction of:
   a. erythrocytes
   b. leukocytes
   c. plastocytes
   d. thrombocytes

3. Which type of blood is considered to be a universal donor?
   a. A
   b. B
   c. AB
   d. O

4. Which cells are most important in the development of immunity?
   a. erythrocytes
   b. lymphocytes
   c. platelets
   d. thrombocytes

5. The most common pulmonary complication resulting from AIDS is:
   a. *Pneumocystis carinii*
   b. pneumococcal pneumonia
   c. Legionnaire's pneumonia
   d. tuberculosis

6. Kaposi's sarcoma is frequently associated with AIDS, and it may affect the:
   a. gastrointestinal system
   b. lymph nodes
   c. skin
   d. all of the above

7. A neoplastic disease of the plasma is:
   a. Hodgkin's disease
   b. leukemia
   c. lymphoma
   d. multiple myeloma

8. Which type of leukemia predominately affects children?
   a. acute lymphocytic
   b. chronic lymphocytic
   c. chronic myelocytic
   d. acute myelocytic

9. Reed-Sternberg cells are associated with what type of neoplastic disease?
   a. leukemia
   b. Hodgkin's disease
   c. multiple myeloma
   d. non-Hodgkin's lymphoma

10. Non-Hodgkin's lymphoma affects what type of blood cells?
    a. erythrocytes
    b. lymphocytes
    c. plastocytes
    d. thrombocytes

11. Explain why researchers currently believe there is an association between viral agents and the development of non-Hodgkin's and Hodgkin's lymphomas.

12. Identify two means of transmission for the AIDS virus.

13. What is the difference in cellular origin between multiple myeloma and leukemia?

14. What is the risk of using radiation or antileukemic drug therapy in treating leukemias?

15. Identify at least three signs and symptoms of Hodgkin's disease.

The Central Nervous System

UPON COMPLETION OF CHAPTER 10, THE READER SHOULD BE ABLE TO:

- Describe the anatomic components of the central nervous system (CNS) and their general function.
- Discuss the roles of the various imaging modalities in evaluation of the CNS, particularly magnetic resonance imaging (MRI) and computed tomography (CT).
- Discuss common congenital anomalies of the CNS.
- Characterize a given condition as inflammatory, degenerative, vascular, or neoplastic.
- Identify the pathogenesis of the pathologies cited and typical treatments for them.
- Discuss the imaging modalities most commonly employed for each type of CNS pathology discussed in this chapter.
- Describe, in general, the radiographic appearance of each of the given pathologies.

ANATOMY AND PHYSIOLOGY

The central nervous system (CNS) comprises the brain and the spinal cord. It is composed of neurons (nerve cells) and neuroglia (the interstitial tissue). The CNS extends peripherally through nerves that carry motor messages through efferent nerves to the muscles and sensory messages from the skin and elsewhere back to the spinal cord and brain through afferent nerves. This chapter concentrates on conditions involving the brain and spinal cord.

The brain consists of the cerebrum (right and left hemispheres), cerebellum, diencephalon (including the hypothalamus), and the brainstem. The brainstem, composed of the midbrain, pons, and the medulla oblongata, serves to connect the cerebrum with the spinal cord. The innumerable motor and sensory nerves pass through the brainstem into the spinal cord. The spinal cord originates as an extension of the medulla oblongata at the foramen magnum in the base of the skull. It extends to approximately the level of the second or third lumbar vertebra to terminate with a cone-shaped area called the conus medullaris (Fig. 10-1). Spinal nerves beyond this point are referred to as the cauda equina.

Both the brain and the spinal cord are invested by the meninges, which consist of three distinct layers (Fig. 10-2). The dura mater

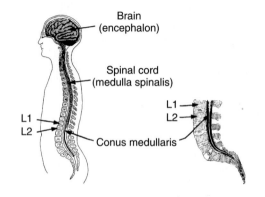

FIG. 10-1 Central nervous system.

is the outermost and is tough and fibrous. It has three major extensions: the falx cerebri, which divides the cerebral hemispheres; the falx cerebelli, which similarly divides the cerebellar hemispheres; and the tentorium cerebelli, which separates the occipital lobe of the cerebrum from the cerebellum. The arachnoid is the middle layer of the meninges and has the appearance of cobwebs. The pia mater is innermost and adheres directly to the cortex of the brain and the spinal cord. The subarachnoid space, at its deepest at the base of the brain, is located between the arachnoid and the pia mater. It is filled with cerebrospinal fluid (CSF) to continuously bathe the brain and spinal cord with nutrients and to cushion them against

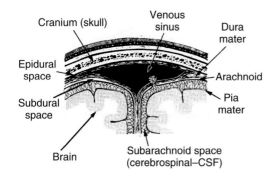

FIG. 10-2 Coronal perspective of meninges and meningeal spaces.

shocks and blows. The CSF is secreted by the choroid plexus, a network of capillaries located in the brain's ventricles.

The ventricles are four interconnected cavities within the brain. As noted, they house the choroid plexus that secretes CSF. The right and left lateral ventricles are located in their respective cerebral hemispheres (Fig. 10-3A,B). They may be further divided into anterior, posterior, and inferior horns, as well as a body and a trigone. The CSF flows from the lateral ventricles into the third ventricle via interventricular foramina (of Monro). The third and fourth ventricles are midline structures connected to each other by the cerebral aqueduct (Fig. 10-3C). From there, it flows through a median and two lateral foramina (Magendie and Luschka, respectively) into the subarachnoid space surrounding the brain and the spinal cord.

Most of the brain's blood is supplied anteriorly via the bilateral internal carotid arteries and posteriorly via the bilateral vertebral arteries. After entering the cranial vault through the foramen magnum, the vertebral arteries converge to form the basilar artery. The basilar

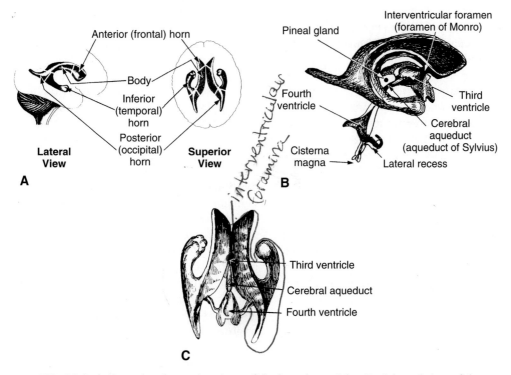

FIG. 10-3 A, Lateral and superior views of the lateral ventricles. **B,** A lateral view of the ventricular system. **C,** A superior view of the ventricular system.

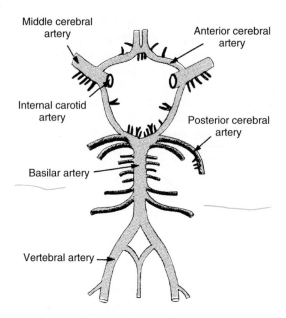

FIG. 10-4 The circle of Willis.

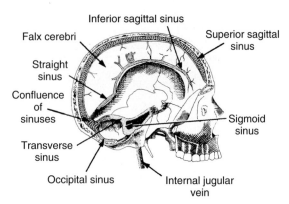

FIG. 10-5 Dura mater sinuses and venous drainage of the brain.

artery and portions of the internal carotid arteries form the circle of Willis (Fig. 10-4) to distribute oxygenated, arterial blood through various branches to all parts of the brain. Venous blood is returned to large venous sinuses in the dura mater, which ultimately drain into the internal jugular veins (Fig. 10-5).

The capillaries that connect the arteries and veins function somewhat differently in the brain than in other organs. Here, they prevent the passage of unwanted substances into the brain through a special function called the **blood-brain barrier.** This is accomplished in a number of ways but especially as a result of these capillary cells having a very tight junction that prevents macromolecules and fluids from leaking out into the brain parenchyma. This protects the brain by keeping toxins out, yet it allows removal of the waste products of brain metabolism. These specialized capillaries are found everywhere in the brain except the pineal and pituitary glands and the choroid plexus. The significance of the blood-brain barrier in terms of imaging is that contrast media enhancement in the brain occurs where the

barrier breaks down from inflammation, ischemia, or neoplastic growth (with its new vascularity). Also, glucose readily passes over this barrier and is the primary agent used so far in positron emission tomography (PET).

Although the intervertebral disks are not part of the CNS, they may impact on it when they herniate and impinge on adjacent spinal nerves. Disks cushion movement of the vertebral column. They are comprised of a tough outer covering, known as the **annulus fibrosus** and a pulpy center called the **nucleus pulposus** (Fig. 10-6).

IMAGING CONSIDERATIONS
Radiography
Conventional radiographic demonstration of the various cranial structures can provide information important in evaluation of the CNS. Its role, however, has largely been reduced to evaluation of cranial trauma because of the rapid ascent of magnetic resonance imaging (MRI) and continued refinements in computed tomography (CT). In addition to visualization of fractures caused by trauma, plain skull films may also reveal normal variants. Blood vessels such as the middle meningeal artery commonly cause radiolucent impressions on the inner table of the cranial vault (Fig. 10-7). Their

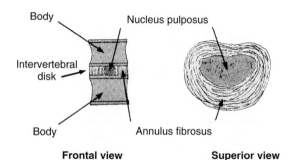

FIG. 10-6 An intervertebral disk.

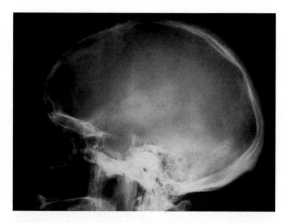

FIG. 10-8 An enlarged sella turcica on this lateral skull radiograph evidences a pituitary macroadenoma.

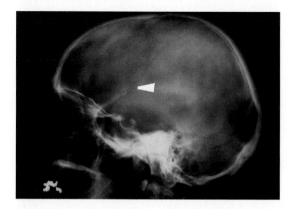

FIG. 10-7 Normal appearance of the middle meningeal artery as indicated on this lateral skull radiograph.

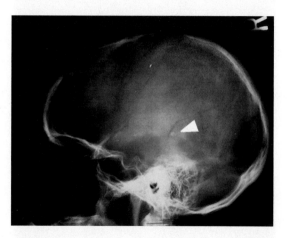

FIG. 10-9 Normal calcification of the pineal gland as seen on this lateral skull radiograph of a 44-year-old man.

linear progression and bilateral appearance help distinguish them from fractures. Visualization of an enlarged or deformed pituitary fossa can provide information concerning the presence of a pituitary tumor or increased intracranial pressure (Fig. 10-8). A calcified pineal gland situated in the midline can be seen on about 60% of all plain skull films (Fig. 10-9). Its displacement can indicate the presence of a pathologic lesion if it is greater than 2 to 3 mm. The choroid plexus (Fig. 10-10), falx cerebri (Fig. 10-11), and falx cerebelli may also be calcified.

The role of plain films in the evaluation of the spine was described in Chapter 2. A number of conditions that impact on the spinal cord can readily be demonstrated (Fig. 10-12).

The fluoroscopic procedure of myelography has been a staple of radiology for years, allowing visualization of conditions (such as herniated disks) that impinge on the spinal cord. Its role, however, is greatly diminishing because of the significant specificity of MRI.

Magnetic Resonance Imaging

For a wide variety of conditions related to the CNS, MRI has emerged as the modality of

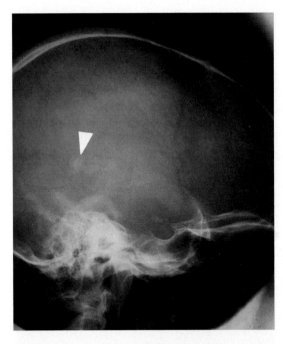

FIG. 10-10 Normal calcification of the choroid plexus in the posterior horn of the lateral ventricle as seen in this lateral skull radiograph of a 60-year-old woman.

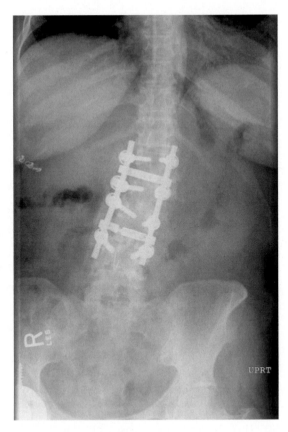

FIG. 10-12 An AP lumbar spine radiograph showing L1 through L4 fusion with stable hardware in place.

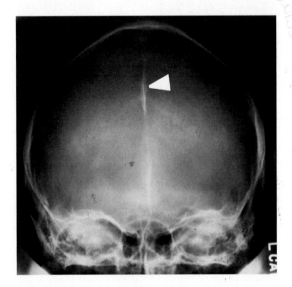

FIG. 10-11 Normal calcification of the falx cerebri as seen in this PA skull projection of a 59-year-old man.

choice (Fig. 10-13). Its sensitivity is excellent in evaluation of all types of spinal disease, including tumors, abscesses, and disk disease. The ability of MRI to evaluate brain tumors and conditions such as stroke, cranial tumors, and infection surpasses that of CT. Because MR does not image the dense petrous bone, it is excellent in evaluating the brainstem and anomalies of the posterior fossa (Fig. 10-14). Evaluation of demyelinating disease such as multiple sclerosis is substantively enhanced by MRI. Despite rapid evolution in technology, it currently has only a small role in the evaluation of trauma, mainly limited to evaluation of spinal cord compression and, in some instances, vertebral fractures.

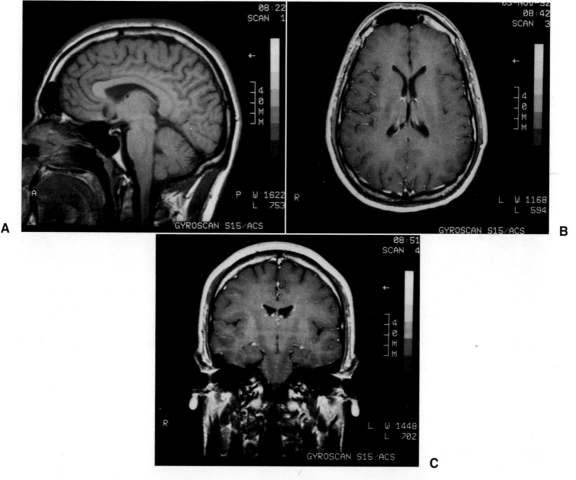

FIG. 10-13 A, Normal MRI of a young woman with a history of seizures as seen in a sagittal, T1-weighted view without gadolinium contrast. **B,** A normal T1-weighted axial view with gadolinium contrast of the same patient. **C,** A normal T1-weighted coronal view with gadolinium contrast of the same patient.

Magnetic resonance angiography (MRA) is used to evaluate vascular anatomy of the head and neck (Fig. 10-15). It has been proven to accurately locate vascular occlusions within the large arteries of the brain, often leading to a stroke. MRA also demonstrates the major veins and dural sinuses within the brain and plays a large role in the diagnosis and treatment of cerebral venous thrombosis. To date, it has not replaced conventional cerebral angiography but is often used as an adjunct modality.

Computed Tomography

CT continues to play a significant role in the evaluation of the CNS. It is rapid, noninvasive, safe, and quite accurate. Because CT has excellent contrast resolution, it readily differentiates among the sulci, ventricles, and gray and white matter within the brain (Fig. 10-16). It is particularly useful in evaluating cerebral bleeding after trauma because it readily reveals the extent of any hematoma present. CT of the brain is performed to evaluate the ventricles, as in the

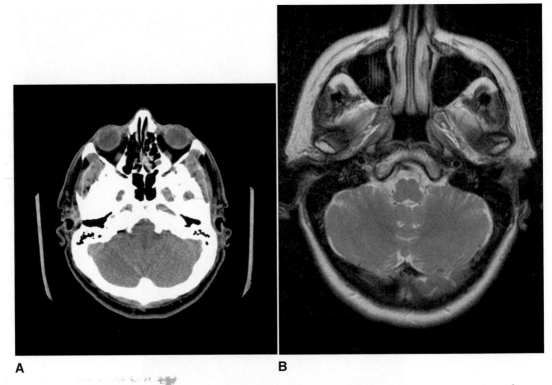

FIG. 10-14 A, CT of the posterior fossa region demonstrating the dense petrous portion of the temporal bone and associated artifacts. **B,** MRI of the posterior fossa region; note how the brain structures are visualized because the bone is not visible.

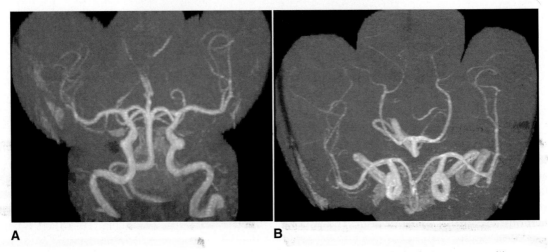

FIG. 10-15 A, Magnetic resonance angiogram (MRA) without contrast enhancement readily showing vasculature within the head and neck. **B,** MRA without contrast enhancement demonstrating the circle of Willis within the brain.

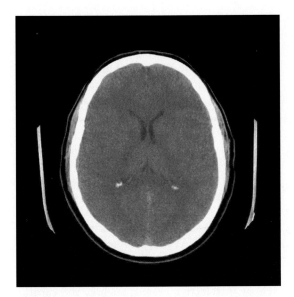

FIG. 10-16 An axial CT of a normal brain distinguishing between white and gray matter and demonstrating ventricular anatomy.

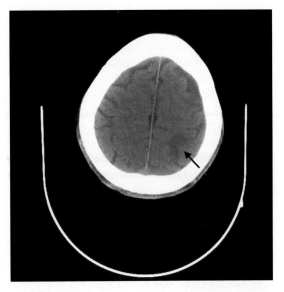

FIG. 10-17 CT of the brain showing a decreased density in brain tissue as a result of infarction.

case of hydrocephalus; to demonstrate cortical atrophy, as in the case of dementia; and to identify neoplasms within the brain, which may or may not create a mass effect or shifting of the midline of the brain. In cases of infarction, edema, abscess, or cyst formation, the tissue density is decreased (Fig. 10-17). The tissue density is increased by fresh blood or recent hemorrhage and calcifications within the brain. Other related roles include any kind of routine anatomic evaluation, such as assessment of shunt functioning and assessment of the bony cerebral and visceral skull. Contrast-enhanced CT of the brain is used to demonstrate anomalies in the cerebral vasculature and to help delineate neoplastic growth within the cranial vault. Postmyelographic CT of the spine is also fairly prevalent but is decreasing with the more widespread use of MRI. CT myelograms can demonstrate encroachments of the spinal cord and nerve roots, as can MR, but bony detail is best visualized with CT. CT is also used to evaluate vertebral fractures, as discussed in Chapter 11.

Ultrasound

Ultrasound is useful in evaluating the brain of neonates before closure of the fontanels because the fibrous tissue covering the fontanels provides a ready window into the brain (Fig. 10-18). It can readily detect cerebral hemorrhage and hydrocephalus. In premature

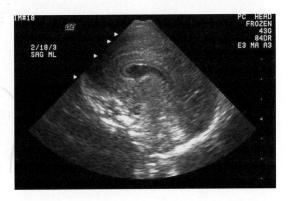

FIG. 10-18 A sonogram of a normal premature neonate head with no evidence of periventricular hemorrhage.

infants the brain tissue around the ventricles (periventricular germinal matrix) is prone to hemorrhage, often resulting in intraventricular hemorrhage. In addition, premature infants are also at an increased risk for periventricular white matter infarction. Portable sonography is a noninvasive method of evaluating cerebral anatomy and can be performed in the neonatal ICU to help evaluate the status of these infants.

Duplex Doppler ultrasound is a noninvasive modality useful in evaluating carotid blood flow. It can demonstrate vascular occlusion and ulceration within the carotid arteries, most commonly at the point of bifurcation. Although it cannot provide the detail present with angiography, it is useful in evaluating patients experiencing carotid artery transient ischemic attacks.

Nuclear Medicine

In nuclear medicine, radionuclide brain scans are primarily utilized to confirm brain death in patients with the appropriate clinical signs, generally following trauma or an intracranial bleed (Fig. 10-19). Technetium-labeled flow agents in combination with single positron emission computed tomography (SPECT) may be used experimentally to assess tumors, areas of stroke and ischemia, and Alzheimer's disease. To complement the more traditional anatomic evaluation of other modalities, PET scanning allows imaging of the body's normal chemical processes and provides physiologic evaluation (Fig. 10-20).

Vascular/Interventional Radiology

Cerebral angiography is used to demonstrate vessel anatomy within the neck and brain (Fig. 10-21). It is used to diagnose neoplastic lesions, stenosis, aneurysms, arterial venous malformations (AVM), and congenital anomalies of the CNS. Cerebral blood flow may be visualized by placing the catheter in the aortic arch or in selective vessels, such as the carotid or vertebral arteries. Angiography can visualize vessels as small as 1 cm using current imaging technology.

Interventional techniques include angioplasty, stent or shunt placement, thrombolysis, or embolization. Percutaneous transluminal angioplasty (PTA) and intraarterial thrombolysis are used to open stenotic vessels to obtain

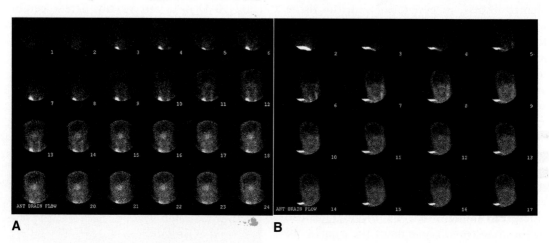

A   **B**

FIG. 10-19 A, A portable radionuclide brain scan confirming brain death by the absence of intracranial blood flow. The brain death occurred following an intracranial hemorrhage from preeclampsia in a postpartum woman. **B,** A portable brain scan also confirming brain death in a patient following a subarachnoid hemorrhage.

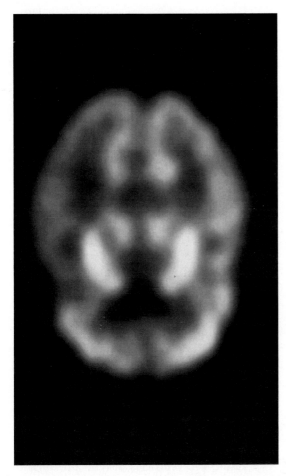

FIG. 10-20 An axial image from a PET scan demonstrating an infarct in the posterior left parietotemporal region, with shunting of blood to hypermetabolic basal ganglia.

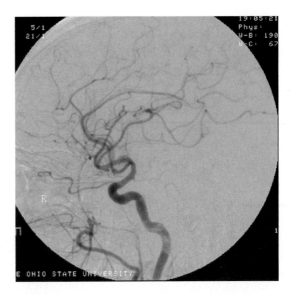

FIG. 10-21 Carotid arteriogram showing vasculature of the head and neck.

an improvement in blood flow. Laser-tipped angioplasty and percutaneous atherectomy may also be performed to open stenotic vessels, especially in the neck. Spheres, coils, or beads are used to embolize or occlude cerebral vasculature, as in the case of an aneurysm or AV malformation. Therapeutic devices such as stents and shunts are also placed by the interventionalist, eliminating the need for surgical intervention.

CONGENITAL AND HEREDITARY DISEASES

Meningomyelocele

As mentioned in Chapter 2, spina bifida is a condition in which the bony neural arch that encloses and protects the spinal cord is not completely closed (Fig. 10-22). It most commonly occurs in the lumbar region, and the spinal cord and its meninges may or may not herniate through the resultant opening. Elevated α-fetoprotein levels in the mother's blood and on amniocentesis may diagnose it prenatally. The defect and soft tissue sac are confirmed with fetal ultrasound. Complications depend on the extent of protrusion and range from treatable to life-threatening. Any opening of the sac to the exterior of the body risks meningeal infection, so surgical closure is critical. If only the meninges protrude, the condition is termed a **meningocele** (Fig. 10-23). These are treated surgically without difficulty and usually with an excellent prognosis. A **myelocele** is a protrusion of the spinal cord, which may be treatable surgically. A **meningomyelocele** is the most serious of possible conditions and consists

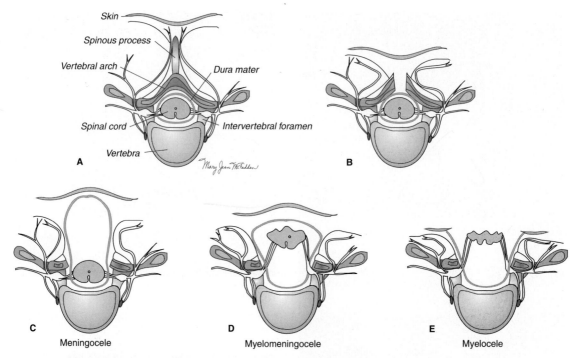

FIG. 10-22 A normal neural arch in comparison to congenital defects: **A,** Normal. **B,** Spina bifida occulta. The median segment of the vertebral arch is missing and covered by skin. **C,** Meningocele. The arch is mostly absent with a bulging dura; however, the spinal cord remains in the vertebral canal. **D,** Myelomeningocele with a deformed spinal cord within the protruding dural sac. **E,** Myelocele: the area is totally exposed.

of a protrusion of both the meninges and the spinal cord into the skin of the back (Figs. 10-24 and 10-25). These patients often present with severe neurologic deficit, the extent of which depends on the level of herniation. Associated neurologic difficulties include paraplegia and diminished control of the lower limbs, bladder, and bowel. Hydrocephalus occurs in most of these patients.

Hydrocephalus

Normally, CSF flows around the spinal cord and over the convexity of the brain before resorption into the venous sinuses. This normal circulation can be interrupted by causes such as an obstruction to flow (noncommunicating hydrocephalus) and impaired absorption (communicating hydrocephalus); increased CSF production can also disturb the normal circulation.

As a result, the ventricles distend proximal to the site of obstruction, resulting in compression atrophy of the brain tissue around the dilated ventricles. In such cases, the sulci are obliterated, and the gyri are flattened. **Hydrocephalus** refers to an excessive accumulation of CSF within the ventricles and can be either congenital or acquired.

In noncommunicating hydrocephalus, an obstruction can result congenitally or from tumor growth, trauma, or inflammation. It interferes with or blocks the normal CSF circulation from the ventricles to the subarachnoid space. It is also commonly associated with malformations of the posterior fossa, such as Arnold-Chiari malformation. An Arnold-Chiari malformation is a congenital defect in which the cerebellar tonsils are displaced downward below the level of the foramen magnum and

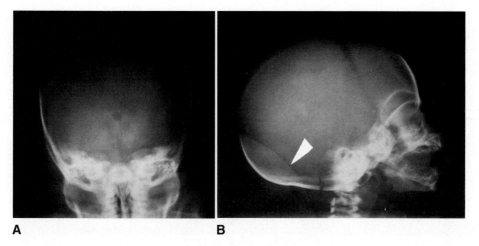

FIG. 10-23 A, Circular defect seen in the middle of the occipital bone of this newborn is the site of a meningocele. **B,** A lateral skull radiograph demonstrates the soft tissue density associated with the meningocele superimposed over the occipital bone.

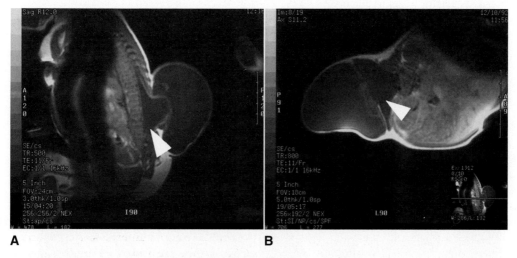

FIG. 10-24 A, A T1-weighted sagittal MRI view without gadolinium in this newborn readily demonstrates a meningomyelocele, with the arrow indicating the herniated spinal cord. **B,** A T1-weighted axial MRI view without gadolinium of the same patient similarly demonstrates the meningomyelocele, with the arrow indicating the herniated spinal cord.

are clearly visible on a sagittal T1 MR examination of the brain.

Poor resorption of CSF by the arachnoid villi results in communicating hydrocephalus. It can arise from a number of factors, including increased intracranial pressure caused by tumor compression, raised intrathoracic pressure impairing venous drainage, inflammation from meningitis, or after a subarachnoid hemorrhage. Hydrocephalus can also occur from overproduction of CSF, although this is the least common cause.

CT provides excellent visualization of hydrocephalus (Fig. 10-26). In neonates, sonography

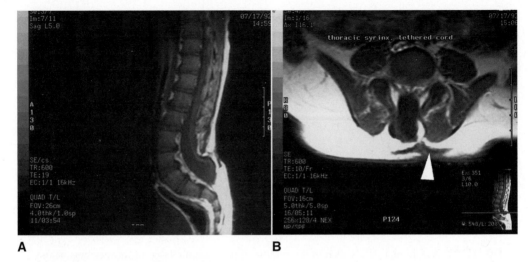

A   B

FIG. 10-25 A, A T1-weighted sagittal MRI view without gadolinium in this infant demonstrates a surgically repaired meningomyelocele. **B,** A T1-weighted axial MRI view without gadolinium similarly demonstrates the surgically repaired meningomyelocele, with the arrow pointing to the surgical site.

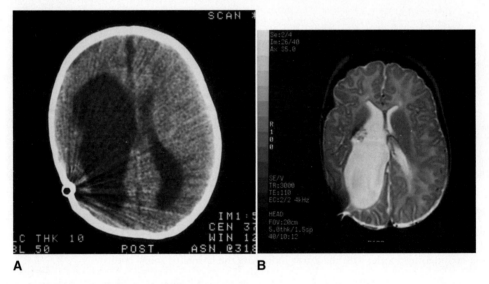

A   B

FIG. 10-26 A, Hydrocephalus as seen on this transverse CT view of a 6-month-old girl with only mild dilatation of the left ventricle. Streaking artifacts originate from the shunt being checked for placement. **B,** A T2-weighted axial MRI view without gadolinium demonstrates the hydrocephalus in the same patient.

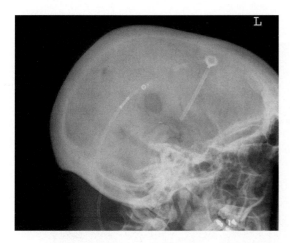

FIG. 10-27 A lateral projection of the skull showing VJ shunt placement.

is used to demonstrate the ventricular system through the infant's fontanels, which permit passage of the beam until their eventual closure. Treatment may consist of surgery. In some cases, a shunt (an artificial passageway) is surgically inserted to divert excess fluids. Placed between the ventricles and either the internal jugular vein, the heart, or the peritoneum, it drains excess CSF. The shunt contains a one-way valve to prevent the backflow of blood into the ventricles. Radiographs are taken to demonstrate shunt placement after insertion (Fig. 10-27), and CT is used to follow up on a periodic basis to evaluate ventricular size, which indirectly assesses shunt function.

INFLAMMATORY DISEASES

Meningitis

An inflammation of the meningeal coverings of the brain and spinal cord is termed **meningitis.** It can be caused by bacteria, viruses, or other organisms that reach the meninges from elsewhere in the body via blood or lymph, as a result of trauma and penetrating wounds, or from adjacent structures (e.g., the mastoids) that become infected. Bacterial infection is the most common cause of meningitis (Fig. 10-28).

Pathogens responsible for acute bacterial meningitis include meningococci, streptococci, and pneumococci. These are pus-forming (pyogenic) types of bacteria, and they may be carried to the meninges via the middle ear or frontal sinus. Meningococcal meningitis is most common in infants, streptococcal meningitis is most common in children, and pneumococcal meningitis is most common in the adult population. In addition, a few cases result from infection by the tubercle bacillus, which is not pus forming. This type of bacterial meningitis is more difficult to diagnose because it does not have the same acute symptoms as the other types of bacterial meningitis. Tuberculous meningitis is usually spread from the lung in association with miliary tuberculosis.

In cases of bacterial meningitis, CSF is under increased pressure and can contribute to hydrocephalus. Acute bacterial meningitis may follow an upper respiratory infection or sore throat. Symptoms include a fever, headache, stiff neck, vomiting, and changes in consciousness, with the patient becoming severely ill within 24 hours. Because bacterial meningitis can be lethal in a short period of time, accurate and immediate diagnosis and treatment are imperative. The primary means of diagnosing meningitis is the increased intracranial pressure detectable via the results of a spinal tap. A brain CT may be performed before the spinal tap to rule out the presence of abnormalities such as a brain mass that would contraindicate performing a lumbar puncture. On laboratory examination, the CSF contains both the bacteria responsible for the infection and a large number of polymorphonuclear leukocytes (pus cells).

Antibiotics, in particular, have been very successful against many forms of meningitis, and antibiotic therapy may begin before a definite diagnosis has been established. If antibiotic therapy is started early, the mortality rate from bacterial meningitis is less than 10%. Contrast-enhanced MR scans can identify subarachnoid inflammation and inflammation of the mastoids or sinuses. CT scans may also be helpful in

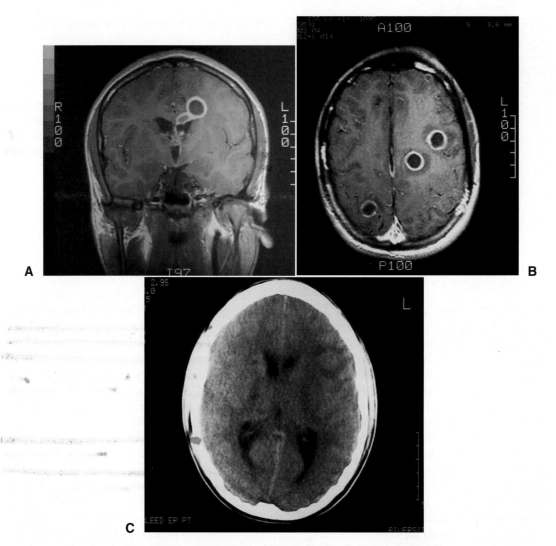

FIG. 10-28 A, A T1-weighted coronal MRI view with gadolinium demonstrates a ring lesion that communicates with the left lateral ventricle in this 17-year-old boy, creating meningitis as a result of transplantation into the brain of a bacterial *(Staph.)* infection. **B,** A T1-weighted axial MRI view with gadolinium of the same patient demonstrates the presence of multiple infectious lesions. **C,** An axial CT view of the same patient demonstrates the presence of an infectious lesion as well as slightly widened ventricles, as characteristic with meningitis.

assessing the presence of skull fractures or a brain abscess.

Chronic meningitis is most commonly caused by fungi and is often seen in AIDS patients or individuals on immunodepressant drug therapy. The symptoms are similar to those associated with acute meningitis; however, unlike acute meningitis, the symptoms occur over weeks rather than days. The treatment of chronic meningitis depends on the infecting agent, with amphotericin B being the preferred drug for all fungal infections. Although the disease may progress at a slower rate, the outcome may still be fatal.

Encephalitis

An infection of the brain tissue is termed **encephalitis.** In contrast to meningitis, which is most frequently a bacterial infection, encephalitis is usually viral in nature (Fig. 10-29) and may also occur subsequent to conditions such as chickenpox, smallpox, influenza, or measles. Primary viral encephalitis may be caused by the arbovirus transmitted by mosquitoes during warm weather or the herpes simplex virus. The symptoms and signs most commonly associated with encephalitis are headache, malaise, and coma. This condition is more serious than meningitis because individuals who acquire encephalitis more frequently develop permanent neurologic disabilities. The viral infection results in cerebral edema with numerous hemorrhagic spots scattered throughout the cerebral hemispheres, brainstem, and cerebellum.

MRI is especially valuable because it can detect brain inflammation earlier than CT, nuclear medicine studies, or EEG evaluation. MR can also rule out other anomalies such as a brain abscess or a subdural empyema or hematoma, which may mimic the clinical signs associated with viral encephalitis. Herpes simplex encephalitis is treated with the antiviral medication acyclovir. Survival rates depend on the etiology of the disease. In some instances, it may be fatal.

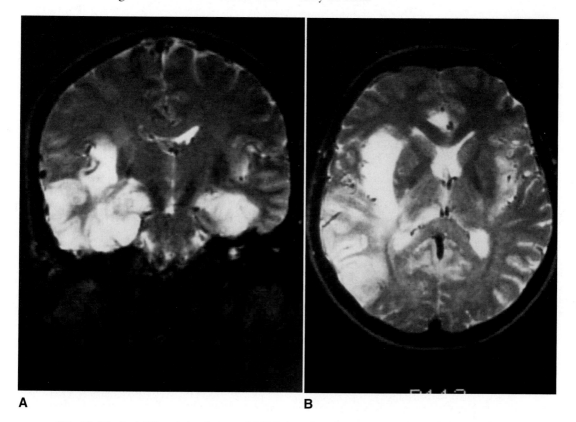

A   **B**

FIG. 10-29 A, A T2-weighted coronal MRI view demonstrates the infectious response in the brain of this boy with herpes encephalitis. **B,** A T2-weighted axial MRI view demonstrates the extent of the infectious process in the same patient with herpes encephalitis.

Brain Abscess

A **brain abscess** is an encapsulated accumulation of pus within the cranium resulting from a cranial infection, a penetrating head wound, or an infection spread through the bloodstream. The symptoms are similar to encephalitis and include fever, headache, nausea and vomiting, seizures, and personality changes. The diagnosis is usually made by CT or MR evaluation of the brain. Brain abscesses are fatal unless they are treated with antibiotic therapy. The specific antibiotic agent depends on the infecting organism and lasts approximately 4 to 8 weeks. Serial CT examinations are often performed during antibiotic therapy to assess the progression of the treatment. In some cases, the abscess may require aspiration or drainage.

If the pus accumulates within the meningeal layers between the dura mater and arachnoid, it is termed a **subdural empyema.** Like a brain abscess, subdural empyemas are diagnosed with CT or MR of the brain. Symptoms are the same as exhibited with a brain abscess; however, subdural empyemas require immediate drainage. Following drainage, the patient is treated with antibiotic therapy similar to those used for brain abscesses.

DEGENERATIVE DISEASES

Degenerative Disk Disease and Herniated Nucleus Pulposus

A **herniated nucleus pulposus,** or herniated disk, may result from either degenerative disease (Fig. 10-30) or trauma. A weakened or

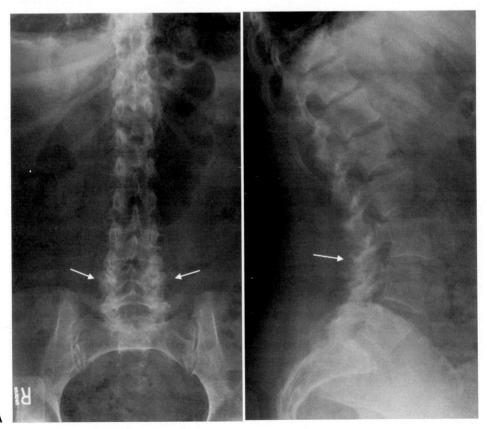

FIG. 10-30 A, An AP projection of the lumbar spine demonstrating degenerative joint disease of the lower lumbar spine. **B,** A lateral lumbar projection of the same patient as in **A.**

torn annulus fibrosus is subject to rupture, which allows the nucleus pulposus to protrude and compress spinal nerve roots. The disk may prolapse in any direction and in some instances may not produce pain. However, pressure may be placed on the spinal cord as the nucleus pulposus spreads beyond its normal confines posteriorly (Fig. 10-31), resulting in pain along the course of adjacent nerve roots and a weakening of the muscles supplied by these nerves. The most common locations for disk herniation are in the lower cervical and lower lumbar regions. In the lumbar region, over 80% occur at the L5–S1 nerve roots, and in the cervical region, C6–C7 herniations are most common.

Symptoms may include a sudden and severe onset of pain in the distribution of the compressed nerve root, in combination with weakened muscles, although at times symptoms may be more insidious. Compression of the nerve roots in the cervical area cause pain in the neck and upper extremities, whereas compression in the lumbar area results in pain in the hip,

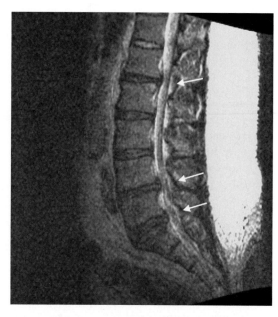

FIG. 10-32 A sagittal MR image demonstrating degenerative disk disease in the lumbar vertebral column.

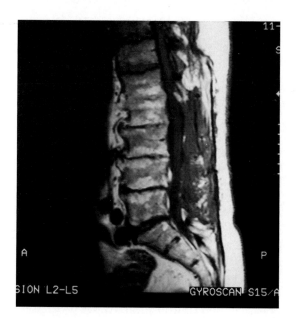

FIG. 10-31 T1-weighted sagittal MRI view of the spine in this 75-year-old man readily demonstrates severe degenerative disk disease as well as fusion of L1 and L2.

posterior thigh, calf and foot. The extent of nerve root compression may be demonstrated through myelography, CT, and MRI. The imaging modality of choice has become MRI (Fig. 10-32), largely supplanting the roles of myelography and CT in diagnosis of disk disease. However, with normal aging, the nucleus pulposus tends to dehydrate, and the change in water content alters the relaxation times on an MR study.

Physical therapy and analgesics are used as treatment, with 95% of patients recovering within 3 months without surgical intervention. If these fail to relieve pain, microscopic diskectomy, surgical decompression, or laminectomy with spinal fusion may be performed.

Cervical Spondylosis

Osteoarthritic conditions may also affect the vertebral column, leading to nerve disorders caused by chronic nerve root compression. These osteoarthritic changes of the neck are referred to as **cervical spondylosis** and are readily visible radiographically, most notably on

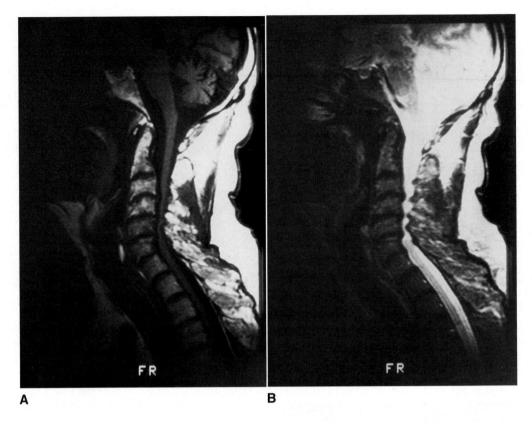

FIG. 10-33 A, A T1-weighted sagittal MRI view demonstrates compression of the spinal cord in this elderly man with cervical spondylosis. CSF is dark adjacent to the gray spinal cord. **B,** A T2-weighted sagittal MRI image indicates the constriction of CSF flow (white) at C2 through C5.

an oblique projection of the cervical spine. Osteophytes (spurs) form in the articular facets of the cervical vertebrae and compress the nerves located in the intervertebral foramina. They may also compress the spinal cord (Fig. 10-33). MRI excels at visualization of spinal cord compression as a result of cervical spondylosis. As with degenerative disk disease, treatment is conservative at first but may include laminectomy and decompression procedures.

Multiple Sclerosis

Multiple sclerosis (MS) is a chronic, progressive disease of the nervous system most commonly affecting individuals between the ages of

20 and 40. It affects women more often than men. The origin of this disease is unknown, but research indicates it may result from a latent herpes virus or retrovirus. It also appears more often in individuals living in a temperate climate than those living in a tropical environment. MS involves degeneration of the myelin sheath covering the nervous tissue of the spinal cord and the white matter within the brain. This demyelination impairs nerve conduction, beginning with muscle impairment and a loss of balance and coordination. As MS progresses, tremors, vision impairment, and urinary bladder dysfunction develop, along with a continued weakening of the muscles. Numerous patchy

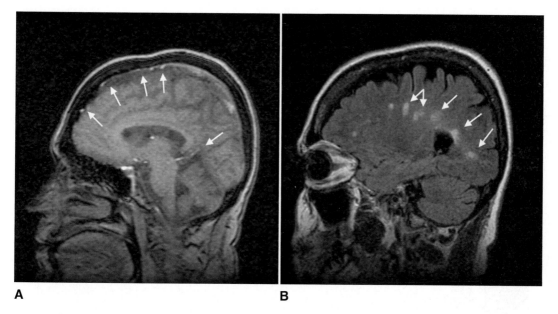

A   **B**

FIG. 10-34 A, A sagittal MR on a patient with known MS. The examination demonstrates
MS plaques on the white matter of the brain. B, A sagittal fluid-attenuated inversion recovery
(FLAIR) MR image of the same patient also demonstrating MS plaque.

areas of demyelinated nerves develop, forming
scar tissue or sclerotic lesions throughout the
nervous system. These scars are termed MS
plaques and are well demonstrated on MRI
examination, making MRI the modality of
choice for evaluating individuals with suspected
MS (Fig. 10-34). In cases of known MS,
contrast-enhanced MR can also differentiate
active inflammation from previous, older brain
plaques.

MS runs a long and unpredictable course,
eventually leading to permanent neurologic disabilities. Except in severe cases, however, the
patient's life span is not shortened by MS.
Patients may be placed on corticosteroids to
shorten the symptomatic periods, but long-
term use of corticosteroids is contraindicated.
Interferon-β is a more promising drug that has
also been used to reduce the frequency of
symptomatic periods, and it may actually delay
the progression of the disease. Most patients
benefit from regular exercise and physical

therapy in conjunction with medication to
reduce muscle spasticity and improve range of
motion.

VASCULAR DISEASES

Cerebrovascular Accident

Atherosclerotic disease affecting the blood
supply to the brain results in a cerebrovascular
accident (CVA) commonly referred to as a
stroke. Strokes are the third leading cause of
death in the United States. There are essentially
two ways a stroke occurs, and they are classified
as either ischemic or hemorrhagic. In an
ischemic stroke, a blood clot blocks a blood
vessel in the brain. In a hemorrhagic stroke, a
blood vessel in the brain ruptures and bleeds
into the brain tissues and structures. This type
of stroke generally has a more sudden onset
than an ischemic stroke. Both CT and MR
(Fig. 10-35) examinations of the brain are able
to distinguish between an ischemic and a

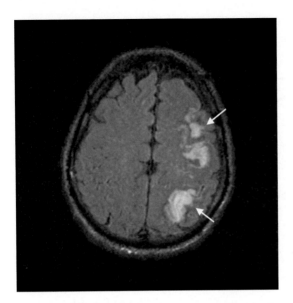

FIG. 10-35 An axial FLAIR MR of the brain demonstrating an infarct in the left parietal lobe.

hemorrhagic cause, with ischemic strokes accounting for the majority of all strokes. MR is especially sensitive to infarction within hours of the onset, whereas CT scans can, at times, appear negative for a day or so following the stroke. Carotid duplex sonograms and MRA are also useful in the diagnosis of a stroke.

Ischemic Strokes

Under normal circumstances, blood clotting slows and eventually stops bleeding and is beneficial. In an ischemic stroke, however, blood clots are dangerous because they can block blood flow and cause vessel occlusion. An ischemic stroke can occur in two ways: infarction caused by thrombosis of a cerebral artery or embolism to the brain from a thrombus elsewhere in the body. A thrombus is a blood clot that obstructs a blood vessel, and an embolus is a mass of undissolved matter (solid, liquid, or gas) present in a blood vessel brought there by blood current. Vessel occlusion or ischemia lasting over 1 hour usually results in development of an infarct and permanent neurologic

damage. These may be easily diagnosed with CT or MRI. Angiography may be performed if the diagnosis with other imaging modalities is questionable. Two types of thrombosis can cause stroke: large vessel thrombosis and small vessel disease, also known as **lacunar infarction.** Large vessel thrombosis most often occurs in the large arteries as a result of long-term atherosclerosis followed by rapid blood clot formation. Typical sites are the bifurcation of the common carotid artery, within the carotid sinus, or the termination of the internal carotid artery, giving rise to the cerebral arteries (Figs. 10-36 and 10-37). An infarct caused by thrombosis of a cerebral artery is termed an **atherothrombic brain infarction** (ABI). Symptoms associated with ABI develop slowly over a period of hours or days and include confusion, hemiplegia, and aphasia. This type of CVA may be preceded by a temporary episode of neurologic dysfunction termed a **transient ischemic attack** (TIA), which includes hemiparesis, hemiparesthesia, or monocular blindness. These symptoms should clear within 2 hours. Patients with a thrombotic stroke are also likely to have coronary artery disease, and heart attack is a frequent cause of death for those who have a thrombotic stroke.

Small vessel disease (i.e., lacunar infarction) occurs when blood flow is blocked to a very small arterial vessel. *Lacune* is French for "hole" and describes the small cavity that remains after products of a deep infarct have been removed by other cells. Although little is known about small vessel disease, it is closely linked to hypertension. About 20% of all strokes are caused by small vessel disease.

An embolism may also cause infarction to the brain from a thrombus elsewhere in the body, most commonly from the left side of the heart. Those CVAs resulting from cerebral embolism have a sudden onset of symptoms without warning.

The mortality rate associated with ischemic strokes is approximately 20%. The prognosis depends on the location and extent of the

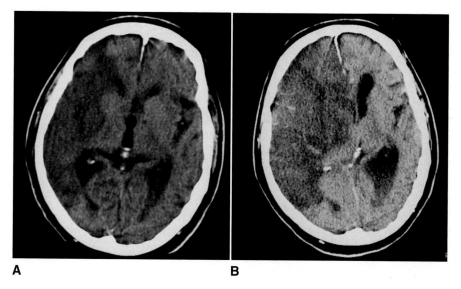

FIG. 10-36 A, An unenhanced CT of the brain of an 83-year-old woman reveals a large infarct along the distribution of the middle cerebral artery on the right side. **B,** A similar unenhanced CT taken 4 days later reveals worsening of the edema with early shift of the right lateral and third ventricles to the left.

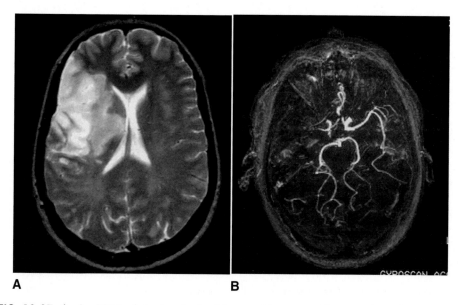

FIG. 10-37 A, An MRI of the head of a 54-year-old woman who experienced sudden left facial paralysis and slumped forward while shopping reveals a large infarct along the distribution of the middle cerebral artery. **B,** An MR angiogram of the same patient demonstrates occlusion of the middle cerebral artery, thought likely to be secondary to an embolus from carotid artery disease.

stroke in addition to the patient's age and general health. Complete recovery is very rare, with deficits remaining 6 months following the stroke most likely remaining permanent. One of the most common treatments involves the administration of recombinant tissue plasminogen activator (tPA) within 3 hours of the onset of symptoms.

Hemorrhagic Strokes

In a hemorrhagic stroke, brain hemorrhage results from a weakening in the diseased vessel wall. Typically, the ruptured vessel has been weakened by arteriosclerosis from hypertension; however, hemorrhage can also result from congenital aneurysms or vascular anomalies. The onset of this type of CVA is sudden and often lethal because it expands rapidly. Brain hemorrhages account for approximately 10% to 15% of all CVAs and are of two types: subarachnoid and intracerebral. Most bleeds occur in the cerebrum and bleed into the lateral ventricle. Most commonly, they are preceded by an intense headache that is often accompanied by vomiting. Loss of consciousness follows within minutes and leads to total contralateral hemiplegia or death. Brain CT is often employed in the case of a hemorrhagic stroke because the fresh blood appears denser than the surrounding brain tissue. Surgical intervention is necessary when the bleed causes brain displacement or when aneurysms must be clipped to reduce fatal bleeding. The prognosis of this type of CVA is very poor, with approximately 35% of patients dying following the stroke and another 15% dying within a few weeks, usually from a subsequent vessel rupture.

NEOPLASTIC DISEASES

Primary tumors of the brain comprise about 10% of the deaths from cancer and may be difficult to classify as purely benign or malignant. In many cases, the location of the brain neoplasm is of equal or greater importance than its malignancy or benignancy because of the complications produced by mass effect. Edema accompanying a tumor causes an increase in intracranial pressure, which can cause headaches, vomiting, blurred vision, and seizures. Hemorrhage and brainstem herniation can occur, resulting in death as brainstem function (e.g., control of respiration) fails.

Other characteristics of primary brain tumors include a greater incidence in young to middle-aged adults and a relative infrequency of metastasis. In children, brain tumors often tend to occur in the posterior fossa, but the anterior portion of the cerebrum is a more prevalent site in adults. In addition, primary brain tumors are among the most common brain neoplasms in children, whereas metastases to the brain from other areas are more common in adults.

Primary brain tumors may be classified according to their site, such as the specific lobe of the brain, or histologic composition. Two categories of brain tumors based on histologic type are glial and nonglial neoplasms. Glial tumors generate from the nonnervous system (i.e., supporting tissues of the brain and spinal cord). **Gliomas** account for about half of all primary brain tumors. Their growth is accomplished through infiltration, making them difficult to treat surgically through resection. Nonglial tumors grow through expansion and are more treatable surgically. Meningiomas are the most frequently occurring nonglial tumor. The modalities of choice in imaging brain tumors of all types are MRI and CT. In addition to surgical intervention, radiation therapy and chemotherapy also play an important role in the treatment of brain tumors.

Gliomas

The most common type of primary brain tumor is the glioma (Fig. 10-38), accounting for approximately 45% of all intracranial tumors. Although derived from glial (supporting) cells, their precise classification is unsettled. However, several growth factors and their receptors have been identified that are associated with the development of gliomas. These tumors may

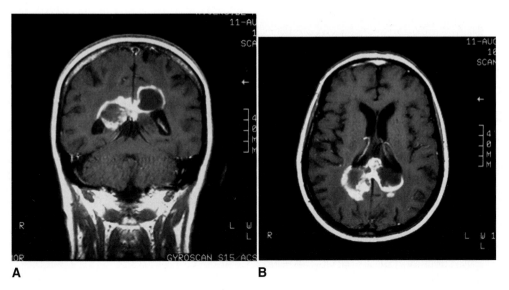

FIG. 10-38 A, A "butterfly" glioma seen in this T1-weighted coronal MRI view with gadolinium in a 54-year-old woman. **B,** A T1-weighted axial MRI view with gadolinium of the same "butterfly" glioma.

contain different types of cells in the same tumor, but one commonality is loss of genetic information from chromosome 17p. Gliomas commonly occur in the cerebral hemispheres and posterior fossa, with nearly half of all gliomas classified as the malignant glioblastoma variety (Fig. 10-39). Other types of glioma include benign astrocytomas, oligodendrogliomas, and ependymomas. In terms of MRI results, gliomas are evaluated based on the associated edema (Fig. 10-40), mass effect, and the amount of contrast enhancement. There is an association between the aggressiveness of the tumor and these three factors. Malignant gliomas may be extremely vascular, demonstrating pathologic vessels on angiographic examination. Low-grade malignant gliomas, however, are relatively avascular. The CT images generally demonstrate an ill-defined area of decreased density (attenuation) with displacement of the midline structures and ventricular compression. Without contrast enhancement, it is difficult to differentiate the surrounding edema from the actual tumor, so the use of an iodinated IV

contrast agent is necessary to enhance the lesion. Surgical biopsy generally provides the final diagnosis of the exact type of glioma. As described above, symptoms include severe headaches, vision impairment, personality changes, and seizures as a result of increased intracranial pressure.

Astrocytomas account for about a third of all gliomas (Fig. 10-41) and are composed of astrocytes, which are star-shaped neuroglial cells with many branching processes. Astrocytomas are white, usually slow-growing, infiltrative tumors with a low grade of malignancy. Early detection leads to a good prognosis. A **glioblastoma multiforme** (an advanced astrocytoma) is highly malignant. An **oligodendroglioma** is a slow-growing astrocytic tumor that is usually histologically relatively benign (Fig. 10-42). It typically calcifies so that its appearance in a punctate or stippled pattern on a skull radiograph is virtually diagnostic. **Ependymoma** is a firm, whitish tumor that arises from the ependyma, the lining of the ventricles (Fig. 10-43). Typically, it derives from the roof

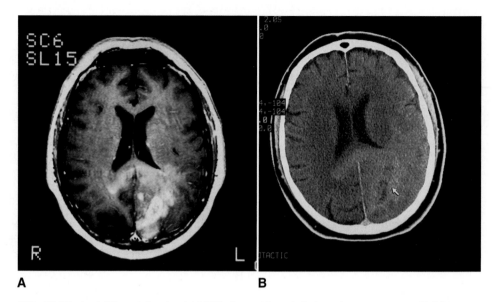

FIG. 10-39 A, A T1-weighted axial MRI view with gadolinium demonstrates a glioblastoma multiforme in a 70-year-old man. **B,** CT study of the brain without contrast demonstrates an intraparenchymal hemorrhage after biopsy in the same patient with the glioblastoma multiforme.

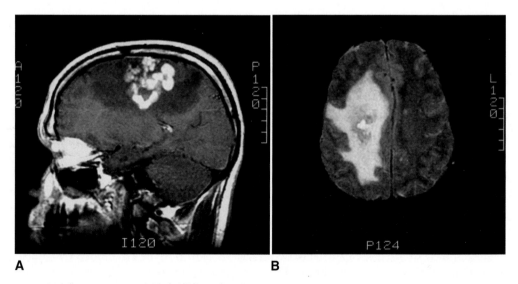

FIG. 10-40 A, A T1-weighted sagittal MRI view with gadolinium of a large glioma with surrounding edema in a 25-year-old man. **B,** a T2-weighted axial MRI view without gadolinium of the same glioma in the right parietal region, again with edema (white on T2) surrounding the tumor.

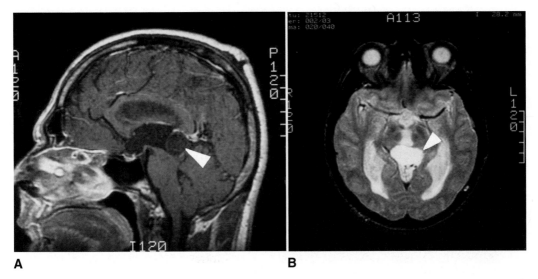

A   **B**

FIG. 10-41 A, A T1-weighted sagittal MRI view with gadolinium demonstrates a pineal gland astrocytoma in this 32-year-old man. **B,** A T2-weighted axial MRI view demonstrates the same pineal gland astrocytoma.

of the fourth ventricle, but it may also appear from the central canal of the spinal cord.

Stereotactic biopsy of the brain lesion is generally used to confirm the diagnosis of a glioma. Treatment of these tumors begins with surgical resection of the tumor followed by radiation therapy and chemotherapy. However, the prognosis is very poor, with only 25% of patients surviving after 2 years.

Medulloblastoma

Like astrocytic tumors, **medulloblastomas** are soft, infiltrating tumors of neuroepithelial tissue. These rapidly growing tumors are highly malignant and most often occur in the cerebellum of children and young adults (Fig. 10-44), usually extending from the roof of the fourth ventricle. They are more common in boys and rarely seen in adults. Because MRI does not image bone or demonstrate artifacts associated with the dense bone within the base of the skull, it is an excellent modality for the demonstration of a medulloblastoma on both enhanced and nonenhanced examination. These

tumors may also be demonstrated on CT examination, with the medulloblastoma visible as a midline lesion that is denser than normal brain tissue, surrounded by edema. In addition, tumor dissemination throughout the subarachnoid space often blocks the flow of CSF, causing hydrocephalus. Shunting is used to relieve the hydrocephalus. Surgical excision of the tumor as possible and radiation therapy to the entire CNS (brain and spinal cord) have improved the 5-year survival rate to over 50% and 10-year survival rate to about 40%. Unfortunately, recurrence is common with this tumor, and chemotherapy regimens have not been found to be consistently effective in controlling the recurrence.

Meningioma

A **meningioma** is a slow-growing, generally benign tumor that originates in the arachnoid tissue. It is the most common nonglial tumor, accounting for about 15% of all intracranial tumors. Meningiomas are more frequent in women than in men, and although menin-

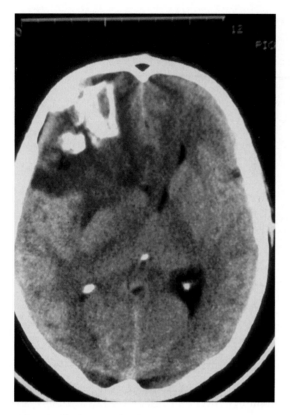

FIG. 10-42 An axial CT view without contrast demonstrates the presence of an oligodendroglioma and surrounding edema.

giomas can affect individuals at any age, they usually arise in adults between the ages of 40 to 60 years. It is most often found adhering to the dura in relation to the intracranial venous sinuses. It does not invade the brain but compresses it with its growth. Resultant neurologic deficits are generally less in proportion to the tumor size than with gliomas.

In some instances, the skull may thicken over the site of the meningioma, with the increased calcification visible on conventional skull radiographs. This area of hyperostosis may be palpable on physical examination. Because these tumors are fed by the meningeal arteries, plain skull films may also demonstrate an enlarged foramen spinosum and increased meningeal vascular markings on the inner table of the skull. Computed tomographic studies demonstrate a well-defined mass of increased attenuation, with calcifications visible in approximately 20% of the lesions. The extent of the meningioma is clearly visible on enhancement with an IV contrast agent. Nonenhanced MRI is not as sensitive as CT at detecting meningiomas because there is not a significant contrast difference between these tumors and normal brain tissue. However, the use of an IV gadolinium contrast agent clearly demonstrates meningiomas on MR examination (Fig. 10-45). Surgical removal is the method of treatment for a symptomatic meningioma. However, if the meningioma is surgically inaccessible, stereotactic radiosurgery using a γ knife may be required.

Pituitary Adenoma

A **pituitary adenoma** is a usually benign tumor of the pituitary gland and comprises about 15% of all intracranial tumors. Hormones produced by the pituitary are affected, with one type of adenoma of the anterior pituitary resulting in gigantism if it develops before puberty and acromegaly if it occurs in adults because of excessive production of growth hormone (GH). Prolactin-secreting adenomas cause amenorrhea-galactorrhea syndrome, in which the breasts spontaneously secrete milk and menstrual periods cease. Pituitary adenomas may grow out of the sella turcica. As they grow, they compress structures such as the optic chiasm, causing visual problems.

A common radiographic demonstration of this growth is an enlargement and erosion of the sella turcica on a lateral skull radiograph. Angiography might demonstrate a displacement of the Sylvian triangle, but generally only after the adenoma has assumed a considerable size. The **Sylvian triangle** is an anatomic landmark created by the middle cerebral artery and its branches. A brain CT is useful to confirm the diagnosis of pituitary adenomas and to detect the extent of these lesions, especially when the tumor extends above the sella turcica. Enlargement of the sella turcica is generally

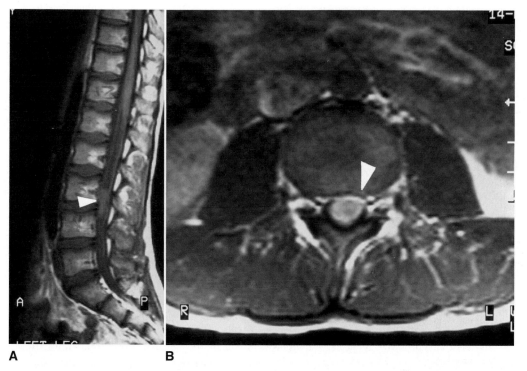

A   B

FIG. 10-43 A, A T1-weighted sagittal MRI view of the lumbosacral spine demonstrates an ependymoma at L3-L4 interspace in this young man. **B,** A T1-weighted axial MRI view with gadolinium demonstrates the same ependymoma.

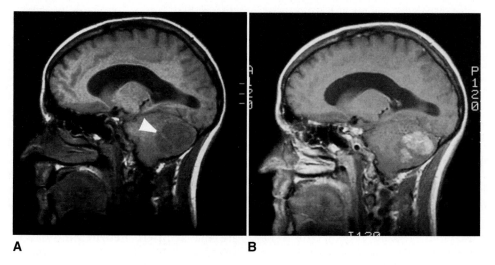

A   B

FIG. 10-44 A, A T1-weighted sagittal MRI view without gadolinium demonstrates a medulloblastoma in the cerebellum of this 25-year-old man. **B,** A T1-weighted sagittal MRI view with gadolinium demonstrates the medulloblastoma, illustrating more of its actual size.

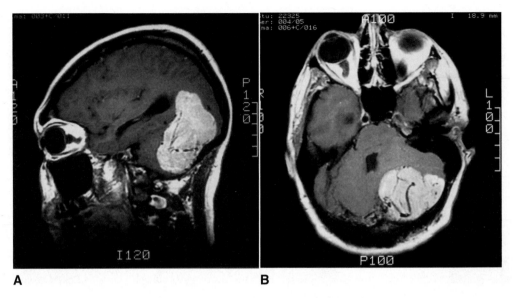

A   **B**

FIG. 10-45 A, A T1-weighted sagittal MRI view with gadolinium of a large meningioma in the posterior occipital area with marked hydrocephalus in this 31-year-old woman. **B,** a T1-weighted axial MRI view with gadolinium of the same meningioma. Displacement of the fourth ventricle is seen, as well as a distortion of the vascular structures within the meningioma.

demonstrated, as well as suprasellar extension into the optic chiasm. These neoplasms are generally slightly denser than the surrounding brain tissue and show obvious enhancement on IV injection of contrast medium. Small micro-adenomas are best demonstrated on thin slice, contrast-enhanced, MR images (Figs. 10-46 and 10-47) or high-resolution CT.

Generally, pituitary adenomas are treatable through surgical extraction, possibly followed by radiation therapy. Small adenomas may also be treated medically by drugs such as bromo-criptine that increase prolactin inhibitory factor (PIF) and suppress the tumor growth.

Craniopharyngioma

A **craniopharyngioma** is a cystic, benign tumor growing from remnants of the development of the pituitary gland. It is thought to be developmental in origin and most commonly presents in childhood. Craniopharyngiomas usually arise above the sella and extend upward into the third ventricle (Fig. 10-48). Occasionally, they are seen within the sella, causing erosion of the sella turcica. Calcification of the wall of the cyst is common and readily identifiable on plain films of the skull. CT examinations show a midline suprasellar mass of low attenuation containing calcification. Angiography may reveal displacement of the Sylvian triangle as caused by a pituitary adenoma if the tumor is large. Although craniopharyngiomas are treated surgically, excision is often difficult because of their location and proximity to structures such as the third ventricle and optic nerves. Radiation therapy is used to enhance the effects of surgery.

Tumors of Central Nerve Sheath Cells

Three tumors of the peripheral nerve sheath are the **acoustic neurilemmoma, acoustic neuroma** (Fig. 10-49), and **schwannoma** (Fig. 10-50). They account for up to 10% of all intracranial tumors and are most common

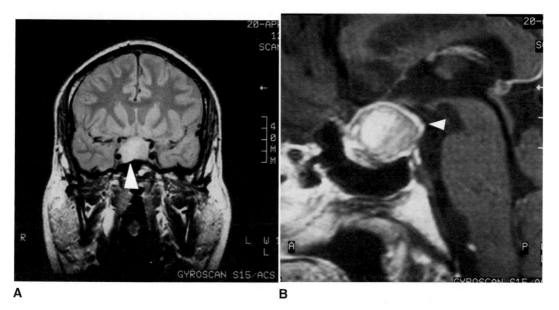

FIG. 10-46 A, A T1-weighted coronal MRI view demonstrates a suprasellar macroadenoma of the pituitary in this 37-year-old man. **B,** A T1-weighted sagittal MRI high-resolution scan with gadolinium demonstrates the same suprasellar macroadenoma of the pituitary.

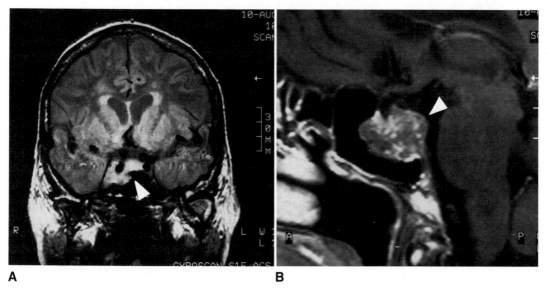

FIG. 10-47 A, Large pituitary adenoma extending downward into the right cavernous sinus in a 79-year-old woman as seen on this MRI T2-weighted coronal scan. **B,** A high-resolution T1-weighted sagittal MRI view of the same pituitary adenoma with gadolinium.

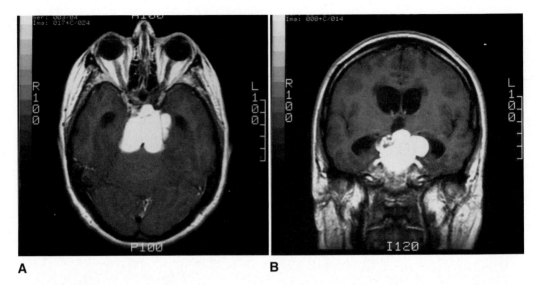

A   **B**

FIG. 10-48 A, A T1-weighted axial MRI view with gadolinium demonstrates a mass, later confirmed by biopsy to be a craniopharyngioma in this 53-year-old woman. **B,** A T1-weighted coronal MRI view with gadolinium demonstrates the relative size of the craniopharyngioma in the same patient.

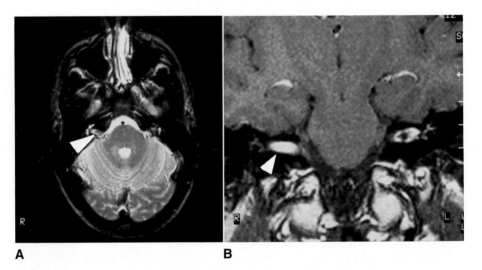

A   **B**

FIG. 10-49 A, A T2-weighted axial MRI view of a right acoustic neuroma that is not readily visible without gadolinium in this 24-year-old man. **B,** A high-resolution, T1-weighted coronal MRI view with gadolinium readily reveals the acoustic neuroma. Compare the appearance of the tumor with the appearance of the normal vasculature and anatomy on the left side.

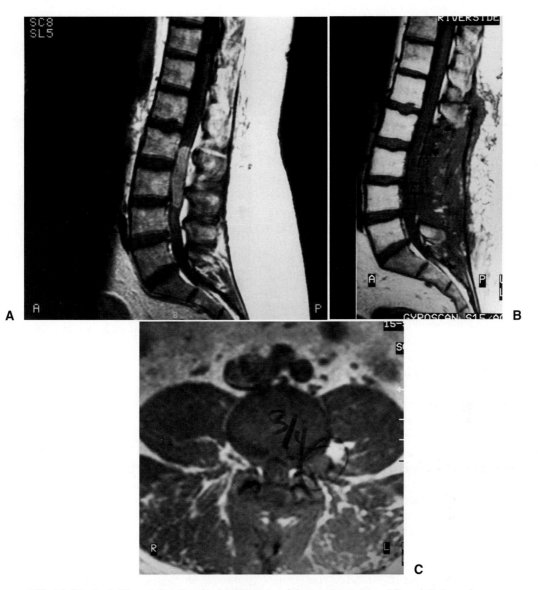

FIG. 10-50 A, A T1-weighted sagittal MRI view of the lumbar spine with gadolinium shows a schwannoma at L3-L4 before surgery in this 27-year-old woman. **B,** A T1-weighted sagittal MRI view of the same lumbar spine without gadolinium after surgery demonstrates apparent total excision of the tumor has been accomplished. Note also the excision of the spinous processes from the surgical site. **C,** A T1-weighted axial MRI view with gadolinium of the L3-L4 interspace demonstrates that some residual tumor is present in the left neural foramina.

in middle-aged and elderly adults. The most common site is the eighth cranial (vestibulo-cochlear or acoustic) nerve. At this location, the tumor compresses the adjacent brain tissue and erodes the temporal bone. Symptoms of acoustic neuromas include facial paralysis, tinnitus, and partial hearing loss on the affected side. Nerve sheath tumors can also be found on other cranial nerves, especially the fifth cranial nerve (trigeminal), and on spinal nerve roots and peripheral nerves. The imaging method of choice for acoustic neuromas is MR. In extreme cases, erosion and expansion of the internal auditory canal may be visible on an AP axial projection of the skull. Stereotactic radiosurgery or conventional surgical excision of the tumor are the methods of treatment.

Metastases from Other Sites

Secondary metastases from another site can involve any intracranial structure and account for about 10% of all brain tumors (Fig. 10-51). The metastatic lesions may be solitary or multiple. Brain metastasis usually arises from lung carcinoma. Other significant causes include adenocarcinoma of the breast, bronchogenic carcinoma, and malignant melanoma. Signs and symptoms of brain metastasis are similar to those for other brain tumors. Patients with metastases from other sites usually present with signs of increased intracranial pressure, especially headache and ataxia; those with primary brain tumors are more likely to present with seizures. Diagnosis and follow-up are done with MR and CT. Treatment includes resection using either conventional surgical techniques or radiosurgery, followed by radiation therapy. Prognosis depends on the number of metastatic lesions and the primary type of malignant disease.

Spinal Tumors

Primary tumors of the spinal cord are less common than those of the brain. They are commonly divided into extradural and intra-

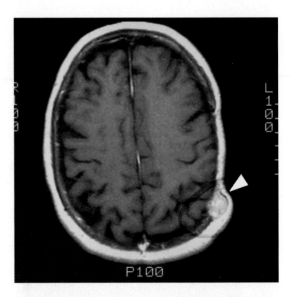

FIG. 10-51 Brain metastases from renal cell carcinoma as seen in this T1-weighted axial MRI view with gadolinium after craniotomy in this 59-year-old woman.

dural groups, with the latter further divided into extramedullary (outside the spinal cord) and intramedullary (within the spinal cord). The most common types (>60%) of primary spinal neoplasms are meningiomas (Fig. 10-52) and **neurofibromas** (Fig. 10-53), both of which are extramedullary tumors. The most common intramedullary tumors are astrocytoma and ependymoma.

Symptoms of these extramedullary tumors may be similar to those of a herniated nucleus pulposus in that spinal tumors also compress the nerve roots, leading to pain and muscular weakness. Intramedullary tumors cause progressive paraparesis and sensory loss. In evaluating spinal cord tumors, MR is the modality of choice and has essentially replaced myelography. Conventional spine radiographs demonstrate bony destruction and widening of the vertebral pedicles. CT myelography may be necessary to identify extradural tumors. Both intramedullary and extramedullary tumors may

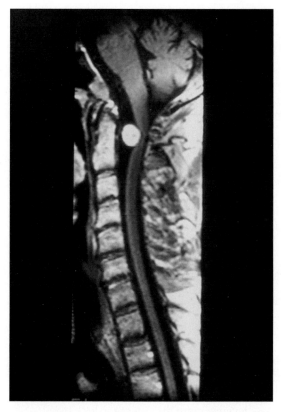

be surgically resected, depending on the location and degree of damage. Approximately 50% of patients undergoing surgery experience a reverse of clinical anomalies resulting from the neoplasm. In cases where surgery is not a viable alternative, radiation therapy is the primary means of treating the tumor.

FIG. 10-52 A T1-weighted sagittal MRI view of the spine with gadolinium demonstrates the presence of a meningioma in this 45-year-old woman with ataxia.

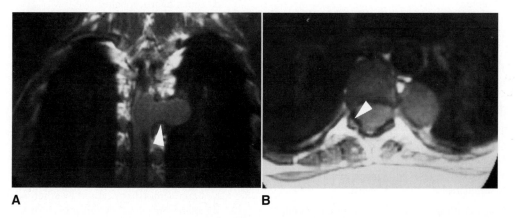

A   **B**

FIG. 10-53 A, A T1-weighted coronal MRI view demonstrates the presence of a "dumbbell" neurofibroma showing clear compression of the spinal cord of this young female with back pain and leg weakness. **B,** An axial T1-weighted MRI image similarly demonstrates the lesion and compression of the spinal cord *(arrow)* into a narrow space.

PATHOLOGY SUMMARY: THE CENTRAL NERVOUS SYSTEM

Pathology	Imaging Modalities of Choice	Additive or Subtractive Pathology
Hydrocephalus	CT, MR, ultrasound in the neonate	
Meningitis	MR	
Encephalitis	MR	
Brain abscess	CT, MR	
Herniated nucleus pulposus	MR, CT, myelography	
Cervical spondylosis	Radiography	Subtractive
Multiple sclerosis	MR	
CVA	MR, CT	
Glioma	MR, CT	
Medulloblastoma	MR, CT	
Meningioma	CT, MR	
Pituitary adenoma	CT, MR	
Craniopharyngioma	CT	
Acoustic neuroma	MR	
Spinal tumor	MR, radiography, CT, myelography	Both
Metastases from other sites	MR, radiography, CT	Subtractive

QUESTIONS

1. Under normal conditions, the central nervous system within the cranial vault is well protected from damage by all of the following except the:
   a. cauda equina
   b. cerebrospinal fluid
   c. diplöe
   d. dura mater

2. The correct order of meninges from outermost to innermost is:
   a. arachnoid, pia, dura
   b. dura, arachnoid, pia
   c. dura, pia, arachnoid
   d. pia, arachnoid, dura

3. The blood-brain barrier prevents passage of unwanted substances into the CNS through the cerebral:
   a. arteries   c. dura mater
   b. capillaries   d. veins

4. Erosion of the sella turcica is most commonly associated with neoplasms of the:
   a. meninges   c. pituitary
   b. pineal gland   d. pons

5. Protrusion of both the spinal cord and the meninges into the skin of the back is a:
   a. meningocele
   b. meningomyelocele
   c. myelocele
   d. spinal hydrocephalus

6. The most typical cause of meningitis is:
   a. bacterial infection
   b. trauma
   c. tumor compression
   d. viral infection

7. The imaging modality of choice for demonstration of herniated nucleus pulposus is:
   a. CT   c. conventional myelography
   b. MRI   d. ultrasonography

8. The term atherothrombic brain infarction denotes:
   a. brain hemorrhage caused by atherosclerosis
   b. infarction caused by thrombosis of a cerebral artery
   c. an embolism to the brain from a left heart thrombus
   d. none of the above

9. Which of the following neoplastic conditions are highly malignant and often occur in the cerebellum of children?
   a. astrocytoma
   b. medulloblastoma
   c. meningioma
   d. pituitary adenoma

10. The most common site for tumors of the peripheral nerve sheath (e.g., schwannoma) is on which cranial nerve?
    a. 4   c. 7
    b. 6   d. 8

11. Where is CSF manufactured and absorbed? Explain the physiologic basis for the development of hydrocephalus.

12. Why is MRI the modality of choice in demonstrating diseases in the posterior fossa?

13. What is the most common cause for CVA and the most common site for it to occur?

14. What are the major differences between meningitis and encephalitis?

15. Explain the differences between glial and nonglial tumors and give an example of each type.

Traumatic Disease

UPON COMPLETION OF CHAPTER 11, THE READER SHOULD BE ABLE TO:

- Differentiate among level I, II, and III trauma centers and the role each plays in the emergency medical system.
- Define common terminology associated with traumatic disease.
- Discuss the role of various imaging modalities in the evaluation and treatment of traumatic injuries.
- Describe, in general, the radiographic appearance of each of the given pathologies.
- Classify skeletal fractures according to the various classifications discussed in this chapter, and describe the healing process associated with skeletal trauma.

KEY TERMS

Atelectasis	Coup lesion	Level II trauma center
Avulsion fracture	Depressed fracture	Level III trauma center
Basilar fracture	Dislocation	Linear fracture
Blowout fracture	Fatigue fracture	Noncomminuted fracture
Closed fracture	Fracture	Occult fracture
Coma	Greenstick fracture	Open fracture
Comminuted fracture	Growth plate fracture	Pneumoperitoneum
Compression fracture	Hematoma	Pneumothorax
Concussion	Impacted fracture	Stress fracture
Contrecoup lesion	Incomplete fracture	Subluxation
Contusion	Level I trauma center	Torus fracture

In the United States, trauma is the most common cause of death for individuals between the ages of 1 and 34 years (Table 11-1), with injury from trauma accounting for approximately 145,000 deaths per year in the United States. The annual medical cost associated with trauma injury is approximately $200 billion. The Committee on Trauma of the American College of Surgeons (ACS) periodically reviews guidelines to ensure optimal patient care by classifying medical centers and hospitals according to their ability to treat various injuries and by publishing guidelines for trauma management. Trauma results primarily from motor vehicle accidents (MVA), unintentional accidents at home and in the workplace, gunshot wounds, stab wounds, physical altercations, domestic violence, and physical abuse. According to the Centers for Disease Control and Prevention (CDC), hospital emergency departments play a critical role in our nation's healthcare system, from treatment of minor trauma to, more recently, the first-line defense against bioterrorism.

Deaths from traumatic injuries have a trimodal distribution (Fig. 11-1), with the first critical period occurring seconds after the injury. Death during this period results from lacerations of the brain and spinal cord or the heart and great vessels. The second critical period occurs during the first 4 hours following the injury, with death generally resulting from intracranial hemorrhage, lacerations of the liver and spleen, or significant blood loss from multiple injuries. The third critical period occurs weeks following the injury, when death results from infection and multiple organ failure.

A well-designed emergency medical system (EMS) provides for prehospital care, acute hospital care, and rehabilitative care. Medical facilities are classified as level I, level II, or level III trauma centers based on the availability of specialized medical personnel and equipment. When patients are medically screened to determine their relative priority for treatment (triaged) at the site of an accident, their injuries are classified as life-threatening, urgent, or nonurgent. Multiple injuries most likely occur in conjunction with severe head injuries. These patients must be treated with utmost care. Before a trauma victim is transported, a clear airway must be established, acute bleeding must be controlled, and the patient must be immobilized to avoid displacing fractures of the skeletal system. Immobilization of the spine is paramount to avoid further injury to the spinal cord, and this is accomplished with the use of splints, backboards with head blocks, and special air splint suits.

TABLE 11-1 DEATHS AND RATES FOR THE 10 LEADING CAUSES OF DEATH IN SPECIFIED AGE GROUPS: UNITED STATES, PRELIMINARY 2000

Rank*	Cause of death and age (based on the Tenth Revision, International Classification of Diseases, 1992)	Number	Rate
	1-4 years		
...	All causes	4,942	32.6
1	Accidents (unintentional injuries) (V01-X59,Y85-Y86)	1,780	11.7
...	Motor vehicle accidents (V02-V04,V09.0,V09.2,V12-V14,V19.0-V19.2, V19.4-V19.6,V20-V79,V80.3-V80.5,V81.0-V81.1,V82.0-V82.1, V83-V86,V87.0-V87.8,V88.0-V88.8,V89.0,V89.2)	630	4.2
...	All other accidents (V01,V05-V06,V09.1,V09.3-V09.9,V10-V11,V15-V18, V19.3,V19.8-V19.9,V80.0-V80.2,V80.6-V80.9,V81.2-V81.9,V82.2-V82.9, V87.9,V88.9,V89.1,V89.3,V89.9,V90-V99,W00-X59,Y85,Y86)	1,150	7.6
2	Congenital malformations, deformations and chromosomal abnormalities (Q00-Q99)	471	3.1
3	Malignant neoplasms (C00-C97)	393	2.6
4	Assault (homicide) (X85-Y09,Y87.1)	318	2.1
5	Diseases of heart (I00-I09,I11,I13,I20-I51)	169	1.1
6	Influenza and pneumonia (J10-J18)	96	0.6
7	Septicemia (A40-A41)	91	0.6
8	Certain conditions originating in the perinatal period (P00-P96)	84	0.6
9	In situ neoplasms, benign neoplasms and neoplasms of uncertain or unknown behavior (D00-D48)	56	0.4
10	Cerebrovascular diseases (I60-I69)	45	0.3
...	All other causes (Residual)	1,439	9.5
	5-14 years		
...	All causes	7,340	18.5
1	Accidents (unintentional injuries (V01-X59,Y85-Y86)	2,878	7.3
...	Motor vehicle accidents (V02-V04,V09.0,V09.2,V12-V14,V19.0-V19.2, V19.4-V19.6,V20-V79,V80.3-V80.5,V81.0-V81.1,V82.0-V82.1, V83-V86,V87.0-V87.8,V88.0-V88.8,V89.0,V89.2)	1,716	4.3
...	All other accidents (V01,V05-V06,V09.1,V09.3-V09.9,V10-V11,V15-V18, V19.3,V19.8-V19.9,V80.0-V80.2,V80.6-V80.9,V81.2-V81.9,V82.2-V82.9, V87.9,V88.9,V89.1,V89.3,V89.9,V90-V99,W00-X59,Y85,Y86)	1,163	2.9
2	Malignant neoplasms (C00-C97)	1,017	2.6
3	Congenital malformations, deformations and chromosomal abnormalities (Q00-Q99)	387	1.0
4	Assault (homicide) (X85-Y09,Y87.1)	364	0.9

Data are based on a continuous file of records received from the States. Rates per 100,000 population in specified group. Figures are based on weighted data rounded to the nearest individual, so categories may not add up to totals. Data are subject to sampling and/or random variation.

... Category not applicable.
*Rank based on number of deaths.

(From National Vital Statistics Report, 49(12), October 9, 2001.)   *(Continued)*

TABLE 11-1 DEATHS AND RATES FOR THE 10 LEADING CAUSES OF DEATH IN SPECIFIED AGE GROUPS: UNITED STATES, PRELIMINARY 2000—cont'd

Rank	Cause of death and age (based on the Tenth Revision, International Classification of Diseases, 1992)	Number	Rate
	5-14 years—cont'd		
5	Intentional self-harm (suicide) (X60-X84,Y87.0)	297	0.7
6	Diseases of heart (I00-I09,I11,I13,I20-I51)	236	0.6
7	Chronic lower respiratory diseases (J40-J47)	130	0.3
8	In situ neoplasms, benign neoplasms and neoplasms of uncertain or unknown behavior (D00-D48)	106	0.3
9	Influenza and pneumonia (J10-J18)	83	0.2
10	Cerebrovascular diseases (I60-I69)	78	0.2
...	All other causes (Residual)	1,764	4.4
	15-24 years		
...	All causes	30,959	80.7
1	Accidents (unintentional injuries) (V01-X59,Y85-Y86)	13,616	35.5
...	Motor vehicle accidents (V02-V04,V09.0,V09.2,V12-V14,V19.0-V19.2, V19.4-V19.6,V20-V79,V80.3-V80.5,V81.0-V81.1,V82.0-V82.1, V83-V86,V87.0-V87.8,V88.0-V88.8,V89.0,V89.2)	10,357	27.0
...	All other accidents (V01,V05-V06,V09.1,V09.3-V09.9,V10-V11,V15-V18, V19.3,V19.8-V19.9,V80.0-V80.2,V80.6-V80.9,V81.2-V81.9,V82.2-V82.9, V87.9,V88.9,V89.1,V89.3,V89.9,V90-V99,W00-X59,Y85,Y86)	3,259	8.5
2	Assault (homicide) (X85-Y09,Y87.1)	4,796	12.5
3	Intentional self-harm (suicide) (X60-X84,Y87.0)	3,877	10.1
4	Malignant neoplasms (C00-C97)	1,668	4.3
5	Diseases of heart (I00-I09,I11,I13,I20-I51)	931	2.4
6	Congenital malformations, deformations and chromosomal abnormalities (Q00-Q99)	425	1.1
7	Cerebrovascular diseases (I60-I69)	193	0.5
8	Influenza and pneumonia (J10-J18)	188	0.5
9	Chronic lower respiratory diseases (J40-J47)	180	0.5
10	Human immunodeficiency virus (HIV) disease (B20-B24)	178	0.5
...	All other causes (Residual)	4,907	12.8
	25-44 years		
...	All causes	128,779	156.4
1	Accidents (unintentional injuries) (V01-X59,Y85-Y86)	24,817	30.1
...	Motor vehicle accidents (V02-V04,V09.0,V09.2,V12-V14,V19.0-V19.2, V19.4-V19.6,V20-V79,V80.3-V80.5,V81.0-V81.1,V82.0-V82.1, V83-V86,V87.0-V87.8,V88.0-V88.8,V89.0,V89.2)	13,261	16.1
...	All other accidents (V01,V05-V06,V09.1,V09.3-V09.9,V10-V11,V15-V18, V19.3,V19.8-V19.9,V80.0-V80.2,V80.6-V80.9,V81.2-V81.9,V82.2-V82.9, V87.9,V88.9,V89.1,V89.3,V89.9,V90-V99,W00-X59,Y85,Y86)	11,556	14.0
2	Malignant neoplasms (C00-C97)	20,200	24.5

(Continued)

TABLE 11-1 DEATHS AND RATES FOR THE 10 LEADING CAUSES OF DEATH IN SPECIFIED AGE GROUPS: UNITED STATES, PRELIMINARY 2000—cont'd

Rank	Cause of death and age (based on the Tenth Revision, International Classification of Diseases, 1992)	Number	Rate
	25-44 years—cont'd		
3	Diseases of heart (I00-I09,I11,I13,I20-I51)	15,267	18.5
4	Intentional self-harm (suicide) (X60-X84,Y87.0)	10,884	13.2
5	Human immunodeficiency virus (HIV) disease (B20-B24)	8,302	10.1
6	Assault (homicide) (X85-Y09,Y87.1)	7,156	8.7
7	Chronic liver disease and cirrhosis (K70,K73-K74)	3,644	4.4
8	Cerebrovascular diseases (I60-I69)	3,122	3.8
9	Diabetes mellitus (E10-E14)	2,416	2.9
10	Influenza and pneumonia (J10-J18)	1,437	1.7
...	All other causes (Residual)	31,534	38.3

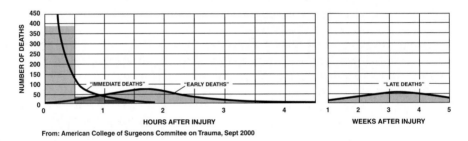

From: American College of Surgeons Commitee on Trauma, Sept 2000

FIG. 11-1 Distribution of trauma deaths.

This system ensures that the trauma victim is taken to the closest appropriate medical facility to receive the proper medical care for the injuries, but not necessarily to the closest hospital. Once the patient arrives at the proper medical facility, another careful assessment is necessary. This secondary triage assessment includes evaluation of the patient's state of consciousness, vital signs (blood pressure, pulse, temperature, and respiration), pupil size and reaction to light, and motor activity of the extremities. A cross-table lateral cervical spine radiograph is necessary to assess damage to the cervical spine before the patient is moved. Additionally, radiographs of the chest, abdomen, and skeletal system must be obtained to evaluate the extent of injuries. Although national vital statistics show that only 5% of all trauma victims have life-threatening injuries, these types of injuries are responsible for 50% of all in-hospital trauma deaths.

LEVEL I, II, AND III TRAUMA CENTERS

The primary hospital in the trauma system is a **level I trauma center.** These medical centers can provide total care for all injuries. A level I center status requires 24-hour per day in-house coverage by a radiographer to perform emergency radiographic and fluoroscopic procedures, surgical imaging procedures, and computed tomographic (CT) examinations. Technologists must be available on call to perform angiographic, sonographic, and nuclear medicine studies as required. Level I trauma centers are generally located in large metropolitan areas and serve as both primary care and tertiary care institutions.

Level II trauma centers are the most common trauma facilities serving as community trauma centers. These institutions can handle the majority of trauma cases and transport patients to level I facilities only when necessary. Level II facilities have a radiographer in house 24 hours per day to perform emergency radiographic, fluoroscopic, and surgical imaging procedures, with technologists on call to perform CT, angiographic, sonographic, and nuclear medicine examinations as needed. These medical centers are generally community hospitals located in smaller cities and towns and provide a valuable service. **Level III trauma centers** are usually located in remote rural areas and serve communities that do not have a level II center. Radiologic technologists are generally in house for most of the day but may be available on call during late evening and nighttime hours.

IMAGING CONSIDERATIONS
Radiography

Conventional radiography is the first imaging modality required in the management of a trauma victim. A cross-table lateral cervical spine radiograph is obtained to evaluate the presence or absence of a fracture before the patient is moved. Portable chest, abdomen, and/or pelvis radiographs are also generally obtained as soon as the patient arrives in the emergency department.

In addition, conventional radiographs are still the primary means of evaluating skeletal trauma. Additional information regarding damage to the muscle, tendons, ligaments, and soft tissue structures is obtained using magnetic resonance imaging (MRI). CT and nuclear medicine studies may also be employed to identify subtle skeletal fractures.

Computed Tomography

The high-energy impact associated with most MVA often results in injury to the neck and head, so CT is an important tool in assessing the trauma victim. CT is excellent for imaging acute cerebral hemorrhage and fractures of the skull and facial bones. Thin slice (2 mm) CT evaluation of the cervical spine is also necessary when conventional cervical spine radiographs do not adequately image the entire spine or when a possible fracture cannot be verified. Axial CT of the cervical spine is performed in conjunction with coronal and sagittal reconstruction to fully assess the areas of interest (Fig. 11-2). According to recent findings, CT evaluation can reduce hospital admission rates and result in more efficient surgical intervention by accurately identifying the presence and extent of injury in the trauma patient. MRI may also be employed to fully assess intracranial injury.

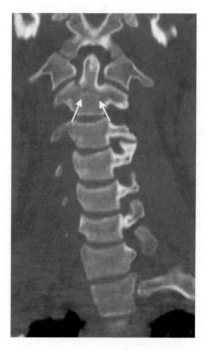

FIG. 11-2 A CT coronal reconstruction of a C2 fracture.

Blunt trauma to the abdomen is best evaluated with CT or abdominal sonography. Trauma to the urinary system occurs in about 10% to 15% of patients experiencing blunt trauma to the lower abdomen and pelvis. In cases of hematuria, CT is preferred over a conventional intravenous pyelogram (IVP) or urogram (IVU) examination. Although the use of oral contrast agents for abdominal CT is debatable, intravenous contrast is routinely employed to allow evaluation of vascular injuries and to better visualize the spleen, pancreas, and kidneys. In addition, in cases of blunt abdominal trauma, CT is able to better visualize fractures of the transverse processes of the lumbar spine, often missed on conventional spine radiographs. CT, in combination with a conventional AP pelvic radiograph, is also used to assess pelvic fractures commonly associated with abdominal injury. In cases of penetrating trauma to the abdomen, angiography may also be used to identify the extent of injury.

TRAUMA OF THE VERTEBRAL COLUMN AND HEAD

The initial management of patients with head and spine trauma is critical. Key items to assess at the scene of the accident include the mechanism of injury and changes in the patient's neurologic status. A neurologic assessment using the Glasgow Coma Scale should be conducted at the scene, and cervical spine injury should be assumed until it is ruled out by radiologic investigation. A cervical spine fracture can be present in up to 20% of patients with a severe head injury.

The head and neck should be immobilized, and care must be taken if intubation is necessary. Hyperextension injuries of the head and neck or direct trauma to the neck can injure the carotid arteries. Bleeding must be controlled to prevent shock, which can worsen the head injury. Once the patient arrives in the emergency department, cervical spine radiographs must be obtained. Computed tomograms of the head and spine may also be indicated, especially if the patient is comatose.

Many studies have been conducted regarding the effectiveness of airbags and seatbelts in preventing head and neck fractures in the event of an MVA. By far, those who do not use any restraining device sustain the most injuries. Those depending only on the airbags sustained the second largest number of injuries to the head and face, followed by those who only used a seatbelt. The most effective protection resulted from the use of both restraining devices. In addition, individuals using only a lap-type seatbelt have a high incidence of lumbar spine injuries, and individuals wearing only a shoulder belt without a lap belt sustain more cervical spine injuries.

Injuries to the Vertebral Column

The causes of vertebral column injuries include direct trauma and hyperextension-flexion injuries (whiplash). Radiographic indications of spinal column injuries include the interruption of smooth, continuous lines formed by the vertebrae stacking on each other (Fig. 11-3). Also, the vertebral bodies may lose some height, or the interspace may narrow. Muscle spasm as a result of trauma may cause a reversal or straightening of the normal spinal curvatures.

Perhaps the most common condition of the vertebral column is generalized back pain, typically in the lumbar area. This may result from injury to the area or from degenerative disease. Such back pain may not always result from bony involvement. Disk disease can cause muscle spasm with pain referral throughout the back. Finally, back pain may be secondary to referred pain from the hip.

Compression fractures are the most frequent type of injury involving a vertebral body. Usually the damage is limited to the upper portion of the vertebral body, particularly to the anterior margin. Such fractures generally occur in the thoracic and lumbar vertebrae

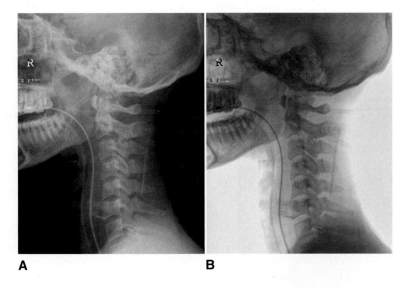

FIG. 11-3 A, A lateral cervical spine radiograph of an individual involved in a motor vehicle accident with an endotracheal tube in place. **B,** The same radiograph as in **A,** but imaged in an inverted mode to assist in evaluation. This is one major advantage of computed radiography.

(Fig. 11-4) with the most common site being T11-T12 in the thoracic spine and T12-L1 in the thoracolumbar juncture.

Cervical spine injuries may involve the odontoid process, usually at the junction of the odontoid and the body of the second cervical vertebra (see Fig. 11-2). A hangman's fracture (Fig. 11-5) is a fracture of the arch of the second cervical vertebra and is usually accompanied by anterior subluxation of the second cervical vertebra on the third cervical vertebra. A hangman's fracture, sometimes referred to as traumatic spondylosis, results from acute hyperextension of the head.

Radiography of the trauma patient with vertebral trauma is critical. Statistically, 5% to 10% of patients with one spine fracture will have another fracture elsewhere in the vertebral column. Fractures and dislocations of the spine are classified as stable or unstable. The spine may be visualized as two columns, with the anterior column composed of the vertebral bodies and intervertebral disks and the posterior column composed of the posterior elements (e.g., spinous processes, lamina). If either the anterior column or the posterior column of the spine is fractured or dislocated, the injury is classified as stable. However, if both columns are involved in the injury, it is classified as unstable. In all cases, the patient should be immobilized until cross-table lateral radiographs have been obtained and cleared by a physician. To rule out possible fractures and dislocations, the lateral cervical spine radiograph must include all seven vertebrae in their entirety, including spinous processes and intervertebral disk spaces. At times, this may require assistance in depressing the patient's shoulders or the use of the specialized cervicothoracic lateral projection (Twining or swimmer's method) to clearly demonstrate the entire seventh cervical vertebra and the upper thoracic vertebra in a lateral projection. Additional trauma projections of the cervical spine such as the pillar projection

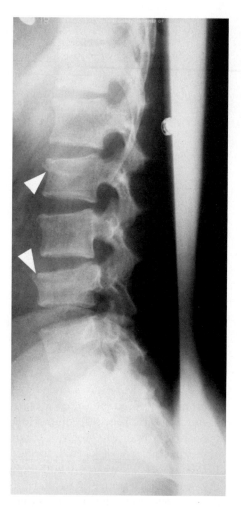

FIG. 11-4 A lateral lumbar radiograph demonstrating compression fractures of the second and fourth lumbar vertebral bodies with no apparent fracture of the posterior elements of the spine.

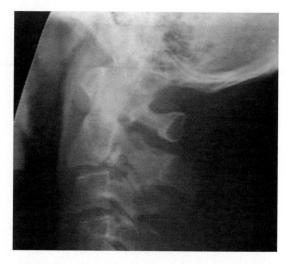

FIG. 11-5 A lateral cervical spine radiograph demonstrating a typical hangman's fracture with disruption of the spinal laminar line at C2 with the spinous process of C2 displaced posteriorly.

or trauma oblique projections may be requested to better demonstrate the complex anatomy of the spine. Trauma cervical spine radiographs are analyzed to evaluate (1) the size, shape, and alignment of the vertebral bodies and spinous processes, (2) the position and integrity of the odontoid process of C2, (3) the orientation and clarity of the facet joints, (4) the relationship of C1 to the occipital bone, (5) the alignment of the spinolaminal lines, and (6) any prevertebral swelling.

Spinal injury often results in a loss of neurologic function. It may be temporary or permanent depending on the cause of the dysfunction. Compression of the spinal cord by contusion or hemorrhage leads to rapid swelling of the spinal cord. This causes a rise in the intradural pressure and causes temporary neurologic dysfunction. This temporary loss of neurologic function usually resolves in several days. However, lacerations of the spinal cord or transection of the cord results in permanent damage because the severed nerves do not regenerate. Laceration of the spinal cord above the fifth cervical vertebra is almost always fatal, and lacerations below this region result in permanent paralysis. Patients with lacerations or transection of the cord develop immediate flaccid paralysis with loss of all sensation and reflex activity, which gradually changes to spastic paraplegia within days.

Fractures or dislocations of the vertebrae may impinge on the spinal cord and cause significant damage. The responsibility of the radiographer

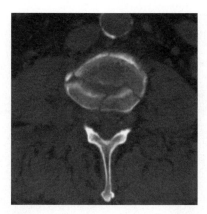

FIG. 11-6 An axial CT demonstrating a comminuted fracture of a vertebral body showing the location of each fragment.

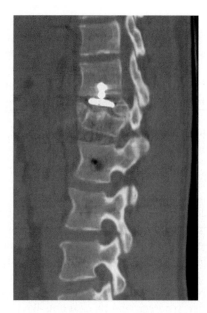

FIG. 11-7 A sagittal reconstruction CT performed postoperatively following the repair of a comminuted fracture of L1.

in terms of proper patient handling and obtaining of diagnostic-quality images cannot be overemphasized. CT plays a vital role in the diagnosis and treatment of vertebral fractures, dislocations, and associated problems (Fig. 11-6). In certain situations, MRI may be used to evaluate the extent of ligamentous and soft tissue injury or injury to the spinal cord.

Stable injuries to the spine are treated with complete bed rest until the swelling and pain subside. Unstable injuries are immobilized with traction until the bone and soft tissue structures have healed. Cervical radiographs are often performed to demonstrate proper alignment while the patient is in traction. Surgery may also be necessary for internal fixation of the fractures or to remove displaced fragments and decompress the spinal cord. CT of the spine is used preoperatively to serve as a road map for the surgeon because this imaging modality clearly demonstrates the size, number, and location of various fracture fragments. It may also be used postoperatively to demonstrate the success of the surgical procedure (Fig. 11-7).

Injuries to the Skull and Brain

The anatomy surrounding the delicate brain generally protects it well under normal condi-

tions. The diploic arrangement of the calvaria, the mechanical buffering action of cerebrospinal fluid (CSF), and the tough dura mater all work to prevent brain injury. Despite this protection, sufficient force to the skull can cause injury to the brain. Head trauma is the major neurologic cause of mortality and morbidity in individuals under 50 years of age.

Head trauma can result in skull fractures, brain injury, or a combination of the two. The role of plain film radiography in evaluation of head trauma is rather limited, as CT allows rapid assessment of the nature of any brain injury. Assessment of the state of the brain following head injury is more crucial than that of the skull. Routine skull radiography on trauma victims may be delayed to allow treatment of the complications of brain injury readily diagnosed by CT. Skull fractures visualized by either modality are often seen with accompanying hematomas. If patients sustain an open skull fracture, they are at risk for development of meningitis or brain abscesses. Regardless of the imaging modality used, the technologist must constantly observe a patient with a head injury while performing an examination. Any change noted in the patient's condition should be reported immediately.

Cerebral Cranial Fractures

Cerebral cranial fractures usually refer to those in the calvaria of the skull. Vascular markings in the skull, either venous or arterial, are routinely demonstrated as linear translucencies and can occasionally be mistaken for cerebral cranial fractures (Fig. 11-8). In most cases, a fracture appears more translucent than a vascular marking because a fracture traverses the full thickness of the skull. Although the edges of the fractures may branch abruptly, they can be seen to fit together, whereas venous channels have irregular edges that cannot be fitted together. The sutures between the individual cranial bones remain visible radiographically even after they become fused. To an untrained eye, these sutures may also resemble a fracture.

In most cases, the location of the skull fracture is more important than the extent of the

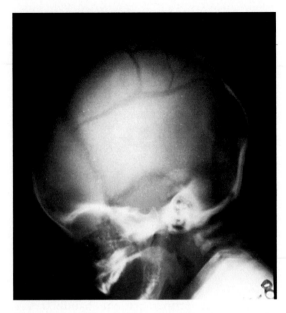

FIG. 11-9 A lateral skull radiograph of a 3-month-old infant with a history of striking his head on a bath tub. The radiograph reveals linear skull fracture of the parietal bone.

fracture. If the fracture crosses an artery, an arterial bleed may occur, resulting in an epidural hematoma. A fracture that enters the mastoid air cells or a sinus communicates with a potentially infected space and can lead to infection, possibly resulting in encephalitis or meningitis.

Fractures visible after skull trauma are generally classified as linear, depressed, or basilar skull fractures. **Linear fractures** appear as straight, sharply defined, nonbranching lines and are intensely radiolucent (Fig. 11-9). Up to 80% of all skull fractures are linear fractures. A **depressed fracture** appears as a curvilinear density because the fracture edges are overlapped (Fig. 11-10). These fractures are caused by high-velocity impact from small objects. Injury to the cerebral cortex may result, causing bleeding into the subarachnoid space. A depressed fracture is best demonstrated when the x-ray beam is directed tangential to the fracture.

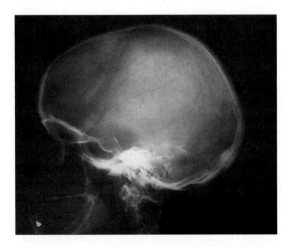

FIG. 11-8 A lateral skull radiograph demonstrating normal vascular markings within the cerebral cranium.

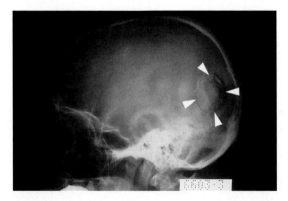

FIG. 11-10 A lateral skull radiograph of a child who was struck in the head with a baseball bat. The radiograph demonstrates a depressed fracture of the occipital bone.

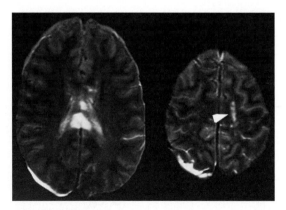

FIG. 11-11 A T2-weighted MRI image demonstrates a shearing injury of the corpus callosum *(arrow)* and a small subdural hematoma on the lateral margins of the brain in this young boy who fell and failed to regain consciousness.

Basilar skull fractures are very difficult to demonstrate radiographically. Air-fluid levels in the sphenoid sinus or clouding of the mastoid air cells is often the only radiographic finding suggesting a fracture. Therefore, it is important to include a cross-table lateral skull radiograph with the trauma skull radiographic series. CT and MR are often used to better identify basilar area fractures and associated soft tissue damage within the skull.

Brain Trauma

In addition to brain injury from a penetration wound (as could happen with a fracture), it can also occur from an acceleration and rapid deceleration of the head, which is termed a closed head injury. With head trauma, the brain is traumatically shaken within the cranium and subjected to forces of compression, acceleration, and deceleration. Brain tissues are injured from compression, tension, and shearing, with the last perhaps most important (Fig. 11-11). The superficial cerebrum in the frontal, temporal, and occipital regions is most often affected.

Following a blow to the head, an individual may experience a temporary loss of consciousness and reflexes. This widespread paralysis of brain function is known as a **concussion** and is characterized by headache, vertigo, and vomiting. Higher mental functions may be impaired for several hours, with the patient remembering little of the events surrounding the concussion. There is a strong tendency toward spontaneous and complete recovery because of the lack of structural damage to the brain. Recovery generally occurs in less than 24 hours. Treatment is conservative once assessment (usually by CT) has ruled out any hemorrhage or fracture. Bed rest and possible admission to the hospital are the usual means of dealing with concussion.

A brain contusion can also result from a direct blow to the head. This bruising of brain parenchyma is more serious than a concussion. A contusion formed on the side of the head where the trauma occurs is called a **coup lesion,** and one formed on the opposite side of the skull in reference to the site of trauma is a **contrecoup lesion** (Fig. 11-12). **Contusions** are characterized by neuron damage, edema, and punctate (pinpoint punctures or depressions) hemorrhaging. On CT, contusions appear as small, ill-defined foci of increased density (Fig. 11-13). Subdural or epidural hematomas can occur in conjunction with a contusion and

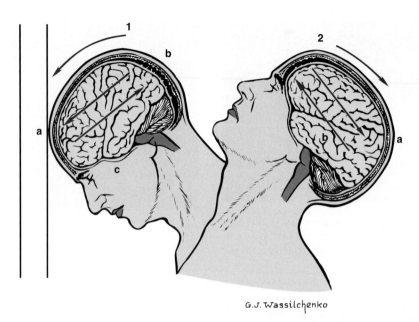

FIG. 11-12 Coup and countrecoup brain injury following blunt trauma. *1,* Coup injury: impact against object. *2,* Contrecoup injury: impact within skull. These injuries occur in one continuous motion—the head strikes the wall (coup) and then rebounds (contrecoup).

result in increased intracranial pressure that can be life-threatening. Signs seen in the patient with a contusion include drowsiness, confusion, and agitation. Hemiparesis and unequal pupil size may also be seen. CT plays a major role in the diagnosis of hematomas resulting from contusions, providing ready visualization of hemorrhagic blood, as described in the following section. Treatment is generally conservative, centering on prevention of shock, control of edema, and drainage of any hematoma present.

Persistence of loss of consciousness for more than 24 hours is known as a **coma.** This is usually a serious condition and may be fatal. Comas result from trauma to the head as well as from nontraumatic metabolic malfunctions or circulatory problems that do not provide sufficient blood flow to the brain. Diagnosis related to a coma may involve use of CT, MR, or both and is centered at determining, if possi-

ble, the cause of the coma. Treatment then rests on success in treating and alleviating the cause of the coma.

Hematomas of the Brain

As noted, brain trauma can result in hemorrhaging of blood from a ruptured artery or vein. Although venous bleeding occurs more slowly than arterial, both types of hemorrhage and resultant edema of the brain cause an increase in the intracranial pressure. Because the skull's structure does not allow expansion, the increased pressure displaces the brain toward its opening, the foramen magnum. This trauma to the brain results in serious neurologic consequences or even death if not treated promptly. CT plays the major imaging role in diagnosis of the hemorrhaging.

A **hematoma** is a collection of blood; four primary types of cerebral hematomas have been

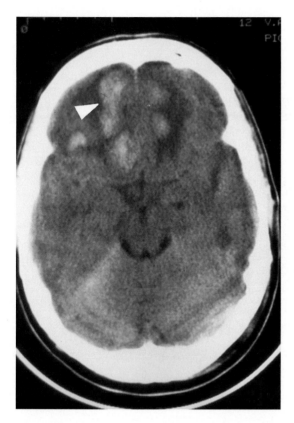

FIG. 11-13 An axial CT scan demonstrates hemorrhagic contusions of the brain as a result of a car accident for this young male patient.

increased density, generally occupying a small area with a sharply convex appearance. Often it is accompanied by a fracture of the skull or facial bones. If not diagnosed and surgically treated quickly, the outcome is fatal as a result of brain displacement and herniation.

A subdural hematoma is positioned between the dura mater and the arachnoid meningeal layers (Figs. 11-16 and 11-17). It usually follows blunt trauma to the frontal or occipital lobes of the skull and results from tearing of subdural veins connecting the cerebral cortex and dural sinuses. As a venous hemorrhage, it bleeds much more slowly than an epidural hematoma. In an acute stage, it is seen on CT as a curvilinear area of increased density on portions or all of the cerebral hemispheres. It pushes the brain away from the skull and causes a mass effect (i.e., brain shift across midline), with accompanying shift of the ventricles. In a subacute stage (up to several days old), it appears on CT as a decreased or isodense fluid collection. In a chronic state (2 to 3 weeks old), the surface of the hematoma becomes concave. Delayed coma can occur with a subdural hematoma.

A subarachnoid hematoma accumulates between the arachnoid layer and the thin pia mater that invests the brain. It occurs most frequently at the vertex where the greatest brain movement occurs in trauma, and it results from tearing of small vessels. In most head trauma cases, a subarachnoid hemorrhage is usually limited to one or two sulci, where it has a dense appearance (Fig. 11-18). Less commonly, the rupture of a major cerebral vessel results in subarachnoid hematoma.

An intracerebral hematoma can result from trauma as well as from nontraumatic causes such as a ruptured hemangioma or stroke (CVA). Common sites following trauma are the frontal, temporal, and occipital lobes of the brain. Small parenchymal vessels tear as a result of coup and contrecoup forces. An intracerebral hematoma is seen on CT as an increased density within the brain causing significant

identified (Fig. 11-14). The highest mortality rate is associated with an epidural (extradural) hematoma (Fig. 11-15). Even when promptly recognized and treated, it has a mortality rate of up to 30%. An epidural hematoma results from a torn artery, usually the middle meningeal artery, with blood pooling between the bony skull and the dura mater. Most commonly, the artery or its branches are torn by a fracture of the thin, squamous portion of the temporal bone. In more than 80% of cases, the skull fracture is visible radiographically. As an arterial bleed, it accumulates rapidly and quickly causes neurologic symptoms, including early coma. It is seen on CT scans as an

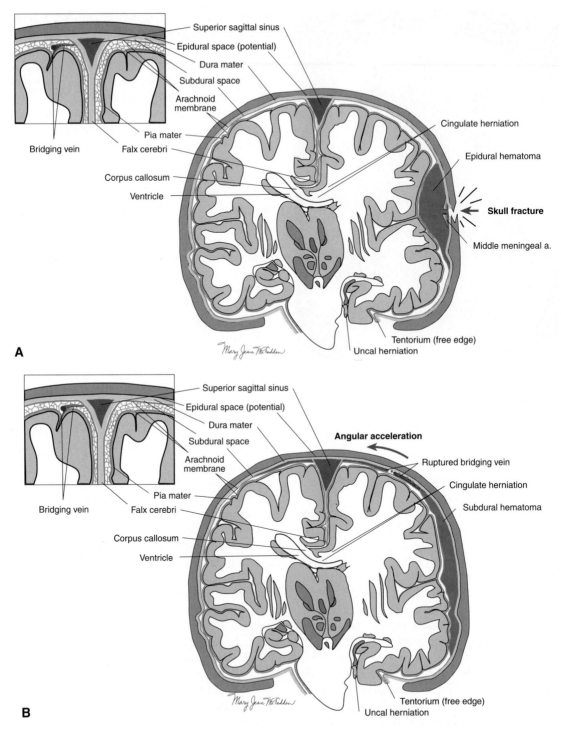

A

Superior sagittal sinus
Epidural space (potential)
Dura mater
Subdural space
Arachnoid membrane
Pia mater
Falx cerebri
Corpus callosum
Ventricle
Bridging vein

Cingulate herniation
Epidural hematoma
Skull fracture
Middle meningeal a.
Tentorium (free edge)
Uncal herniation

B

Superior sagittal sinus
Epidural space (potential)
Dura mater
Subdural space
Arachnoid membrane
Pia mater
Falx cerebri
Corpus callosum
Ventricle
Bridging vein

Angular acceleration
Ruptured bridging vein
Cingulate herniation
Subdural hematoma
Tentorium (free edge)
Uncal herniation

FIG. 11-14 Diagram of an epidural hematoma (**A**) and subdural hematoma (**B**).

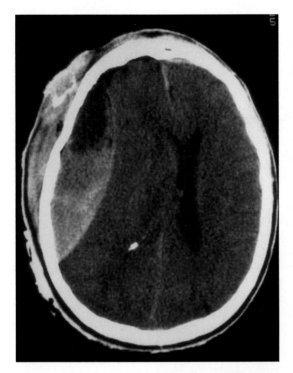

FIG. 11-15 A noncontrast axial CT view of this young male patient injured in an auto accident readily demonstrates a large epidural hematoma.

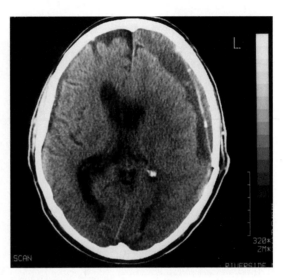

FIG. 11-16 CT demonstration of a large subdural hematoma outside the brain tissue in the left frontoparietal area of this 76-year-old man.

mass effect (Fig. 11-19) and may have an accompanying subarachnoid component. These hematomas develop edema around them as time passes and are slowly resorbed if the patient survives.

Diagnosis of hematomas is made primarily through clinical history and neurologic signs and symptoms. As noted, CT and MR play a major role in ready visualization of bleeding. Angiography may be used to visualize any defects in the cerebral vasculature. Treatment is often conservative unless active bleeding or significant mass effect is present, in which event an opening in the skull may be created surgically to allow drainage of blood and prevent complications. Prevention of infection and meningitis is important in the case of a fractured skull.

SKELETAL TRAUMA

Fractures

A fracture is a discontinuity of bone caused by mechanical forces either applied to the bone or transmitted directly along the line of a bone. When a fracture occurs, blood vessels are broken as a result of the break in the endosteum and periosteum. As blood and lymph and tissue fluids infiltrate this area, swelling and pain result. Such soft tissue swelling is a major clue to diagnosis (Fig. 11-20). Computed radiography (CR) is an asset in evaluating the soft tissue structures surrounding a skeletal fracture because one image can be manipulated to demonstrate both soft tissue and bony detail.

General radiography is extremely important in the evaluation of skeletal trauma and serves several purposes. The most obvious of these is to diagnose the presence of a fracture or dislocation. If a fracture is present, for example, a determination can be made as to whether the underlying bone is normal or whether the fracture is pathologic in nature. Before the fracture is stabilized, radiographs are taken to show the

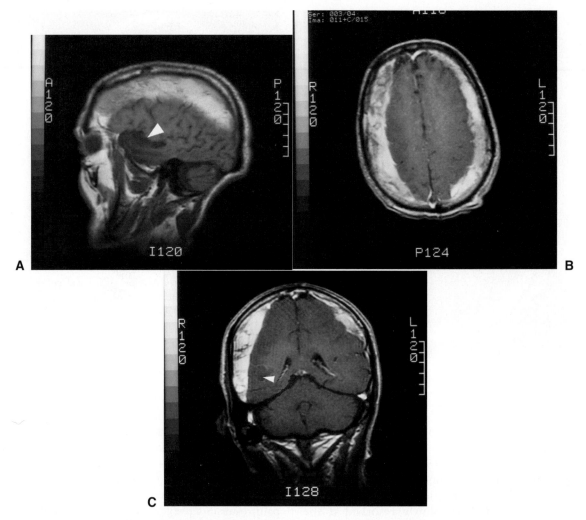

FIG. 11-17 A, A T1-weighted sagittal MRI view demonstrates a large subdural hematoma as well as a temporal lobe infarct *(arrow)*. The white versus gray appearance of the hematoma distinguishes subacute (fresh) from older blood. **B,** A T1-weighted axial MRI view with gadolinium demonstrates a large, bilateral subdural hematoma in this 67-year-old man. **C,** A T1-weighted coronal MRI view with gadolinium demonstrates the same bilateral subdural hematoma. The arrow indicates the right-sided temporal lobe infarct.

position of the bone ends. Fractures are in "good alignment" when there is no perceptible angulation or displacement in frontal and lateral projections. Postreduction films indicate the success of the fracture reduction (Fig. 11-21). Remember, if the fracture is placed in a cast, the exposure factors must be increased differ-

ently to penetrate the wet or dry cast. Finally, subsequent radiographs are taken to assess healing and any possible complications of fractures.

In any case of trauma, it is essential to have at least two projections of the part, preferably taken at right angles to one another. A minimum of

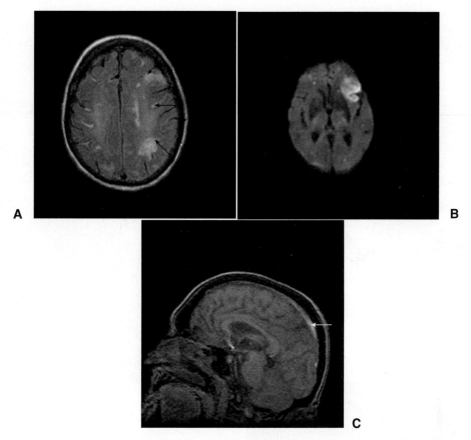

FIG. 11-18 A, B, Axial MR images demonstrating a subarachnoid hemorrhage as indicated by the sulci opacified by blood. **C,** A sagittal fluid-attenuated inversion recovery (FLAIR) MR image of the same patient.

two projections is also necessary to adequately determine fracture alignment (Fig. 11-22). These radiographs should demonstrate the joint above and below the area of trauma because there may be dislocation and because the injury may transfer force to a point distal or proximal to the point of injury. An example is a fracture or dislocation of the fibular head concurrent with an ankle or distal tibial fracture.

Frequently, fractures are obvious by clinical examination, but radiographic changes in appearance may be subtle. Fractures usually appear as a radiolucent line, but they may be thin and easily overlooked. Occasionally a fracture appears as a radiopaque line if the frag-

ments overlap. A step in the cortex, as indicated by a break in the normal bony contour, is a second radiographic indication (Fig. 11-23). Other signs include interruption of the bony trabeculae, bulging or buckling of the cortex, soft tissue swelling, and joint effusion. Also, the relationship of the end of a bone to its shaft is an important sign, as in the loss of normal volar tilt to the distal radial articular surface with an impacted distal radial fracture. CT (Fig. 11-24) and nuclear medicine bone scan are often used in combination with conventional radiography to assess skeletal fractures. MR is used as an adjunct to conventional radiography to assess soft tissues, muscles, ligaments, and tendons.

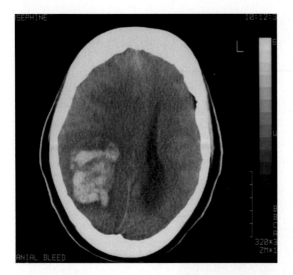

FIG. 11-19 A massive intracerebral hematoma that occurred spontaneously in this 63-year-old woman. The patient expired within a few hours after the bleed began.

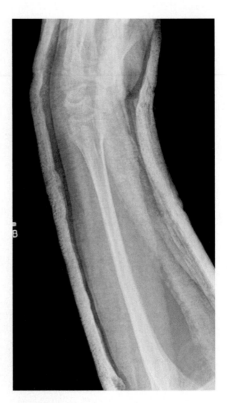

FIG. 11-21 A postreduction lateral wrist image showing proper alignment in the cast.

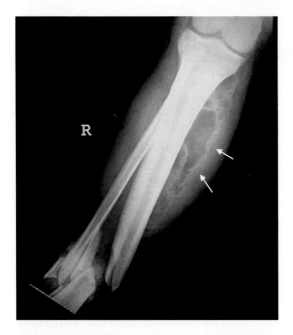

FIG. 11-20 A computed radiographic image of a comminuted fracture of the tibia and fibula with associated soft tissue edema.

Skeletal trauma usually causes significant soft tissue injuries, including neurovascular damage, capsular and ligamentous tears, cartilage injury, and hemarthroses. Such injury may be assessed in several ways, but the primary modality for assessing damage is MRI. Stress radiographs may also be utilized to determine ligamentous stability. Radiographs of both extremities are often used to compare epiphyseal appearance. Arteriography is used to assess any vascular damage as a result of skeletal trauma.

When performing radiography of the skeletal system, it is critical for the technologist to choose the appropriate exposure factors to produce a radiograph demonstrating good soft tissue definition in addition to achieving good penetration of the bony anatomy. If the soft tissue is too dark or the associated bony

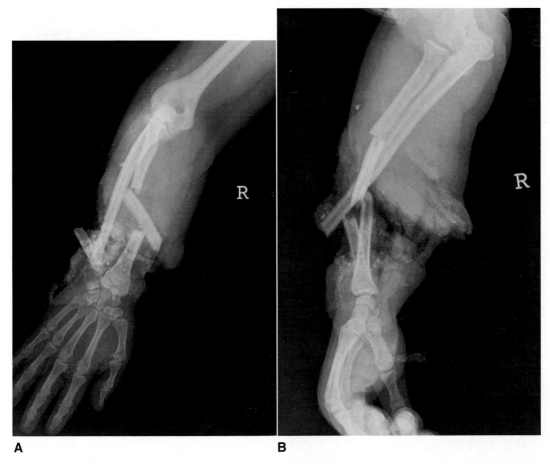

A   **B**

FIG. 11-22 A, An AP projection of an open comminuted fracture of the forearm caused by a machine injury. **B,** A lateral projection of the same forearm demonstrating anterior and posterior displacement of the fractured bones.

anatomy too light (i.e., no trabecular pattern), then the radiograph is of compromised diagnostic quality. As mentioned earlier, this is one advantage of using CR or direct radiography (DR) because by altering the image contrast (window width) and density (window level), the clinician can evaluate both soft tissue and bony structures on the same image. Additionally, it is often helpful to the radiologist if the radiographer notes, through film markers or as written on the requisition, areas of point tenderness. This is a highly specific indication of a

fracture that may be subtle. Larger body parts such as the hip, thigh, and knee are less assessable for point tenderness; instead, inability to bear weight is suggestive of a fracture. Again, an important role of the radiographer is to assess the patient regarding such symptoms and signs and to provide the radiologist with as much information as possible, both on the radiographs and verbally or in writing on the requisition.

Bone tissue is unique in its ability to repair itself in that it reactivates processes that nor-

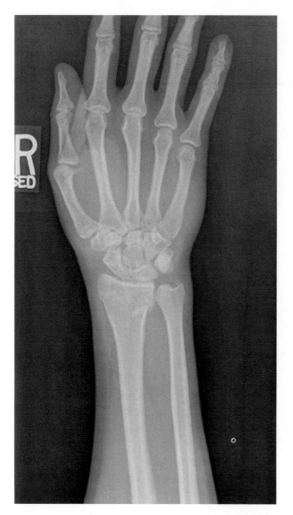

FIG. 11-23 A PA projection of the wrist demonstrating a subtle fracture of the radius. Notice a break in the bony cortex and discontinuity of the cortical bone.

mally occur during embryogenesis (Fig. 11-25). Initially, the break in the bone is filled by a large clot that temporarily bridges the fracture. Within 2 to 3 days, osteoblasts slowly begin to appear around the injured bone. Immobilization of the injured site is critical because any unnatural movement interferes with the deposition of the calcified matrix necessary for permanent union of the fracture. Provisional callus is mainly composed of cartilage and begins to form approximately 1 week after the fracture. As calcium continues to be deposited within the provisional callus, it is replaced by bony callus (Fig. 11-26), which is responsible for rigidly uniting the fracture site. Although the break is rigidly united within 4 to 6 weeks, excess bone still encircles the external fracture site, and excess bone is still found within the marrow space at this time. Remodeling of the bone and total healing require months. Weight-bearing force on the fracture site tends to guide the modeling process, so in many cases the patient may be instructed to begin using the affected limb in a limited fashion at this point in the healing process. If everything goes well during the healing process, the bone may repair to the point that the fracture site is no longer visible on subsequent radiographs. Proper healing greatly depends on the initial immobilization (casting, splinting, pinning, or plating), proper alignment or reduction of the fracture, and proper metabolic activity, which includes good vascularity and blood supply, proper nutrition, and normal hormone levels. Bacterial infections of the fracture site may inhibit callus formation, thus complicating the healing process.

Delayed union is a term referring to a fracture that does not heal within the usual time. If a fracture is not reduced properly or is not properly immobilized, malunion may occur. Malunion refers to a fracture that heals in a faulty position, thus impairing the normal function or cosmetic appearance of the affected body part (Fig. 11-27). The most serious complication is nonunion. Nonunion refers to a fracture in which healing does not occur and the fragments do not join (Fig. 11-28). This is often a result of lack of vascularization. Injuries to other soft tissue structures or organs can be associated with skeletal fractures, such as a rib fracture that penetrates the lung and results in a pneumothorax. Additional complications of skeletal fractures include muscular ossification and fat emboli occurring in bones containing yellow bone marrow.

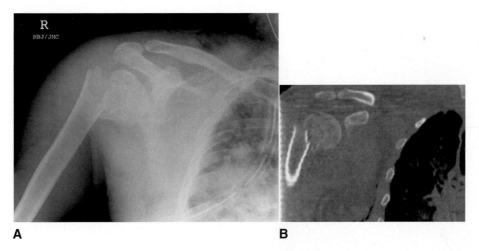

FIG. 11-24 A, A conventional AP projection of a shoulder demonstrating a fracture of the humeral neck sustained in a motor vehicle accident. **B,** A CT coronal reconstruction of the same patient.

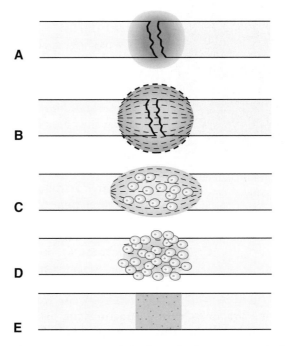

FIG. 11-25 A schematic representation of the bone healing process. **A,** Bleeding at broken ends of the bone with subsequent hematoma formation. **B,** Organization of hematoma into fibrous network. **C,** Invasion of osteoblasts, lengthening of collagen strands, and deposition of calcium. **D,** Callus formation; new bone is built up as osteoclasts destroy dead bone. **E,** Remodeling is accomplished as excess callus is resorbed and trabecular bone is laid down.

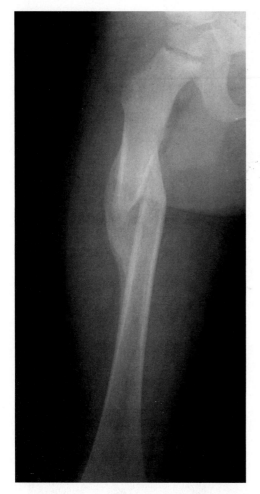

FIG. 11-26 A femoral radiograph demonstrating advanced callus formation following a transverse fracture of the femur.

Fracture Classifications

Several means of classifying fractures exist (Fig. 11-29). One distinction is whether the fracture is open or closed. An **open fracture** is one in which the bone has penetrated the skin (Fig. 11-30). This type of fracture leaves an open route for bacteria to enter from outside the body, which may lead to possible infection.

As described earlier, the intrusion of bacteria can alter the healing process, and precautions must be taken to prevent infection from setting into the bone or surrounding soft tissue structures. A **closed fracture** (formerly referred to as a simple fracture) is one in which the skin is not penetrated, thus reducing the chance of infection (Fig. 11-31).

Fractures may be classified according to the mechanics of stress that produce the break or the appearance of the fracture line. This includes torsion (twisting), transverse, linear, and spiral fractures. When one of the fractured bone ends is jammed into the cancellous tissue of another fragment, it is called an **impacted fracture** (Fig. 11-32).

Fractures may also be classified according to their location, such as intertrochanteric (transcervical) (Fig. 11-33), supracondylar, or transcondylar fractures. Often they may not fit into a specific classification because they may demonstrate mixed features. The following pages discuss the appearance of common types of fractures.

Comminuted Fractures

Sometimes one or more fragments separate along the edges of the major fragment in addition to the major line of the fracture. Such fractures are said to be comminuted (Fig. 11-34). **Comminuted fractures** differ from multiple fractures as follows. In the case of a multiple fracture, each fracture is complete, leaving a fragment of intact shaft between them. Comminuted fractures do not represent a complete thickness of bone as do multiple fractures. Occasionally, the bone involved in a comminuted fracture may be extensively shattered, as might occur from a gunshot wound. Such fractures are also particularly apt to be open fractures (Figs. 11-22 and 11-30).

A butterfly fracture is a comminuted fracture in which there are one or two butterfly wing or wedge-shaped fragments split off from the main fragments. A splintered fracture is a comminuted fracture with long, sharp-pointed fragments.

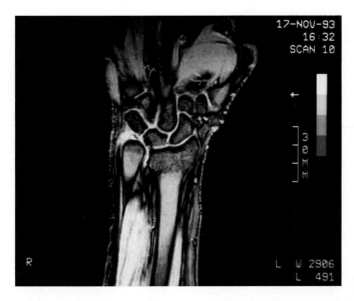

FIG. 11-27 An MRI of the wrist after fracture on a 55-year-old woman with a 2-month history of increasing pain and disability. There is malunion of the distal radial fracture with loss of palmar inclination and reversal with subsequent dorsal inclination.

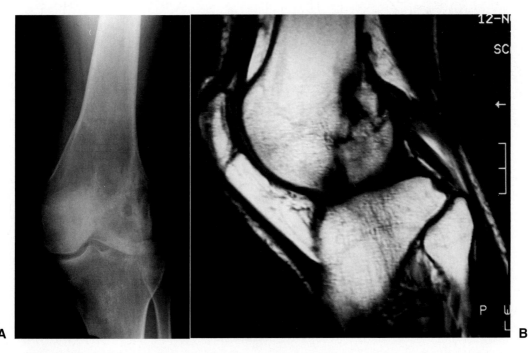

FIG. 11-28 A, A knee radiograph of a 32-year-old man who sustained a gunshot wound to the left knee 3 years previously. Nonunion of the lateral femoral condyle is demonstrated. **B,** An MRI of the same patient demonstrating nonunion of the posterior lateral femoral condyle with large subchondral defects.

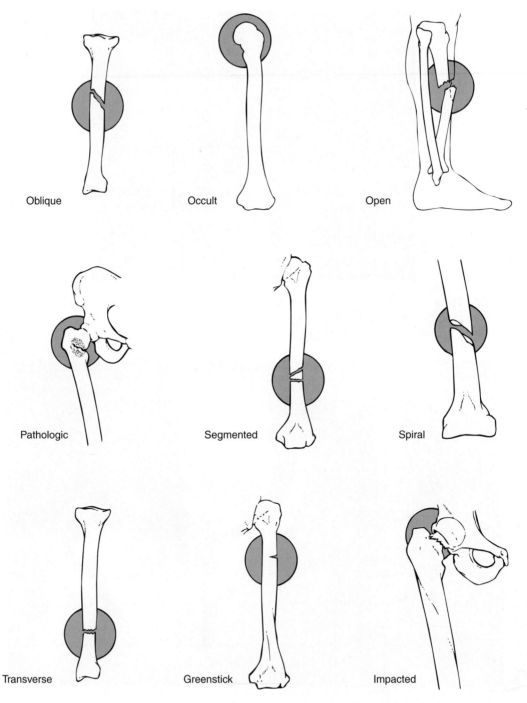

FIG. 11-29 Examples of types of bone fractures.

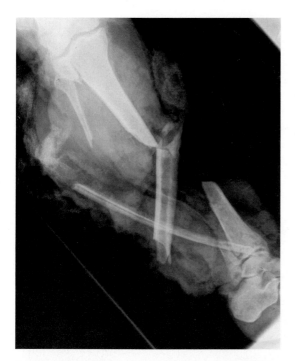

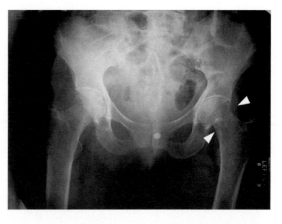

FIG. 11-32 A radiograph of the pelvis on an elderly woman with trauma to her left hip. The radiograph demonstrates an impacted fracture of the left hip.

FIG. 11-30 An open, comminuted fracture of the tibia and fibula with amputation.

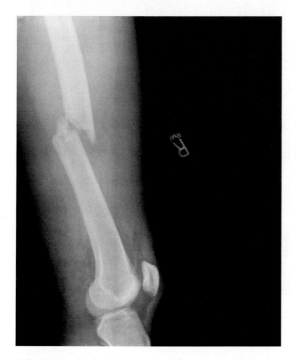

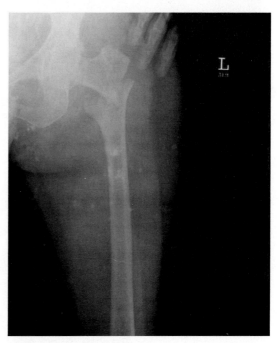

FIG. 11-33 An AP projection demonstrating an intertrochanteric fracture of the femur.

FIG. 11-31 A closed transverse fracture of the femur.

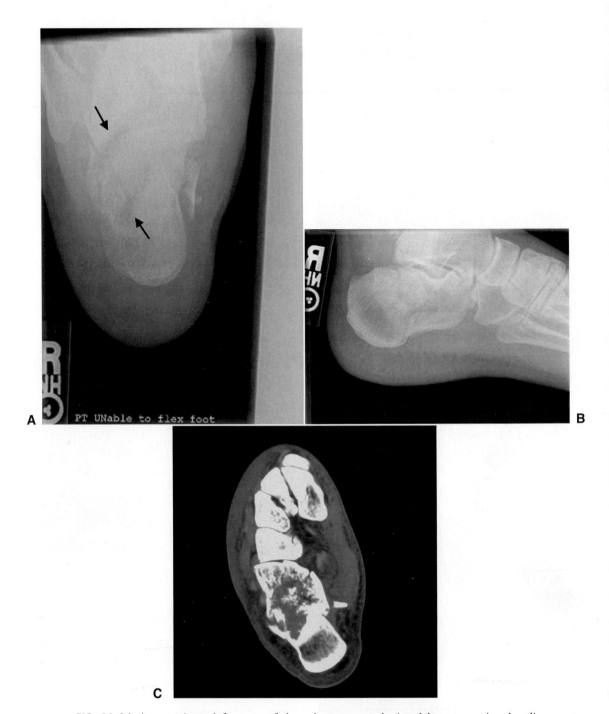

FIG. 11-34 A comminuted fracture of the calcaneous as depicted by conventional radiographs. **A,** An AP axial projection. **B,** A lateral projection. **C,** An axial CT of the same patient.

Complete, Noncomminuted Fractures

Complete, **noncomminuted fractures** are those in which the bone has separated into two fragments. The fractures may be recognized according to the direction of the fracture line. A spiral or oblique fracture is an example of this type. Such a fracture usually results from a rotary type of injury that twists the bone apart and is particularly common in the shafts of long bones (Fig. 11-35). A transverse fracture (Figs. 11-36, 11-37, and 11-38) is another type of complete, noncomminuted fracture. Demonstrated radiographically, such a fracture through normal bone is invariably ragged along the fracture line. A pathologic fracture is commonly a transverse fracture occurring in abnormal bone that is weakened by various

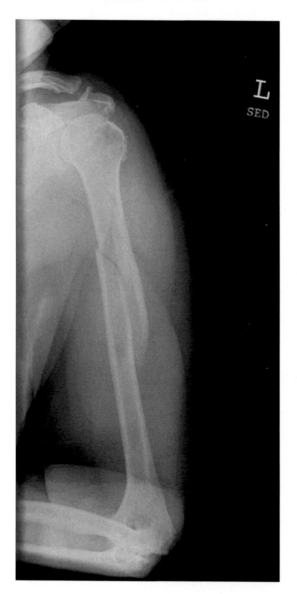

FIG. 11-35 A humerus radiograph of an individual who sustained a twisting injury of the humerus. The radiograph demonstrates a spiral fracture of the humerus.

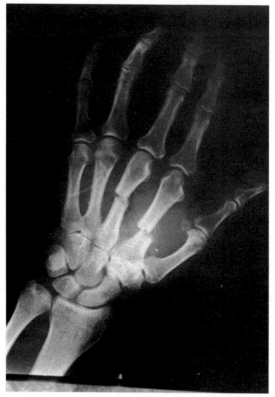

FIG. 11-36 A hand radiograph of a 32-year-old man involved in an industrial accident, demonstrating transverse fractures of the second and third metacarpals.

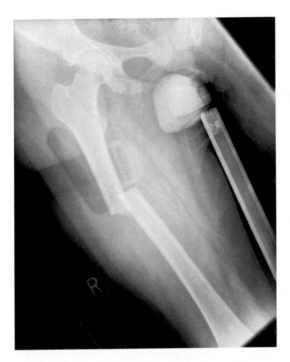

FIG. 11-37 An AP projection of a transverse fracture of the femur.

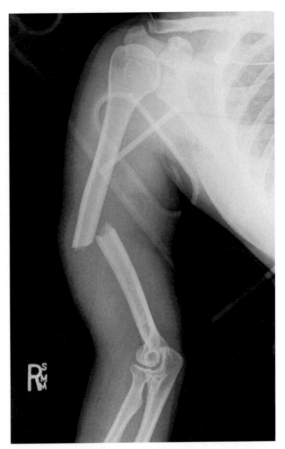

FIG. 11-38 An AP projection of a transverse fracture of the humerus sustained in a motor vehicle accident. Notice the backboard visible on the image.

diseases, such as a bone cyst or metastatic bone neoplasm (Fig. 11-39). It may result from the disease process itself or from a relatively minor trauma. Often, pathologic fractures may be the first indication of the presence of pathology. Multiple fractures are another type of complete, noncomminuted fracture in which two or more complete fractures occur involving the shaft of a single bone (Fig. 11-40).

Avulsion Fractures

Avulsion fractures occur when a fragment of bone is pulled away from the shaft. These usually occur around joints because of ligament, tendon, and muscle tearing, as associated with a sprain or dislocation (Fig. 11-41). A chip fracture is an avulsion fracture of a small fragment or chip of bone from the corner of a phalanx or other long bone. These are very common in the fingers and are often tiny.

Incomplete Fractures

Incomplete fractures are those in which only part of the bony structure gives way, with little or no displacement. A common example is the **greenstick fracture,** in which the cortex breaks on one side without separation or breaking of the opposing cortex (Fig. 11-42). The effect is similar to that of trying to break a green twig; hence its name. Greenstick fractures are found almost exclusively in infants and children under the age of 10 years because of the softness of the cancellous bone. A **torus fracture** is a greenstick fracture in which the cortex bulges

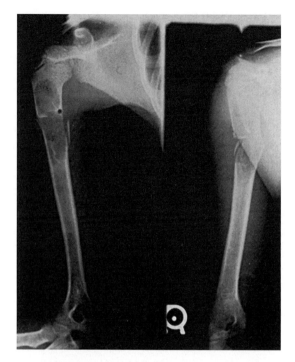

FIG. 11-39 A humerus radiograph demonstrating a pathologic fracture through a bone cyst. The patient had complained of pain and denied a history of trauma associated with this fracture.

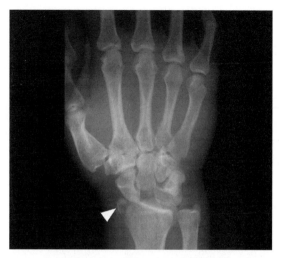

FIG. 11-41 A wrist radiograph obtained following trauma to the wrist resulting in perilunate dislocation with an associated avulsion fracture of the distal radius.

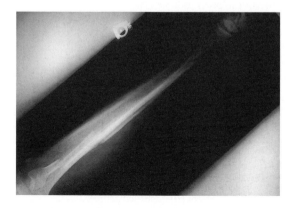

FIG. 11-40 A forearm radiograph of an individual involved in a motor vehicle accident. The radiograph revealed multiple fractures of the forearm.

outward, usually in the metaphysis, producing only a slight irregularity (Fig. 11-43).

Incomplete fractures may also occur in demineralized bone, such as occurs with osteoporosis. The bone in question breaks only part of the way through, resulting in a sharp angular deformity without displacement.

Penetrating fractures are a type of incomplete fracture resulting from penetration by a sharp object such as a bullet or a knife. Frequently there is a comminution at the site of the injury.

Growth Plate Fractures

Growth plate fractures involve the end of a long bone of a child (Fig. 11-44). The fracture may be limited to growth plate cartilage and is thus not directly visible unless displacement occurs, or it may extend into the metaphysis, epiphysis, or both. Crush injuries of the growth plate can also occur. Comparison projections are often used with such fractures to compare growth plate appearances, and MR may be used

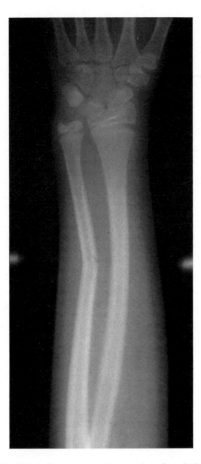

FIG. 11-42 A forearm radiograph of a child who sustained a fall. It demonstrates a greenstick fracture of the middle portion of the ulna. Notice the incomplete break of the cortex of the ulna.

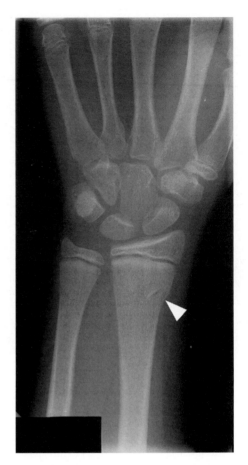

FIG. 11-43 A forearm radiograph of a 14-year-old girl who fell on her hand, resulting in a torus fracture of the distal radius.

to further evaluate epiphyseal separations. Healed injuries of this type may result in an alteration of the length of the involved bone.

Stress and Fatigue Fractures

Stress fractures usually occur as a result of an abnormal degree of repetitive trauma. They are generally found at the point of muscular attachments, such as in the fibula of a runner. Stress fractures may not be clearly visible on plain radiographs, especially initially on injury, but may be diagnosed with a nuclear medicine bone

scan or an MR of the affected area (Fig. 11-45). **Fatigue fractures** occur at sites of maximal strain on a bone, usually in connection with unaccustomed activity. Most frequently, fatigue fractures are found in the metatarsals, particularly the second metatarsal—the classic "march" fracture. Other common names for fatigue fractures include stretch or insufficiency fractures.

Occult Fractures and Bone Bruise

An **occult fracture** gives clinical signs of its presence without radiologic evidence. Follow-up examination within 10 days reveals bone

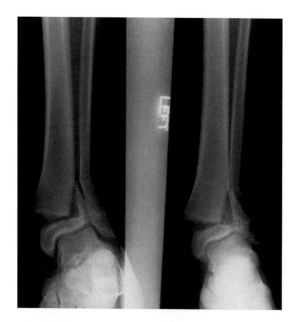

FIG. 11-44 A lower leg radiograph demonstrating an epiphyseal-metaphyseal fracture of the tibia with a transverse diaphyseal fracture of the distal fibula.

resorption or displacement at the fracture site (Fig. 11-46). The most common sites for occult fractures are the carpal navicular and the ribs. A bruise to the bone may be revealed on MR examination (Fig. 11-47) and is presumed to represent hemorrhage and edema, usually beneath an adjacent joint surface. Nuclear medicine bone scans may also be helpful in assessing subtle rib fractures.

Fractures in Specific Locations

Some fractures occur in selected areas and are usually easily recognized. One of these is the Colles' fracture (Fig. 11-48), which is a fracture through the distal inch of the radius. The distal fragment is usually angled backward on the shaft with impaction along the dorsal aspect. An avulsion fracture of the ulnar styloid process occurs in more than half of all Colles' fractures. This is the most common wrist fracture, and it usually results from falling on an outstretched hand. The external skin contour of a Colles' fracture displays a "dinner fork" deformity. A Smith's fracture is a reverse Colles' fracture with displacement toward the palmar aspect of the hand. A direct blow or fall with the wrist in hyperflexion is the usual mechanism of injury.

A boxer's fracture occurs when the fifth metacarpal (and occasionally the fourth metacarpal) fractures as a result of a blow to or with the hand (Fig. 11-49). It is the most common type of metacarpal fracture and may be immobilized with or without reduction, as it is difficult to maintain the reduction in this type of fracture. A Bennett's fracture is a fracture and dislocation of the first carpometacarpal joint. This fracture results in an avulsion fracture of the base of the first metacarpal in association with a dislocation of the trapezium from the pulling action of the abductor pollicus longus tendon in the hand. The injury occurs when the thumb is forced backward while in partial flexion and is commonly seen in basketball players and skiers. It may be repaired with a closed pinning technique if the fracture displacement is less than 3 mm or with an open reduction in cases of displacement greater than 3 mm. A Monteggia's fracture is one of the proximal third of the ulnar shaft, with anterior dislocation of the radial head (Fig. 11-50). With both proximal and distal injuries to the forearm, it is important to ensure that both joints are included on the radiograph.

In the ankle, the most common injuries are to the malleoli. A Pott's fracture involves both malleoli, with dislocation of the ankle joint (Fig. 11-51). Less common fractures may seem more like minor sprains, requiring the radiologist to examine every aspect of the bony anatomy. A Maisonneuve fracture (Fig. 11-52) is a less frequent ankle injury. It consists of a severe ankle sprain with a fracture of the proximal third of the fibula. This fracture may be easily overlooked because the more painful ankle injury may cause the proximal fibular injury to be missed.

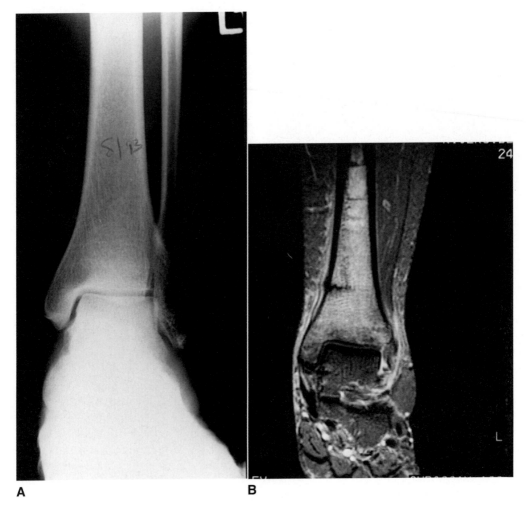

FIG. 11-45 A, An ankle radiograph on a 55-year-old woman complaining of pain in the medial aspect of the distal tibia. The radiograph appears normal with no evidence of fracture. **B,** An MRI of the same patient demonstrating a stress fracture of the distal tibia.

As mentioned earlier, radiographic signs of some fractures are subtle at best. Such is sometimes the case with the elbow. The elbow "fat pad sign" can be an indicator of a nonvisualized, underlying fracture of the bones of the elbow. In the elbow, there is normally a small accumulation of fat adjacent to the anterior surface of the distal humerus. This radiolucency is normally visible radiographically on a lateral

projection of the elbow. A similar pad is found along the posterior surface but is normally not visualized radiographically. If the joint capsule is distended by fluid as a result of a fracture, the posterior fat pad becomes displaced from the bone and is visible on the lateral projection of the elbow. Visualization of a posterior fat pad is considered to be a sign of a possible underlying fracture. The anterior fat pad may also be

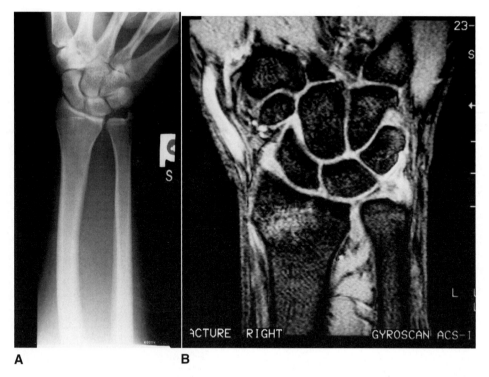

A   **B**

FIG. 11-46 A, A right wrist radiograph of a 31-year-old man who sustained an injury by falling while ice skating. No definite fracture or dislocation is demonstrated. **B,** An MR of the right wrist of the same patient as in **A** demonstrating an occult, oblique, intraarticular distal radial fracture beginning just proximal to the styloid and extending to the middle third of the radius.

displaced, giving a sail-shaped appearance. This is a prime example of how soft tissue demonstration can assist in making a diagnosis.

Visceral Cranial Fractures

Visceral cranial fractures refer to fractures of the facial bones and generally result from a blow to the face. As discussed earlier, facial or head trauma may also indicate a possible cervical spine fracture or injury. In addition, soft tissue injury of the eyes, nose, and mandible is often accompanied by bony fractures. CT has largely replaced the use of conventional radiographs in evaluating fractures of the maxillofacial bones and orbits (Fig. 11-53).

A zygomatic arch fracture may be difficult to recognize initially because of the edema. However, a fracture may be indicated by clinical signs, which include black eyes, flattening of the cheek, and a restriction of the movement of the mandible. Careful examination by palpation is performed by the physician because a fracture of the zygomatic arch may be present without accompanying facial fractures. A depressed fracture of the zygomatic arch may also be difficult to demonstrate radiographically (Fig. 11-54). If radiographs are requested, an oblique submentovertical projection may be used to best demonstrate the extent of the fracture. A parietoacanthal (Waters' method) is also of value in

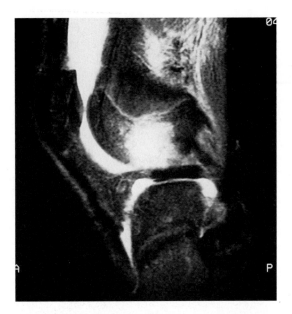

FIG. 11-47 An MRI of the right knee of a 17-year-old boy who suffered a rotary injury while playing basketball. The image demonstrates extensive bone bruising of the lateral meniscocondylar notch and femoral condyles.

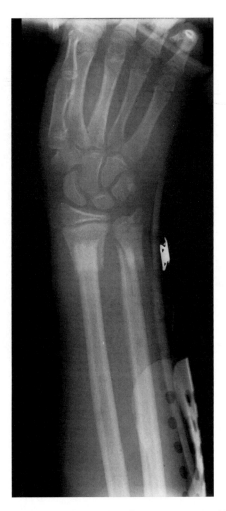

FIG. 11-48 A radiograph of a wrist on an elderly woman who fell on an outstretched hand. The radiograph demonstrates a classic Colles' fracture.

examining the fractures of the zygomatic arch. The mandible is very prone to fracture because of the prominence of the chin; therefore, any patient suffering a head or face injury should be clinically examined for a mandibular fracture. Anatomically, the mandible is strongest at the center and weakest at the ends, with the most common site for fracture at the angle, followed by the condyles. Mandibular fractures (Fig. 11-55) are generally detected by the patient's inability to open the mouth and pain when moving the mandible. These fractures also cause a misalignment of the patient's teeth. Care must be taken to demonstrate all areas of the mandible (body, ramus, and symphysis) when ruling out mandibular fractures. The mandible is the slowest healing bone in the body and will show clinical union much sooner than radiographic union.

Fractures of the maxilla are serious because of the adjacent nasal cavity, paranasal sinuses, and orbit and the close proximity of the brain. The maxilla also transmits cranial nerves and major blood vessels. Maxillary fractures may be divided into three major classifications: horizontal, pyramidal, and transverse. A horizontal fracture of the maxilla (LeFort I) refers to a separation of the body of the maxilla from the base of the skull above the palate and below the zygomatic process. This type of fracture results in a freely movable jaw. A pyramidal fracture (LeFort II) involves vertical fractures through

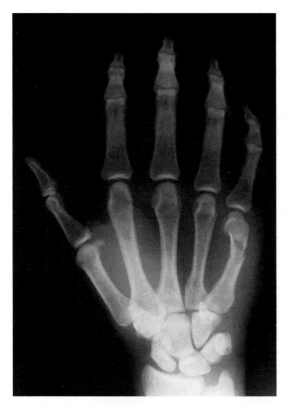

FIG. 11-49 A radiograph demonstrating a boxer's fracture of the fifth metacarpal head of the right hand.

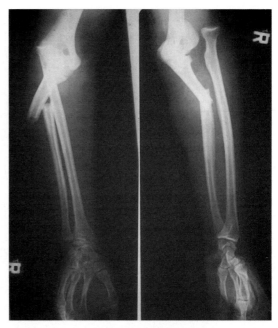

FIG. 11-50 A forearm radiograph of an individual who fell off a cliff, landing on an outstretched hand with the elbow partially flexed. The radiograph demonstrates a Monteggia's fracture of the forearm.

the maxilla at the malar and nasal bones, forming a triangular separation of the maxilla. A transverse fracture (LeFort III) is the most extensive and serious type of maxillary fracture; it extends across the orbits and results in separation of the visceral and cerebral cranium.

A **blowout fracture** results from a direct blow to the front of the orbit that transfers the force to the orbital walls and floor. This fracture occurs in the thinnest, weakest portion of the orbit, the orbital floor just above the maxillary sinuses (see Fig. 11-53C,D). If this condition is not diagnosed and treated, impairment of extraocular movements develops. A parietoacanthal projection (modified Waters' method) provides the most information in terms of conventional radiographic diagnosis of blowout

fractures. Again, CT is the best modality for imaging the orbits.

A tripod fracture occurs when the zygomatic or malar bone is fractured at all three sutures: frontal, temporal, and maxillary (Fig. 11-56). The patient with a tripod fracture complains of restricted jaw movement because the mandible's coronoid process is trapped by the zygoma. This fracture results in a free-floating zygoma and may cause facial disfigurement if not diagnosed and properly treated.

The nasal bone is the most frequently fractured facial bone. The fracture is usually transverse and depresses the distal portion of the nasal bones. A nasal bone fracture may be accompanied by a fracture of the ascending process of the maxillae or of the nasal septum. The nasal septum is composed of the vomer and the perpendicular plate of the ethmoid

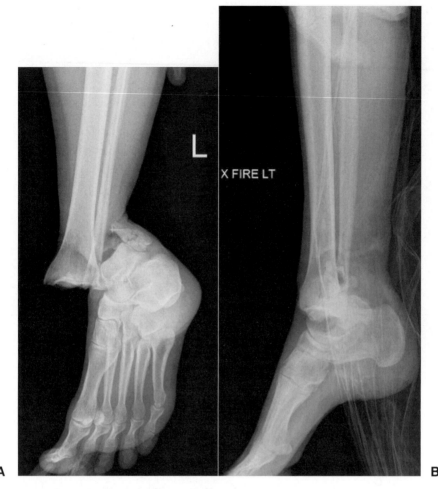

FIG. 11-51 Ankle radiographs (**A,** AP projection; **B,** lateral projection) depicting a Pott's fracture of the ankle. Notice the trimalleolar fracture and dislocation of the joint. The injury was sustained in an MVA between a car and semi-truck.   *Continued*

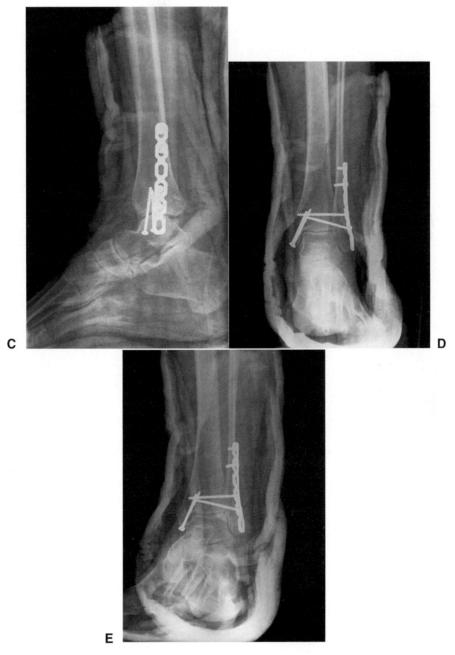

FIG. 11-51, cont'd C-E, Postreduction images obtained following surgical repair of the fracture.

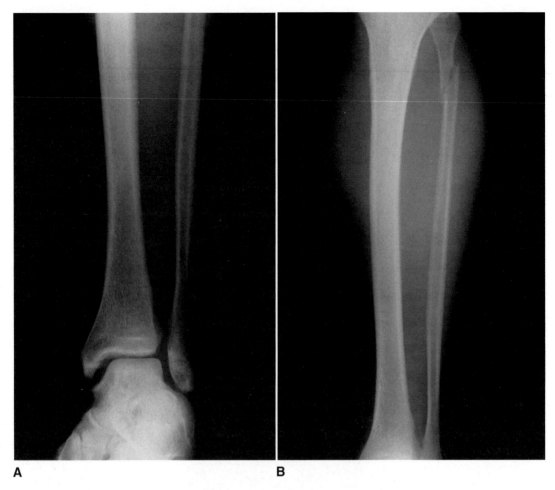

A   **B**

FIG. 11-52 A, A left ankle radiograph on a patient sustaining a twisting injury demonstrates a widening ankle mortise on the medial aspect with marked soft tissue swelling indicative of a Maisonneuve fracture. **B,** A left tibia-fibula radiograph on the same patient demonstrating a Maisonneuve fracture with minimal angulation and external rotation of the proximal fragment.

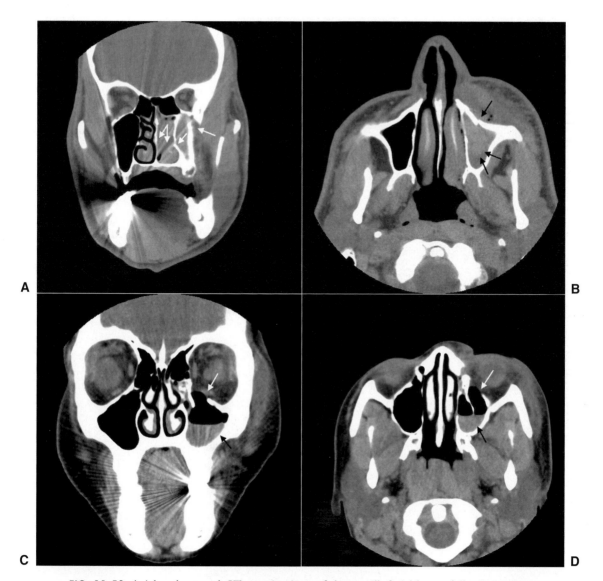

FIG. 11-53 Axial and coronal CT examinations of the maxillofacial bones following trauma to the face. **A,** A coronal CT of a patient complaining of a nosebleed after being hit in the face. The CT demonstrates blood in the nasal and sinus cavities with associated facial bone fractures and displacement of the nasal septum. **B,** An axial projection of the same patient as in **A. C,** A coronal CT of a patient sustaining a direct blow to the right orbit resulting in a blowout fracture of the floor of the right orbit. Notice the blood in the maxillary sinus. **D,** An axial CT of the same patient as in **C.**

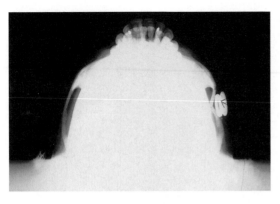

FIG. 11-54 A submentovertical projection of the zygomatic arch demonstrating a depressed fracture of the zygomatic arch resulting from a direct blow to the left cheek.

bone. A nosebleed, or epistaxis, is usually present with a nasal bone fracture. As discussed earlier, CT is the best method of assessing fractures of the facial bones (see Fig. 11-53A,B); however, radiographs of nasal bone fractures may be obtained in addition to a clinical examination to confirm a fracture (Fig. 11-57).

Dislocations

A joint **dislocation** results when a bone is out of its joint and not in contact with its normal articulation (Fig. 11-58). Common sites for joint dislocations are the shoulder, hip, and acromioclavicular joints. A **subluxation** is a partial dislocation, often occurring with a fracture (Fig. 11-59). The vertebral column, especially the cervical spine, is a common site of subluxations.

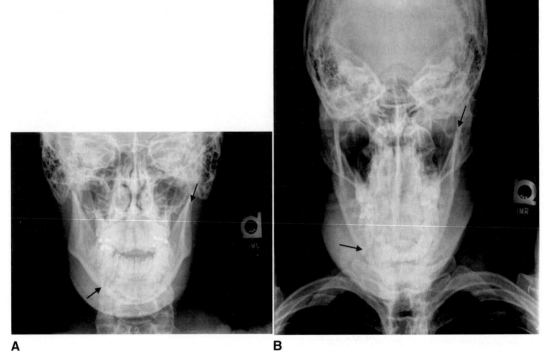

A   **B**

FIG. 11-55 PA **(A)** and AP axial, Towne method **(B)** projections of the mandible demonstrating a mandibular fracture.

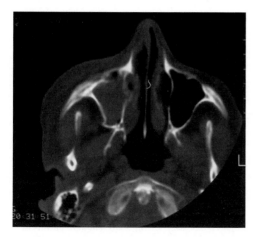

FIG. 11-56 A CT image demonstrating a tripod fracture of the right zygomatic bone.

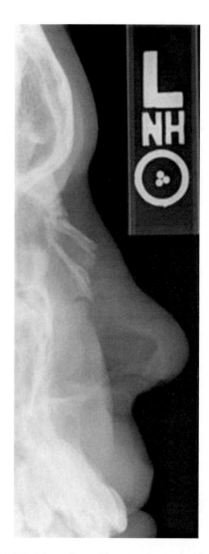

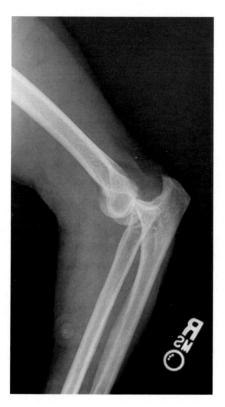

FIG. 11-57 A lateral nasal bone radiograph of a man who was struck in the face. The radiograph demonstrates a nasal bone fracture.

FIG. 11-58 A lateral projection of a dislocated elbow.

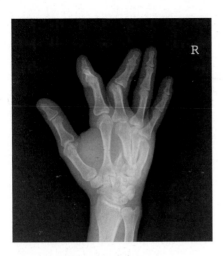

FIG. 11-59 An AP hand demonstrating a metacarpal fracture and subluxation of the PIP, third digit.

Shoulder joints most commonly dislocate anteriorly (Fig. 11-60). Such dislocations are readily detectable radiographically because the humeral head usually locates below the glenoid fossa and coracoid process. Often an avulsed greater tuberosity is present with anterior dislocations. A Hills-Sachs deformity is a compression fracture of the humeral head. It occurs on the superior and posterior head of the humerus due to impaction of the humeral head against the glenoid labrum during dislocation. If undetected by the clinician, this defect can increase the chance of subsequent dislocations of the same shoulder. Posterior dislocations of the shoulder (Fig. 11-61) are more difficult to diagnose, as they may appear normal on an AP radiograph. A transscapular (Y) projection, as well as a posterior oblique projection, is useful in locating the humeral head in a suspected posterior dislocation. Other than trauma, seizure disorders and electric shock are the major causes for shoulder dislocations. In fact, a posterior dislocation may be the first sign of a seizure disorder.

With traumatic dislocation of the hip, the femoral head is most commonly displaced posteriorly to lie against the sciatic notch (Fig. 11-62). It may also displace anteriorly and lie adjacent to the pubis or obturator foramen. Congenital hip dislocations are not caused by trauma, are usually unilateral, and are recognized by a shortening of the extremity. If the condition is not recognized until the child begins to walk, conservative therapies may be replaced by surgical intervention.

Acromioclavicular joint separations (Fig. 11-63) are more common in children than adults. The typical film sequence for this diagnosis involves radiographs taken with and without weights. Determining the alignment between the acromial end of the clavicle and the acromion process of the scapula assesses a joint separation.

Battered Child Syndrome

Battered child syndrome is a term associated with a physical form of child abuse and was first described in 1860. Physical child abuse often coexists with both emotional and sexual abuse. This syndrome affects boys and girls equally, generally under the age of 4 years. Approximately 25% of cases involve children under the age of 2 years. In addition, about 20% of the children who survive physical abuse suffer permanent injuries. An accurate incidence of child abuse is difficult to ascertain, but statistics from the National Child Abuse and Neglect Data System indicate that approximately 1200 children died of neglect or abuse in 2000. It has been shown that family history is a strong predictor of child abuse because adults who were abused as children often abuse their own children, primarily because they do not know how to handle their anger. Statistics also indicate a higher incidence of abuse in homes with single parents, young parents, families where substance abuse is prevalent, or families living in poverty. Radiographs are often used as evidence in cases of suspected child abuse.

Physical signs of battered child syndrome include bruises, burns, abrasions, and fractures in various stages of healing. Active children who are not abused often have bruises over the

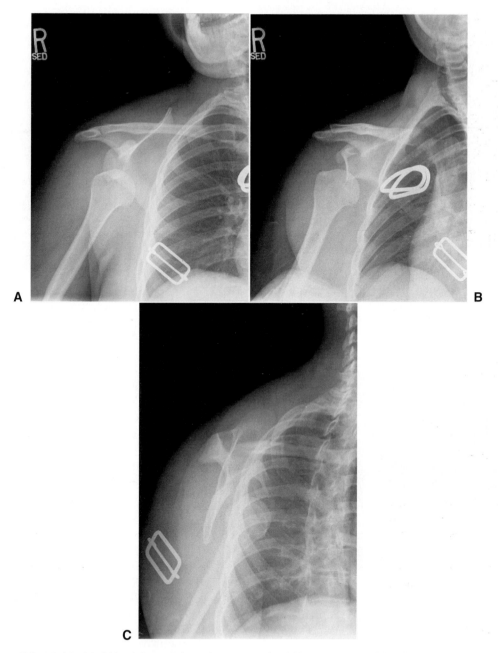

FIG. 11-60 AP (**A**), oblique (**B**), and transscapular (**C**) projections of the shoulder demonstrating an anterior dislocation of the humeral head. Note the location of the humeral head below the glenoid fossa and coracoid process of the scapula.

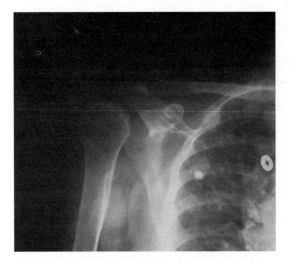

FIG. 11-61 A shoulder radiograph demonstrating a posterior dislocation of the humerus with the humeral head overlapping the rim of the glenoid fossa. The humeral head is also displaced slightly superolaterally.

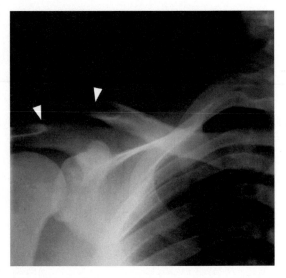

FIG. 11-63 A weight-bearing acromioclavicular radiograph demonstrating a dislocation as evidenced by uneven alignment of the acromial end of the clavicle and the acromion process of the scapula.

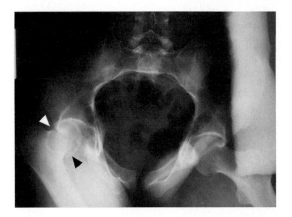

FIG. 11-62 A pelvis radiograph of a 25-year-old man whose right knee struck the dashboard in a motor vehicle accident, resulting in a posterior dislocation of the right femoral head.

bony areas of their body, such as their knees and elbows. However, bruises or injury around the eyes, cheeks, mouth, buttocks, or thighs; bite marks; certain bone fractures; and cigarette burns are suspicious. In most cases, the expla-nation for the injury is inconsistent with the actual injury.

Radiographic skeletal surveys to include bones of the upper extremities, lower extremi-ties, skull, spine, and ribs should be performed on initial inspection of the child if abuse is suspected. In some cases the bone survey may be repeated 2 weeks later to better identify new fractures not visible on the initial series. Radiographic signs of child abuse include hematomas and single or multiple fractures of varying ages, especially in areas where it is diffi-cult for the child to self-inflict the injury (Fig. 11-64). Often, fractures may indicate that an extremity has been twisted or turned until it breaks, or multiple rib fractures indicate repeated traumatic injuries, generally inflicted by a parent or guardian.

Shaken baby syndrome is a severe type of physical abuse that affects the child's head and neck. Shaking of the child causes whiplash injury to the neck as well as brain trauma, such as a subdural or subarachnoid hematoma, with

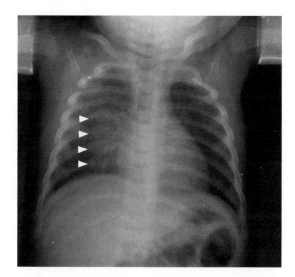

FIG. 11-64 A pediatric chest radiograph revealing numerous rib fractures with adjacent soft tissue masses resulting from hemorrhage surrounding the fracture sites.

no evidence of trauma to the external cranium. Shaken baby syndrome is associated with a high morbidity and mortality rate, with over 25% of cases resulting in death. CT and MR of the brain are excellent modalities for diagnosing this syndrome.

All emergency room personnel should be familiar with signs of child abuse and are ethically required to report suspected cases of child abuse to the proper authorities. In addition, children may be admitted to the hospital or transferred to a specialized crisis intervention facility for further evaluation.

Avascular Necrosis

Avascular necrosis is a term used to denote bone death resulting from inadequate blood supply. It frequently affects the hip, knee, shoulder, or carpal scaphoid and is most common in men between the ages of 30 and 60 years. It can occur idiopathically or following trauma to a joint (posttraumatic avascular necrosis), especially in cases of joint dislocation involving a tear of the joint capsule. The symptoms are nonspecific but may include pain up to 1 year following the trauma. If the lower extremity is affected, a limp may also be present.

MR is the modality of choice for evaluating avascular necrosis of the bone because it can demonstrate abnormalities associated with early-stage necrosis. Additional information is obtained with a nuclear medicine bone scan or CT. Conventional radiography is not sensitive enough to demonstrate early signs of avascular necrosis but does demonstrate the later stages of the disease. The radiographic appearance of avascular necrosis at a later stage includes sclerosis in combination with a collapse of the bone and narrowing of the joint space. Treatment consists of analgesics for pain and exercise to maintain range of motion. If diagnosed early, surgical intervention to provide cortical bone grafts or core decompression may help provide support and relieve pressure to allow revascularization of the bone.

Legg-Calvé-Perthes Disease

Legg-Calvé-Perthes disease is a common form of avascular necrosis affecting the femoral head. The etiology of this disorder is unknown, and the disease process is fairly quiet. Perthes refers specifically to ischemic necrosis of the head of the femur. It tends to occur in boys between the ages of 5 and 10 years. It can be idiopathic or follow injury or trauma to the affected hip. Clinically, these patients present with a limp that is accompanied by little or no pain. Radiographically, the bone in the center of the epiphysis is fragmented, and the head of the femur is flattened (Fig. 11-65) and contains areas of both sclerotic bone and osteolytic regions. Magnetic resonance images normally demonstrate low signal intensity from the affected hip in Legg-Calvé-Perthes disease (Fig. 11-66). In many cases, the patient develops a secondary degenerative osteoarthritis (see Chapter 2). This condition is treated with casting, traction, and bed rest or a surgical osteotomy with internal fixation.

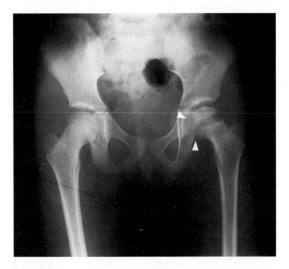

FIG. 11-65 An AP pelvis radiograph of a young man demonstrating Legg-Calvé-Perthes disease of the left femoral head. Notice the asymmetry of the femoral heads.

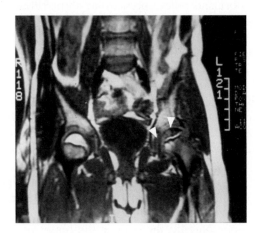

FIG. 11-66 An MRI of the patient in Fig. 11-65. The image demonstrates low signal intensity in the left femoral epiphysis, consistent with Legg-Calvé-Perthes disease.

TRAUMA OF THE CHEST AND THORAX

Approximately 25% of all trauma deaths occurring annually result from chest injuries. Diagnosis of the cause of the respiratory distress and the extent of the injury must be made

quickly. For patients with acute respiratory distress with suspected hemothorax or pneumothorax, a chest tube may be inserted in the fourth or fifth intercostal space without waiting for a chest radiograph. A portable chest radiograph is then obtained to further evaluate the thorax following the placement of the "blind" chest tube. Bony injuries such as rib fractures, clavicular fractures, scapular fractures, and sternal fractures may penetrate the lungs and damage the heart and great vessels. Pulmonary contusion may also result from other penetrating, compressive, or decelerating trauma to the chest. Radiographically, changes in the lungs from contusion appear 4 to 6 hours following the trauma. The radiographic appearance changes frequently during the first 24 to 48 hours, so multiple chest radiographs may be necessary to assess the damage to the lung tissue because pulmonary contusions are usually much larger than apparent on the initial chest radiograph.

Pneumothorax

A **pneumothorax** occurs when free air is trapped in the pleural space and compresses the lung tissue. This air may enter the pleural space from perforation of the visceral pleura, allowing gas to enter from the lung, penetration of the chest wall, or by generation of gas by gas-forming organisms in an empyema.

Common causes of a pneumothorax (Fig. 11-67) include penetrating chest trauma, such as stab wounds, gunshot wounds, fractured ribs, or a thoracocentesis needle, or a spontaneous blowout of a bleb (a flaccid vesicle, like a blister), resulting from some other pulmonary disease (Fig. 11-68). A pneumothorax may occur spontaneously from trauma or as the result of some pathologic process. The typical manifestation of a spontaneous pneumothorax is sudden, one-sided chest pain followed by dyspnea.

Radiographically, a pneumothorax appears as a strip of radiolucency devoid of vascular lung markings, with separation of the visceral and parietal pleura (Fig. 11-69). It is best demon-

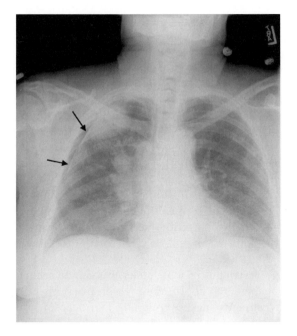

FIG. 11-67 A portable AP chest image demonstrating a traumatic pneumothorax and atelectasis of the right upper lobe of the lung.

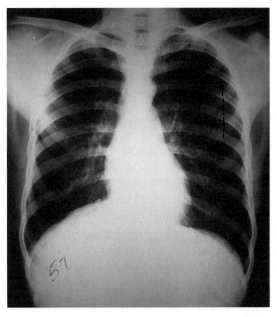

FIG. 11-69 Pneumothorax seen as thin white line around the periphery of the left lung, with an absence of lung markings in the periphery.

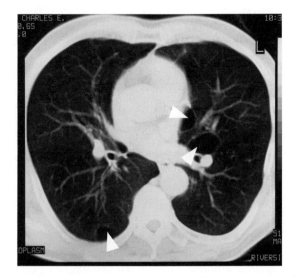

FIG. 11-68 Large emphysematous blebs as seen on CT. Spontaneous blowout of these could result in a pneumothorax.

strated on an erect expiration PA chest radiograph. Occasionally, wrinkles in the patient's skin produce artifacts that can mimic a pneumothorax. Such an artifact is called a pseudopneumothorax.

A tension pneumothorax occurs when air enters the pleural space but cannot leave the space because of a check valve mechanism in the fistula. This results in a complete collapse of the lung and a shift of the mediastinum to the side opposite the pneumothorax (Fig. 11-70). A tension pneumothorax requires immediate medical attention to prevent life-threatening circulatory collapse.

Treatment of a pneumothorax depends on the amount of lung collapse and the type of pneumothorax. A collapse of 30% or less is usually treated by bed rest and needle aspiration. Immediate treatment of a tension pneumothorax might involve insertion of a needle

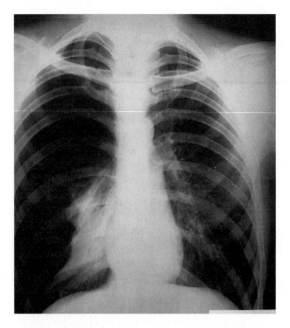

FIG. 11-70 Tension pneumothorax of the right lung following a stab wound in this 25-year-old man. The collapsed lung has almost no air in it and is seen as a soft tissue density adjacent to the heart.

into the chest wall to equalize air pressure. Otherwise, many pneumothoraces are treated through decompression by a closed-tube thoracostomy attached to a water-seal drain.

Atelectasis

Atelectasis means incomplete expansion of the lung as a result of partial or total collapse. In trauma situations, this often occurs in combination with a penetrating wound to the chest. Atelectasis itself is not a disease, but it is a sign of an abnormal process. One common manifestation is bibasilar atelectasis, which is also seen following trauma to the thorax following surgical procedures. A chest radiograph reveals the airless area of the lung, which may be segmental or lobar. If an entire lobe is affected, the mediastinum shifts to the affected side because of loss of volume of the affected lung. The chest radiograph can also demonstrate a decrease in the intercostal interspace, elevation

of the hemidiaphragm of the affected side, and depression or elevation of the hilum, depending on which lobe is affected. If the atelectasis is segmental, the radiographic shadow is triangular, with the apex of the triangle pointing toward the hilum of the affected lung.

Compression atelectasis occurs when blood, pleural effusions, pneumothoraces (Fig. 11-67), or other space-occupying lesions cause collapse (Fig. 11-71). Air that is completely absorbed from alveoli beyond an obstructed bronchus results in absorption atelectasis. Plate-like atelectasis describes the radiographic appearance of one or more linear opacities, usually at the lung bases and parallel to the diaphragm (Fig. 11-72).

Treatment of acute atelectasis can be accomplished by appropriate respiratory therapy treatments such as coughing and deep breathing. Bronchoscopy can also be used to allow suctioning of secretions that are causing an obstruction. Thoracocentesis can be used to relieve the compression caused by an effusion.

ABDOMINAL TRAUMA

Traumatic injuries to the abdomen result from gunshot wounds, stab wounds, and blunt abdominal trauma. Although abdominal injuries account for only approximately 15% of trauma deaths, most occur more than 48 hours following trauma and usually result from sepsis. As mentioned earlier in this chapter, the severity of injuries sustained in an MVA are greatly reduced by wearing both shoulder and lap belts whether the individual is in the front or back seat of a motor vehicle; however, chest and abdomen contusions and abdominal trauma can result from a rapid deceleration into the seatbelt, even when it is worn properly. Many patients with serious abdominal injuries from MVA initially have very minimal symptoms and physical findings. Abdominal trauma can cause serious injury not only to the GI tract but also to abdominal organs such as the liver, spleen, kidneys, and pancreas; the retroperitoneum;

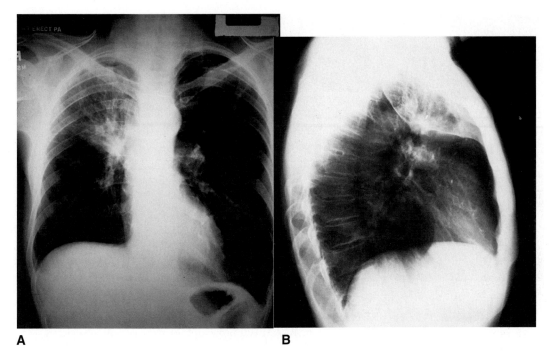

A   B

FIG. 11-71 A, Absorption atelectasis caused by the obstructive effects of carcinoma of the bronchus supplying the upper lobe of the right lung. **B,** The lateral projection of the same patient clearly demonstrates atelectasis of the right upper lobe secondary to bronchogenic carcinoma.

and the pelvic organs. Blunt trauma from steering wheel injuries often damages the liver and spleen because the energy of deceleration and compression frequently damages the parenchyma of these structures.

Supine and erect abdominal radiographs and erect chest radiographs are most desirable following abdominal injury. Chest radiographs are important to assess diaphragmatic injury. In addition, free air is best demonstrated radiographically with the patient in an erect position. Often, it is well seen on a chest radiograph because of the proximity of the central ray to the diaphragms. Free air ascends and accumulates under the diaphragm on one or both sides, and as little as 1 cc of air can be demonstrated radiographically on an erect projection. Much larger amounts of air must be present to

be visualized on a supine radiograph. However, placing the patient erect is not always possible because of the patient's condition. Left lateral decubitus radiographs of the abdomen can be substituted for the erect projection, with any free air present accumulating over the lateral aspect of the liver and the lateral aspect of the pelvis. Optimally, the patient should remain on the left side for approximately 10 minutes before the exposure to allow sufficient time for the air to ascend.

Supine abdominal radiographs help to identify foreign objects such as bullets, separation in the bowel loops, or loss of the psoas muscle shadow as a result of fluid or blood within the peritoneum and air around the right kidney or psoas muscle margins. The initial inspection of the abdominal trauma may be followed by

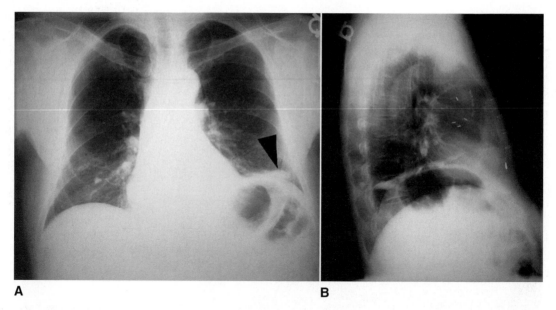

A   **B**

FIG. 11-72 A, Plate-like atelectasis seen as a linear opacity in the base of the left lung as indicated by the arrow in this PA projection. **B,** A lateral projection of same patient also clearly demonstrates plate-like atelectasis.

specific studies involving the urinary tract (Fig. 11-73). Intravenous urograms may be indicated if injury to the urinary system is suspected; however, CT examination of the abdomen following an injection of an iodinated contrast agent provides a much clearer view of renal anatomy and organ injury.

CT has also proven to be the best means of diagnosing GI trauma and is capable of visualizing lacerations, hematomas, and ruptures. Even small amounts of intraabdominal hemorrhage can be readily detected. The duodenum is the portion of the GI tract most often damaged by blunt trauma. Because of its relationship to the spine, the duodenum can be compressed between the abdominal wall and the spine, resulting in a duodenal hematoma. Often CT evaluation of liver and spleen injuries helps in evaluating surgical versus nonsurgical management of these injuries.

Penetrating abdominal wounds, as occur with a gunshot, may produce free air if the bowel has been injured. Some of the common conditions seen radiographically after trauma are fractures of the spine, pelvis, or ribs; obliteration of normal fat planes and visceral margins; accumulation of peritoneal fluid such as blood; and the presence of free peritoneal air (Fig. 11-74).

Intraperitoneal Air

In the normal patient, the peritoneum is a closed cavity (except for the female reproductive system) containing only small amounts of serous fluid. The presence of free air in this cavity, a **pneumoperitoneum,** is usually abnormal and can indicate perforation of the GI tract. Large amounts of air likely indicate colon perforation, whereas small amounts of air are more indicative of duodenal perforation.

The common causes of a pneumoperitoneum (Fig. 11-75) include traumatic rupturing of the stomach or intestines or nontraumatic bowel perforations as described in Chapter 4. In

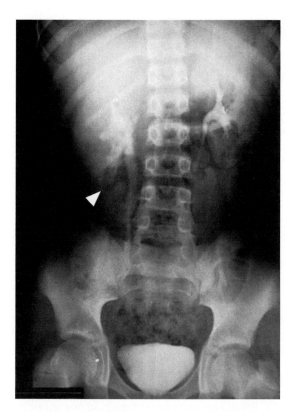

FIG. 11-73 An intravenous urogram demonstrating a fractured right kidney following a football injury.

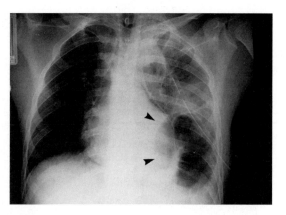

FIG. 11-74 A chest radiograph demonstrating a traumatic diaphragmatic hernia resulting from a motor vehicle accident.

response to perforation, an intense inflammatory response develops and may eventually wall off the perforation into an abscess.

On an AP radiograph with the patient in a supine position, the football sign may be demonstrated as an indicator of a pneumoperitoneum. This is a lucent, oval gas collection that corresponds to the anterior peritoneal cavity. The pattern of gas resembles the shape of a football with the seam of the football being the falciform ligament outlined by free air. Visualization of this sign requires a relatively large amount of free air to be present.

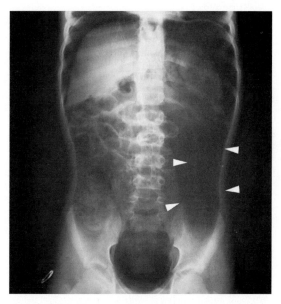

FIG. 11-75 An abdominal radiograph of a 5-year-old child with a passive pneumoperitoneum resulting from perforation of the stomach during anesthesia. Note how the free air outlines the outer border of the bowel, liver, and spleen.

1. A contusion formed on the side of the head where trauma occurs is called a:
   a. concussion
   b. contrecoup lesion
   c. coup lesion
   d. spondylosis

2. A fracture of the skeletal system in which the bone has penetrated the skin is termed:
   a. closed
   b. comminuted
   c. noncomminuted
   d. open

3. Fractures that occur at sites of maximal strain on a bone, usually in connection with unaccustomed activity, are classified as _____ fractures.
   a. avulsion
   b. fatigue
   c. growth plate
   d. stress

4. A fracture that heals in a faulty position is termed:
   a. callus
   b. delayed union
   c. malunion
   d. nonunion

5. Shoulder dislocations are most commonly displaced:
   a. anteriorly   c. interiorly
   b. posteriorly   d. exteriorly

6. Avascular necrosis commonly affects the:
   1. shoulder
   2. hip
   3. fingers
   a. 1 and 2
   b. 1 and 3
   c. 2 and 3
   d. 1, 2, and 3

7. Incomplete expansion of a lung as a result of partial or total collapse defines:
   a. atelectasis   c. pleurisy
   b. empyema   d. pneumothorax

8. Penetrating chest trauma could lead to a:
   a. coma
   b. coup lesion
   c. pneumoperitoneum
   d. pneumothorax

9. Demonstration of a pneumothorax is best accomplished by making the exposure:
   a. in an erect, lateral position
   b. in a lateral decubitus position
   c. in an erect PA position on expiration
   d. in an erect PA position on inspiration

10. Which portion of the GI system is most frequently damaged by blunt trauma of the abdomen?
    a. cecum   c. ileum
    b. duodenum   d. jejunum

11. Define the term "shaken baby syndrome" and explain its effect on the CNS.

12. Spinal cord compression results in neurologic dysfunction, which may be temporary or permanent. Explain the mechanism for each type of dysfunction described in the text.

13. Differentiate among the four types of hematomas to the brain and specify which type has the highest mortality rate. Why?

14. What imaging modality or modalities best demonstrate stress or fatigue fractures? Why?

15. Describe the difference between comminuted and noncomminuted fractures of the skeletal system.

Answer Key

Chapter 1
1. C
2. B
3. B
4. B
5. B
6. C
7. B
8. A
9. D
10. D

Chapter 2
1. B
2. B
3. B
4. A
5. D
6. A
7. C
8. B
9. B
10. C
11. D
12. D
13. B
14. B
15. D

Chapter 3
1. C
2. C
3. B
4. B
5. C
6. C
7. A

8. D
9. B
10. B

Chapter 4
1. A
2. C
3. C
4. C
5. C
6. C
7. D
8. D
9. D
10. A

Chapter 5
1. B
2. B
3. B
4. D
5. F
6. B
7. D
8. D
9. B
10. C

Chapter 6
1. D
2. A
3. D
4. A
5. B
6. C
7. C
8. E

9. B
10. D
11. D
12. B
13. A
14. B

Chapter 7
1. D
2. D
3. D
4. B
5. A
6. B
7. D
8. D
9. C
10. B

Chapter 8
1. D
2. A
3. B
4. B
5. B
6. E
7. B
8. C
9. C
10. B
11. D
12. C
13. A
14. D
15. B

Chapter 9
1. C
2. A
3. D
4. B
5. A
6. D
7. D
8. A
9. B
10. B

Chapter 10
1. A
2. B
3. B
4. C
5. B
6. A
7. B
8. B
9. B
10. D

Chapter 11
1. C
2. D
3. B
4. C
5. A
6. A
7. A
8. D
9. C
10. B

Glossary

Abruptio Placentae   Condition in which a normally implanted placenta prematurely separates from the uterus.

Absorption Atelectasis   Type of atelectasis that occurs when air is completely absorbed from alveoli beyond an obstructed bronchus.

Achalasia   A neuromuscular abnormality of the esophagus that results in failure of the lower esophageal sphincter to relax.

Achondroplasia   A hereditary, congenital disturbance that causes inadequate bone formation and results in a peculiar form of dwarfism.

Acquired Immune Deficiency Syndrome (AIDS)   An acquired viral infection that paralyzes normal human immune mechanisms.

Acromegaly   A disease marked by progressive enlargement of the head, hands, and feet caused by abnormal secretion of growth hormone.

Acute   Having a quick onset and lasting a short period of time with a relatively severe course.

Additive Pathologies   A radiographic term used to describe diseases that are more difficult than normal to penetrate.

Adenocarcinoma   Carcinoma derived from glandular tissue.

Adenomatous Polyp   A saccular projection into the bowel lumen.

Air-Bronchogram Sign   Radiographic sign seen in various respiratory diseases where air-filled bronchi become visible when surrounded by nonaerated alveoli.

Albers-Schönberg Disease   A form of osteosclerotic osteopetrosis; this is a benign skeletal anomaly that involves increased bone density in conjunction with fairly normal bone contour.

Alimentary Tract   Extending from the mouth to the anus, the major portion consists of the gastrointestinal system, which digests and absorbs food.

Anemic   Condition in which level of hemoglobin in blood is less than 12 g per 100 ml.

Anencephaly   Congenital absence of the cranial vault.

Aneurysm   A localized ballooning or outpouching of a vessel wall as a result of weakening from atherosclerotic disease, trauma, infection, or congenital defects.

Ankylosing Spondylitis   A form of rheumatoid arthritis of unknown etiology that affects the spine in a progressive fashion, eventually fusing the spine into a rigid block of bone.

Anomaly   Any marked deviation from the norm, especially as a result of congenital or hereditary defects.

Anthracosis   Pneumoconiosis caused by inhalation and deposition of coal dust.

Appendicitis   An inflammation of the appendix.

Arthritis   Inflammation in which lesions are confined to the joints.

Asbestosis   Pneumoconiosis caused by inhalation and deposition of asbestos dust.

Ascites   An accumulation of fluid in the peritoneal cavity.

Aspiration Pneumonia   Pneumonia caused by entrance of foreign particles (e.g., vomitus) aspirated into the lower respiratory tract.

Astrocytoma   A glioma composed of astrocytes, which are star-shaped neuroglial cells with many branching processes.

Asymptomatic   Showing or causing no identifiable symptoms.

Atelectasis   Loss of air in a lung resulting from a partial or total collapse of a lung.

Atheroma   A mass of plaque occurring in atherosclerosis.

Atherosclerosis   A common form of arteriosclerosis in which deposits of fibrofatty plaque or thickenings form within the intima or intermedia of large and medium-sized arteries.

Autoimmune Disorder   Disease in which antibodies form against and injure the patient's own tissues, in contrast to the normal process in which antibodies form in response to foreign antigens.

Autosome   The 22 pairs of chromosomes found in a typical cell, other than the sex chromosomes.

Avascular Necrosis   Bone death as a result of inadequate blood supply.

Avulsion Fracture   A fracture in which a fragmented bone is pulled away from the shaft, usually occurring around a ligament or tendon, and often with muscle-tearing, as is associated with a sprain or dislocation.

Benign   Refers to a localized and generally noninvasive lesion.

Bennett's Fracture   Oblique fracture of the first metacarpal below the thumb.

Bicornuate Uterus   A uterus with paired uterine horns extending to the uterine tubes.

Bleb   A flaccid vesicle.

Blood-Brain Barrier   The special functioning of the cerebral capillaries that prevents the passage of unwanted substances into the brain.

Blowout Fracture   A fracture of the orbital floor resulting from a direct blow to the front of the orbit, with the force of the blow transferred to the orbital walls and floor.

Bone Bruise   An indication of an occult fracture, revealed by MRI, and presumed to represent hemorrhage and edema, usually beneath an adjacent joint surface.

Bone Cyst   A benign lesion consisting of a wall of fibrous tissue filled with fluid.

Bowel Sounds   The normal sounds of the bowel in motion as heard on auscultation.

Boxer's Fracture   A fracture of the fifth metacarpal bone as a result of a blow to or with the hand.

Bradycardia   A very slow heart rate.

Bronchial Adenoma   A glandular tumor, either benign or malignant, situated in the submucosal tissues of large bronchi.

Bronchiectasis   Chronic dilatation of the bronchi, with inflammation and destruction of bronchial walls and cilia.

Bronchitis   Inflammation of one or more bronchi.

Bronchogenic Carcinoma   Carcinoma of the lung that arises from the epithelium of the bronchial tree.

Bruise   Bleeding into the tissue spaces as a result of capillary rupture; also known as a contusion.

Bulla   A large vesicle, usually 2 cm or more in diameter, filled with air.

Bursitis   Inflammation of the bursae of the tendons, with the subdeltoid bursa as the most common site.

CAD   Coronary artery disease, resulting from deposition of atheromas in the arteries supplying blood to the heart muscle.

CVA   Cerebrovascular accident, generally resulting from a loss of blood supply to the brain or from a cerebral bleed.

Callus   An unorganized meshwork of woven bone formed following a fracture, ultimately replaced by hard, adult bone.

Cancellous   Refers to the spongy, latticelike structure of bone filled by bone marrow.

Cancer   A general term used to denote various types of malignant neoplasms.

Cantor Tube   A single-lumen, mercury-weighted gastric tube used for intestinal intubation and decompression.

Carcinoma   A malignant growth comprised of epithelial cells that tends to invade surrounding tissues and give rise to metastases.

Cardiomegaly   The appearance of an enlarged heart, as indicative of many cardiovascular disorders.

Celiac Disease   A malabsorption syndrome that occurs as a result of sensitivity to gluten, an agent found in wheat products.

Cervical Spondylosis   Degenerative joint disease affecting the cervical vertebrae, vertebral disks, and surrounding ligaments and connective tissue.

Chest Tube   Tube inserted through the chest wall between the ribs to allow for drainage of air and/or fluid from the thoracic cavity.

Chip Fracture   An avulsion fracture consisting of a small fragment or chip of bone from the corner of a phalanx or other long bone.

Cholecystitis   An acute inflammation of the gallbladder most frequently caused by obstruction.

Cholelithiasis   The presence of gallstones.

Chondrosarcoma   A malignant bone tumor composed of atypical cartilage.

Chronic   Presenting slowly and persisting over a long period of time.

Chronic Obstructive Pulmonary Disease (COPD)   Designation applied to conditions that result in pulmonary obstruction, most commonly chronic bronchitis and pulmonary emphysema.

Cirrhosis   Liver condition in which the parenchyma and architecture are destroyed and replaced by fibrous tissue and regenerative nodules.

Closed Fracture   A fracture that does not produce an open wound.

Clubfoot   Deformity of the foot involving the talus.

Coarctation   A narrowing or compression.

Coccidioidomycosis   Systemic, fungal infection caused by a fungus that thrives in semiarid soil and is particularly endemic in the southwestern United States and northern Mexico.

Colles' Fracture   A fracture through the distal 1 inch of the radius in which the distal fragment is displaced posteriorly.

Colonic Atresia   Congenital failure of development of the distal rectum and anus to a variable extent, frequently accompanied by fistula formation to the genitourinary system.

Coma   A state of unconsciousness from which the patient cannot be aroused.

Comminuted Fracture   A fracture in which the bone is splintered or crushed.

Communicating (External) Hydrocephalus   Type of hydrocephalus caused by poor resorption of cerebrospinal fluid (for a variety of reasons) by the arachnoid villi.

Compact   Refers to the dense, outer portion of bone.

Complete Noncomminuted Fracture   A fracture in which the bone separates into two fragments.

Compound Fracture   A fracture in which the bone ends penetrate the soft tissue and skin; also termed open fracture.

Compression Atelectasis   Type of atelectasis that occurs when pleural effusions, pneumothoraces, or other space-occupying lesions cause collapse.

Compression Fracture   A fracture produced by compression.

Concussion   Brief loss of consciousness as a result of a blow to the head.

Congenital   Existing at, and usually before, birth and resulting from genetic or environmental factors.

Congenital Megacolon   Hirschprung's disease, consisting of an absence of neurons in the bowel wall, typically in the sigmoid colon.

Congestive Heart Failure   Condition existing when the heart is unable to propel blood at a sufficient rate and volume to prevent congestion of circulatory subsystems.

Consolidation   The process of tissue or fluid accumulation.

Contrecoup Lesion   A contusion formed on the opposite side of the skull in reference to a trauma site.

Contusion   An injury in which the tissue is bruised but not broken.

Cor Pulmonale   Hypertension in the pulmonary artery and an enlargement of the right ventricle of the heart.

Corpus Luteum Cyst   A cyst that develops in the yellow endocrine body formed in the ovary in the site of a ruptured ovarian follicle.

Coup Lesion   A contusion formed on the side of the head in which trauma occurs.

Craniopharyngioma   A cystic, benign tumor that usually grows above the sella and upward into the third ventricle of the brain.

Craniosynostosis   Premature or early closure of the sutures of the skull.

Crohn's Disease   A chronic granulomatous inflammatory disease of unknown etiology involving any part of the gastrointestinal tract, but commonly involving the terminal ileum; also known as regional enteritis.

Crossed Ectopy   A condition in which one kidney lies across the body midline and is fused to the other kidney.

Cryptococci   Yeastlike organisms of a fungal origin.

CVP Line   Specialized catheter inserted usually via the subclavian vein to the level of the right atrium to compensate for loss of peripheral infusion sites or to allow for fluid infusion in significant amounts.

Cystadenoma   Adenoma associated with cystoma.

Cystadenocarcinoma   Malignant neoplasm of the ovary; generally occurs in women over the age of 40 years.

Cystic Fibrosis   Congenital disorder affecting exocrine gland function, with respiratory effects including excessive secretions, obstruction of the bronchial system, infection, and tissue damage.

Cystitis   Inflammation of the bladder as a result of its infection.

Degenerative   Refers to deterioration of the body usually associated with the aging process.

Degenerative Disk Disease   The gradual, degenerative changes to the spine associated with aging.

Delayed Union   Refers to a fracture that does not heal in the usual amount of time.

Depressed Fracture   A fracture of the skull in which a fragment is depressed inward.

Dermoid Cysts (Cystic Teratomas)   Cystic masses arising from unfertilized ova, containing hair, fat, or bone, and located in an ovary.

Diagnosis   The name of a disease an individual is believed to have.

Diastole   The phase of the heart cycle in which the myocardium is relaxing.

Diploë   The spongy bone tissue found between the two tables of the cranial bones.

Disease   Any abnormal disturbance of the normal function or structure of a body part, organ, or system that may display a variety of manifestations.

Dislocation   The displacement of any part out of contact with its normal articulation.

Dissecting Aneurysm   An aneurysm resulting from hemorrhage that causes longitudinal splitting of the arterial wall.

Diverticulum   A pouch or sac of variable size occurring normally or created by herniation of a mucous membrane through a defect in its muscular coat.

Diverticulitis   Inflammation of a diverticulum.

Diverticulosis   The presence of diverticula in the absence of inflammation.

Dobhoff Tube   An enteral tube used to deliver a liquid diet directly to the duodenum.

Dominant   In relation to hereditary diseases, refers to a disease transmitted by a single gene from either parent.

Dysphagia   Difficulty in swallowing.

Ectopic Kidney   A kidney that is out of its normal position, usually found lower than normal.

Embolus   A mass of undissolved matter (solid, liquid, or gas) present in a blood vessel brought there by blood current. Vessel occlusion by an embolus usually results in development of an infarct.

Embolization   Interventional angiography procedure in which devices such as coils are used to intentionally clot off vessels, often before surgery to prevent excessive bleeding.

Emphysema   A lung condition characterized by an increase in the air spaces distal to the terminal bronchioles and with destruction of alveolar walls.

Empyema   An accumulation of pus in the pleural cavity.

Emergency Medical System (EMS)   A system for trauma care that provides prehospital care, acute hospital care, and rehabilitative care.

Encephalitis   Inflammation of the brain.

Enchondroma   A benign growth of cartilage arising in the metaphysis of a bone.

Endemic   Term given to disease of high prevalence in an area where the causative organism is commonly found.

Endometriosis   A condition in which endometrial tissue implants in aberrant pelvic locations.

Endoscopy   The use of lighted instruments with optic connections to visualize disease of the esophagus and stomach, or rectum and distal colon (e.g., sigmoidoscopy).

Endotracheal Tube   Tube inserted via the nose or mouth into the trachea for purposes of airway management, suctioning, or mechanical ventilation.

En Face   A radiographic descriptor referring to visualization of a pathology in a "head-on" or "straight-on" fashion, as compared to a profile-like image.

Ependymoma   A glial tumor that is firm and whitish and arises from the ependyma, the ventricle lining.

Epidemiology   The investigation of disease in large groups.

Epidural Hematoma   A hematoma positioned between the bony skull and the dura mater.

Epididymoorchitis   A testicular condition that may result in benign masses of the testes.

Epiphrenic Diverticulum   A pulsion diverticulum of the distal esophagus just above the hemidiaphragm.

Erythrocytes   Red blood cells.

Esophageal Atresia   Congenital lack of esophageal development past some point, commonly associated with tracheoesophageal fistula.

Esophageal Varices   Varicose veins of the esophagus that occur in patients with portal hypertension.

Etiology   The study of the cause and origin of disease.

Ewald/Edlich Tube   A large-bore gastric tube used to evacuate the contents of the stomach.

Ewing's Sarcoma   A primary malignant bone tumor arising in medullary tissue, occurring more often in cylindrical bones.

Exostosis   A benign bone growth, projecting outward from the bony cortex.

Expectoration   Expulsion of mucus or phlegm from the throat.

Fallopian Tube   The tube extending laterally from the uterus to the ovary, serving as a conduit for the ova.

Fat Pad Sign   A radiographic indicator of a nonvisualized, underlying fracture of the bones of the elbow that displays as a tear-shaped radiolucency adjacent to the anterior and sometimes posterior surface of the distal humerus.

Fecalith   A hardened ball of stool that forms in the intestine.

Fibroadenoma   Adenoma containing fibrous tissue.

Fibrocystic Disease   A benign, generally bilateral breast condition characterized by various-sized cysts located throughout the breasts.

Filling Defect   An area of total or relative radiolucency within a column of barium.

Fistula   An abnormal, tubelike passage from one structure to another.

Foley Catheter   A catheter that is placed through the urethra and retained in the urinary bladder by a balloon that is inflated with air or fluid.

Follicular Cyst   A cyst arising from the ovum.

Fracture   The breaking or rupturing of bone caused by mechanical forces either applied to the bone or transmitted directly along the line of a bone.

Fusiform Aneurysm   An arterial aneurysm in which the entire circumference of the vessel wall is affected.

Gallstone Ileus   A condition in which gallstones erode from the gallbladder, creating a fistula to the small bowel that may cause a bowel obstruction.

Ganglion   Cystic swelling that develops in connection with a tendon sheath, usually on the back of the wrist.

Gastritis   Inflammation of the stomach mucosa.

Gastroenteritis   General grouping of a number of inflammatory disorders of the stomach and intestines.

Gastroesophageal Reflux Disease   An incompetent cardiac sphincter allowing the backward flow of gastric acid and contents into the esophagus.

Giant Cell Tumor   A neoplastic growth of the skeletal system consisting of numerous multi-nucleated osteoclastic giant cells; also called osteoclastoma.

Glioma   A tumor composed of tissue that represents neuroglia, commonly occurring in the cerebral hemispheres of the posterior fossa.

Glomerulonephritis   An inflammatory reaction of the renal parenchyma caused by streptococcal infection.

Gouty Arthritis   An inherited, metabolic disorder with excess amounts of uric acid produced and deposited in the joint and adjacent bone, most commonly in the metatarsophalangeal joint of the great toe.

Greenstick Fracture   A fracture in which the cortex breaks on one side without separation or breaking of the opposing cortex.

Growth-Plate Fracture   A fracture that involves the end of a long bone of a child, and that may be limited to growth-plate cartilage or extend into the metaphysis, epiphysis, or both.

Hangman's Fracture   A fracture of the arch of the second cervical vertebra, usually accompanied by anterior subluxation of the second cervical vertebra on the third cervical vertebra; also known as atraumatic spondylosis, these usually result from acute hyperextension of the head.

Harris Tube   A single-lumen gastric tube using mercury as a weight that is used as a decompression and diagnostic aid.

Heartburn   Burning symptoms experienced substernally as a result of the reflux of gastric acids into the esophagus.

Hematocrit   A common laboratory test that determines the body's total number of red blood cells.

Hemangioma   A benign tumor of dilated blood vessels.

Hematoma   A localized collection of blood in an organ, space, or tissue as a result of a break in the wall of a blood vessel.

Hemorrhagic Stroke   A stroke in which a blood vessel in the brain breaks or ruptures.

Hemothorax   Pleural effusion containing blood.

Hepatitis   An inflammation of the liver resulting from a variety of causes.

Hepatocellular Adenoma A benign tumor of the liver most frequently associated with oral contraceptives.

Hepatocellular Carcinoma A primary malignant tumor of the liver.

Hepatomegaly Enlargement of the liver as might be seen with viral hepatitis.

Hereditary Genetically transferred from either parent to child and derived from ancestors.

Hernia The protrusion of a part of an organ (e.g., bowel loop) through a small opening in the wall of a cavity.

Herniated Nucleus Pulposus Herniation of the nucleus pulposus of the disk through a rupture in the annulus fibrosus.

Herpes An inflammatory skin disease caused by a virus.

Hiatal Hernia Protrusion of any structure, especially some portion of the stomach, into the thoracic cavity through the esophageal hiatus of the diaphragm.

Hickman Catheter Specialized catheter inserted via the subclavian vein to allow for multiple tapping for injection of various agents, especially tissue-toxic chemotherapeutic agents.

Hirschprung's Disease An absence of neurons in the bowel wall, typically in the sigmoid, preventing relaxation of the colon and normal peristalsis; congenital megacolon.

Histoplasmosis Systemic, fungal infection caused by a fungus that thrives in soil, especially that fueled by bird or bat excreta; especially endemic to the Ohio and Mississippi River valleys.

Hodgkin's Disease A malignant condition of lymphoid tissue associated with Reed-Sternberg cells.

Homeostasis The body's normal, internal resting state of equilibrium.

Horseshoe Kidney A condition where the lower poles of the kidney are joined across midline by a band of soft tissues, resulting in a rotation anomaly on one or both sides.

Human Immunodeficiency Virus (HIV) The virus associated with acquired immune deficiency syndrome.

Hyaline Membrane Disease Also known as respiratory distress syndrome, it is a disorder of prematurity caused by incomplete maturation of the alveoli that makes proper gas exchange difficult.

Hydatidiform Mole Represents an abnormal conception where there is usually no fetus, and the uterus is filled with cystically dilated chorionic villi that resemble a bunch of grapes.

Hydrocele A benign testicular mass consisting of a collection of fluid in the testis or along the spermatic cord.

Hydrocephalus A congenital or acquired condition resulting from accumulation of cerebrospinal fluids in the ventricles of the brain and leading to ventricular enlargement, compression of brain tissue, and increased intracranial pressure.

Hydronephrosis An obstructive disease of the urinary system that causes a dilatation of the renal pelvis and calyces with urine.

Hypernephroma The most common malignant tumor of the kidney.

Hyperparathyroidism Abnormally increased activity of the parathyroid glands, causing excess hormone production, which overstimulates osteoclasts, which are responsible for bone removal.

Hyperplasia Overdevelopment.

Hypertrophic Pyloric Stenosis A congenital anomaly of the stomach in which the pyloric canal is greatly narrowed because of hypertrophy of the pyloric sphincter.

Hypoplasia   Less than normal development.

Hysterosalpingogram   A radiographic examination for screening of the nongravid woman; injection of contrast into the uterus and the flow into the uterine tubes reveals their patency, which may affect the ability to become pregnant.

Iatrogenic   Pertains to any adverse condition in a patient occurring as a result of medical treatment.

Idiopathic   No identifiable causative factor.

Ileal Atresia   A congenital absence of the ileum portion of the small intestines.

Imperforate Anus   Congenital disorder characterized by lack of an anal opening to the exterior.

Incarcerated Hernia   A hernia in which the bowel is trapped by tissues that prevent it from being reduced, possibly causing an obstruction.

Incidence   A statistical measure that refers to the number of new cases of a disease found in a given time period.

Incompetency (Valvular)   Regurgitation of blood through the heart valves as a result of improper closure.

Incomplete Fracture   A fracture in which only part of the bony structure gives way, with little or no displacement.

Infarct   An area of ischemic necrosis.

Infection   An inflammatory process caused by exposure to some disease-causing organism.

Inflammatory   Refers to the body process of destroying, diluting, or walling off a localized injurious agent.

Inguinal Hernia   Hernia in which a bowel loop protrudes through a weakness in the inguinal ring, with descension into the scrotum.

Insufficiency (Valvular)   Regurgitation of blood through the heart valves.

Intraaortic Balloon Pump   Specialized catheter with a balloon at its distal end; inflation and deflation from a pump provides mechanical support of the left ventricle and the systemic circulation.

Intracerebral Hematoma   Bleeding within the brain tissue, commonly in the frontal lobe, which results from trauma or a ruptured hemangioma.

Intrathoracic Stomach   Condition in which all of the stomach slides above the diaphragm into the thoracic cavity.

Intussusception   The prolapse of a segment of bowel into a distal segment.

Involucrum   A shell or sheath of new supporting bone laid down by periosteum around a sequestrum of necrosed bone.

Ischemia   A local and temporary impairment of circulation caused by obstruction of circulation.

Ischemic Stroke   A stroke in which a blood clot blocks a blood vessel in the brain.

Jaundice   Yellowish discoloration of the skin and whites of the eyes caused by bilirubin accumulation in the body tissues.

Kaposi's Sarcoma   A sarcoma present in the connective tissues of about one fourth of all AIDS patients.

Lacunar Infarction   Small vessel disease that results in a thrombotic stroke.

Le Fort Fracture   Bilateral, horizontal fractures of the maxillae, subcategorized as Le Fort I, II, or III fractures, depending on the extent of injury.

Left Ventricular Failure   Congestive heart failure that results when the left ventricle cannot pump an amount of blood equal to the venous return in the right ventricle.

Legionnaire's Disease   Severe, bacterial pneumonia named for its outbreak at an American Legion Convention in Pennsylvania in 1976.

Leiomyoma   A benign tumor derived from smooth muscle.

Lesion   General term used to describe the various types of cellular change that can occur in response to a disease.

Leukemia   A malignant disease of the leukocytes and their precursor cells in the blood and bone marrow.

Leukocytes   White blood cells.

Levacuator Tube   A wide double-lumen tube used for evacuation of gastric contents and irrigation of stomach.

Levin Tube   A gastroduodenal catheter of a small enough caliber to allow transnasal passage, often termed a nasogastric tube.

Linear Fracture   A fracture that extends lengthwise through a bone.

Maisonneuve Fracture   An infrequent ankle injury consisting of a severe ankle sprain with a fracture of the proximal one third of the fibula.

Malabsorption Syndrome   Group of diseases of various causes in which there is interference with normal digestion and absorption of food to the small bowel.

Malignant   Refers to a lesion that grows, spreads, and invades other tissues.

Malrotation   Unnatural position of the intestines caused by failure of normal rotation during embryologic development.

Malunion   Union of fragments of a fractured bone in a faulty position, impairing normal function or cosmetic appearance.

Manifestation   Observable changes resulting from cellular changes in the disease process.

Mantoux Text   Injection of purified protein derivative (PPD) under the skin for purposes of diagnosing tuberculosis.

Mastitis   Inflammation of the breast, most often caused by *Staphylococcus* bacteria.

Mechanical Obstruction   Refers to a bowel obstruction that occurs as a result of blockage of the bowel lumen.

Mediastinal Emphysema (Pneumomediastinum)   The presence of air or gas in the mediastinum as a result of leakage of air from the bronchial tree.

Medical Jaundice   Jaundice that results from hemolytic disease, in which excessive amounts of red blood cells are destroyed, or when the liver is damaged as a result of cirrhosis or hepatitis.

Medullary Canal   Inner spongy or cancellous portion of a long bone where bone marrow is produced.

Medullary Sponge Kidney   A congenital anomaly of the urinary system in which the only visible abnormality is the dilatation of the medullary and papillary portions of the collecting ducts, usually bilaterally.

Medulloblastoma   Soft, infiltrating tumors of neuroepithelial tissue that are highly malignant.

Meningioma   A hard, usually vascular tumor that occurs mainly along meningeal vessels and the superior longitudinal sinus.

Meningitis Inflammation of the meninges caused by bacteria or virus.

Meningocele Hernial protrusion of the meninges through a defect of the skull or vertebral column.

Meningomyelocele Protrusion of the spinal cord and meninges through a defect of the vertebral column, as is commonly associated with spina bifida.

Metabolic Pertaining to the normal physiologic function of the body.

Metastasis The spread of cancer cells.

Miliary Tuberculosis Type of tuberculosis caused by hematogenous spread of the disease, with a characteristic appearance similar to millet seeds, which are small, white grains.

Milk of Calcium A semiliquid sludge seen radiographically in the gallbladder; it results from the settling of bile caused by an obstruction at the neck of the gallbladder.

Miller-Abbott Tube A double-lumen intestinal tube with an inflatable balloon at the distal end, used in the treatment of bowel obstructions.

Monteggia Fracture A fracture in the proximal third of the ulnar shaft with dislocation of the radius.

Morbidity Rate The incidence of illness in the population sufficient to interfere with an individual's normal daily routine.

Morphology The form and structure of disease.

Mortality Rate The number of deaths from a particular disease averaged over a population.

Multiple Myeloma A malignant neoplasm of plasma cells characterized by skeletal destruction, pathologic fractures, and bone pain.

Multiple Sclerosis A chronic, slowly progressive disease of the central nervous system, characterized by demyelination of the nerve sheath.

Mycoplasma Pneumonia The most common form of primary atypical pneumonia, occurring most frequently in young adults.

Myelocele Protrusion of the spinal cord through the normally closed bony neural arch of the spine.

Mycobacterium avium A type of tubercle bacillis that may cause tuberculosis; rare in humans, but most common in chickens and swine.

Necrosis Tissue death.

Neoplastic Pertaining to new, abnormal tissue growth.

Nephroblastoma (Wilms' Tumor) A rapidly developing malignancy of the kidneys, usually affecting children before age 5.

Nephrocalcinosis A condition characterized by precipitation of calcium in the tubules of the kidney, resulting in renal deficiency.

Nephroptosis Prolapse of a kidney.

Nephrosclerosis Intimal thickening of predominantly the small vessels of the kidney as a result of reduced blood flow through arteriosclerotic renal vasculature.

Nephrostomy Tube A tube inserted through the abdominal wall into the renal pelvis to drain urine.

Neurofibroma A tumor of peripheral nerves caused by abnormal proliferation of Schwann cells.

Neurogenic Bladder   A bladder dysfunction caused by interference with the nerve impulses concerned with urination.

Nidus   An area of sclerosis with a radiolucent center associated with an osteoid osteoma.

Noncommunicating (Internal) Hydrocephalus   Type of hydrocephalus in which obstruction occurs congenitally, from tumor growth, trauma, and inflammation; interferes or blocks normal CSF circulation.

Non-Hodgkin's Lymphoma   A malignancy of the lymphoid cells found in the lymph nodes, bone marrow, spleen, liver, and gastrointestinal system.

Nonunion   Complication of a fracture when healing does not occur and fragments do not join.

Nosocomial   Refers to diseases acquired in or from a health care environment.

Occult Fracture   A fracture that gives clinical signs of its presence without radiologic evidence; follow-up within 10 days reveals bone resorption or displacement at the fracture site.

Oligodendroglioma   A glioma, it is a slow-growing astrocytic tumor that is usually relatively benign.

Oligohydramnios   The presence of too little (less than 300 ml) amniotic fluid at term, generally associated with renal disorders in the fetus.

Osteoarthritis   Noninflammatory degenerative joint disease occurring mainly in older persons, producing gradual deterioration of the joint cartilage.

Osteoblasts   The bone-forming cells responsible for bone growth, ossification, and regeneration.

Osteochondroma   A benign tumor of adult bone capped by cartilage.

Osteoclastoma   A tumor that is usually benign and characterized by osteolytic areas, most commonly found around the knee and wrist of young adults comprised of numerous, multinucleated osteoclasts; also called giant cell tumor.

Osteoclasts   Cells which are associated with absorption and removal of bone.

Osteogenesis Imperfecta   A congenital disease in which the bones are abnormally brittle and subject to fractures.

Osteoid Osteoma   A benign tumor of bonelike structure developing on a bone and sometimes other structures.

Osteomalacia   A condition marked by softening of the bones, caused by lack of calcium in the tissues and a failure of bone tissue to calcify.

Osteomyelitis   Infection of bone, most often caused by staphylococcus, which may localize or spread to the bone to involve the marrow and other bone tissues.

Osteopenia   A softening of bone demonstrated radiographically as a decreased bone density such as in the case of osteoporosis or osteomalacia.

Osteopetrosis   A hereditary disease characterized by abnormally dense bone, likely as a result of faulty bone resorption.

Osteophytes   An osseous outgrowth (spur).

Osteoporosis   Metabolic bone disorder resulting in demineralization of bone, most commonly seen in women past menopause.

Osteosarcoma   A primary malignancy of bone usually arising in the metaphysis, most commonly around the knee.

Paget's Disease   A metabolic disorder of unknown etiology, most common in the elderly, characterized by an early, osteolytic stage and a late, osteoblastic stage.

Pancreatitis   Acute or chronic, asymptomatic or symptomatic, inflammation of the pancreas caused by autodigestion by pancreatic enzymes.

Paraesophageal Hiatal Hernia   A hiatal hernia in which the stomach or adjacent structures herniate above the diaphragm, while the gastroesophageal junction remains below the diaphragm.

Paralytic Ileus   A failure of bowel peristalsis, often seen following abdominal surgery, that may result in bowel obstruction.

Patent Ductus Arteriosis   Abnormal persistence of an open ductus arteriosis after birth, resulting in recirculation of arterial blood through the lungs.

Pathologic Fracture   A fracture which occurs in abnormal bone weakened by a disease process.

Pathology   The study of structural and functional manifestations of disease.

Palliative   Treatment designed to relieve pain without the goal of curing the disease.

Peau d'Orange Appearance   Appearance of multiple small depressions on the skin surface as a result of hair follicles becoming visible from skin edema, as might occur with breast cancer.

Pedunculated Polyp   A polyp attached to the bowel wall by a narrow stalk.

Pelvic Inflammatory Disease (PID)   A bacterial infection of the female genital system, most often caused by bacteria.

Penetrating Fracture   A type of incomplete fracture resulting from penetration by a sharp object, frequently with comminution at the site of injury.

Peptic Ulcer   Ulceration of the mucous membrane of the esophagus, stomach, or duodenum.

Percutaneous Transluminal Angioplasty (PTA)   Use of a specialized catheter, typically equipped with an inflatable balloon, to perform vessel repair from within the artery or vein during angiography.

Permanent Catheterization   Interventional angiography procedure in which a catheter is placed in the subclavian or jugular vein and tunneled under the skin to allow for improved dialysis access.

Pessary   A device inserted into the vagina to provide proper support to a uterus that lacks proper support.

Phlebitis   Inflammation of a vein, often associated with venous thrombosis.

Placenta Accreta   An abnormal adhesion of the placenta to the uterine wall.

Placenta Previa   The condition in which the placenta develops in the lower half of the uterus, encroaching or on, and completely or partially covering, the internal cervical os.

Plate-like Atelectasis   Radiographic appearance seen in atelectasis in which one or more linear opacities are seen, usually at the lung bases and parallel to the diaphragm.

Pleural Effusion   A collection of excess fluid in the pleural cavity.

Pleurisy   Inflammation of the pleura with exudation into the pleural cavity and on its surface.

Pneumatocele   A thin-walled, air-containing cyst that is a characteristic radiographic lesion seen in staphylococcal pneumonia.

Pneumococcal Pneumonia   The most common bacterial pneumonia, generally affecting an entire lobe of a lung.

Pneumoconioses   A group of occupational diseases characterized by permanent deposits of particulate matter in the lungs and by resultant pulmonary fibrosis.

Pneumocystitis carinii **Pneumonia**   Life-threatening infection of the lungs most commonly associated with AIDS.

Pneumonia   The most frequent type of lung infection, resulting in an inflammation of the lung with compromised pulmonary function.

Pneumoperitoneum   The presence of air or gas in the peritoneal cavity.

Pneumothorax   An accumulation of free air or gas in the pleural space that compresses the lung tissue.

Polycystic Kidney Disease   A familial kidney disorder in which innumerable tiny cysts that are present congenitally gradually enlarge during aging to compress and eventually destroy normal tissues.

Polycystic Ovaries   Ovaries that contain multiple small cysts.

Polydactyly   The presence of more than five digits.

Polyhydramnios   An excess of amniotic fluid; it may be associated with anencephaly or gastro-intestinal disturbances in the fetus.

Polyp   A small mass of tissue arising from mucous membrane to project inward into the lumen of the bowel.

Pott's Fracture   A fracture of the lower part of the fibula involving both malleoli with dislocation of the ankle joint.

Prevalence   A statistical measure that refers to the number of cases of a disease found in a given population.

Prognosis   The prediction of course and outcome for a given disease.

Provisional Callus   An early indication of fracture healing, mainly composed of cartilage that begins to form approximately 1 week after a fracture.

Pseudocyst   An abnormal or displaced space resembling a cyst.

Pseudopneumothorax   A radiographic artifact produced by a wrinkle in the skin that mimics a pneumothorax.

Pseudopolyps   Islands of unaffected mucosa that are visible when surrounded by the affected mucosa of ulcerative colitis.

Pulsion Diverticulum   A diverticulum created by herniation of the mucous membrane through the muscular coat of the esophagus as a result of pressure from within.

Punctate   Pinpoint punctures or depressions; commonly used in reference to the appearance of a type of hemorrhaging.

Pyelonephritis   Bacterial infection of the kidney and its pelvis.

Pyogenic Arthritis   Joint inflammation that occurs secondary to other infections.

Pyuria   The presence of pus in the urine created by its drainage from renal abscesses into the kidney's collecting tubules.

Rales   An abnormal sound heard on auscultation of the chest.

Recessive   In relation to hereditary disease, refers to a disease transmitted by both parents to an offspring.

Reed-Sternberg Cells   A specific cell type that helps differentiate Hodgkin's lymphomas from other types of lymphatic disease.

Reflux Esophagitis   The backward flow of gastric acids into the esophagus.

Regeneration   Process in which damaged tissues are replaced by new tissues that are essentially identical to those replaced.

Regional Enteritis   A chronic granulomatous inflammatory disease of unknown etiology involving any part of the gastrointestinal tract, but commonly involving the terminal ileum.

Renal Agenesis   The absence of the kidney on one side, with an unusually large kidney on the other side.

Renal Colic   Severe, agonizing pain that refers along the course of a ureter toward the genital and loin regions in response to the movement of a renal calculus.

Renal Failure   The end result of a chronic process that gradually results in lost kidney function.

Reticuloendothelial System   Specialized cells found in the liver, bone marrow, and spleen, whose function is phagocytosis.

Rheumatoid Arthritis   A chronic, systemic disease primarily of joints, characterized by an overgrowth of synovial tissues and articular structures, and progressive destruction of cartilage, bone, and supporting structures.

Rh Factor   Blood factor first discovered in the blood of the rhesus monkey; contained by approximately 85% of the population who are said to be "Rh positive."

Rickets   Osteomalacia that occurs before growth-plate closure, caused by deficiency of vitamin D, especially in infants and children.

Right Ventricular Failure   Congestive heart failure that results when the right ventricle cannot pump as much blood as it receives from the right atrium, slowing venous blood flow.

Saccular Aneurysm   A localized sac affecting only a part of the circumference of an arterial wall.

Sail sign   Radiographic appearance of an enlarged thymus in an infant, so described because of its characteristic sail-like appearance.

Sarcoma   A type of tumor, often highly malignant, composed of a substance like embryonic connective tissue.

Schatzki's Ring   A ring or web of mucosa that protrudes into the lumen of the esophagus, thought to develop as a defense mechanism against gastric reflux.

Scoliosis   Abnormal lateral curvature of the spine.

Seminoma   A malignant neoplasm of the testis, usually occurring in males between the ages of 30 and 40 years.

Sequestrum   A piece of dead, devascularized bone that separates from living bone during the process of necrosis.

Sessile Polyp   A polyp with a wide base attached directly to the bowel wall.

Shunt   An artificial passageway used to drain excess fluids (e.g., from the ventricles into the internal jugular vein, the heart, or the peritoneum in the case of excess CSF).

Sign   An objective manifestation of disease perceptible to the managing physician, as opposed to subjective symptoms perceived by the patient.

Silicosis   Pneumoconiosis caused by inhalation of silica dust, as is common among miners, grinders, and sand blasters.

Sinoatrial (SA) Node   The heart's "pacemaker," this is a bundle of nerve fibers located in the upper portion of the right atrium near the superior vena cava. From this node, an electrical current is transmitted through the myocardium, resulting in a heartbeat.

Sinusitis   Inflammation of a sinus, which may be purulent or nonpurulent, acute or chronic.

Situs Inversus   Complete reversal of the viscera of the thorax and abdomen.

Sliding Hiatal Hernia   A hiatal hernia in which a portion of the stomach and gastroesophageal junction are both situated above the diaphragm.

Somatic Cells   Those body cells other than the germ cells of the egg in the female and spermatozoa in the male.

Spermatocele   A cystic dilatation of the epididymis

Spina Bifida   A developmental anomaly characterized by incomplete closure of the vertebral canal, through which the choriomeninges may or may not protrude.

Spiral (Oblique) Fracture   A fracture in which the bone has been twisted apart, usually resulting from a rotary-type injury.

Spondylolisthesis   Forward displacement of one vertebra over another (commonly occurring at the L5-S1 junction), usually caused by a developmental defect in the pars interarticularis.

Spondylolysis   A condition marked by a cleft or breaking down of the body of a vertebra between the superior and inferior articular processes.

Staghorn Calculus   A large renal calculus that assumes the shape of the pelvicalyceal junction, resembling the horn of a stag.

Staphylococcal Pneumonia   Pneumonia caused by infection with *Staphylococcus* that localizes in and/or around the bronchi.

Stent   A specialized device placed to provide patency, usually in a vessel or duct.

Strangulated Hernia   Herniation in which the bowel loop passes through a constriction tight enough to cut off its blood supply, leading to necrosis of that portion of the bowel without prompt surgical intervention.

Strangulation   A constriction that cuts off blood supply.

Stress Echocardiography   Echocardiography combines an exercise test with an echocardiogram to check the heart's contraction ability and its pumping efficiency; in patients where exercise is not possible, certain drugs may be given to create the effect of exercise on the heart.

Stress Fracture   A fracture that occurs at a site of maximal strain on a bone, usually connected with some unaccustomed activity (also known as march, stress, or insufficiency fractures).

Subarachnoid Hematoma   A hematoma that accumulates between the brain's arachnoid layer and its pia mater.

Subcutaneous Emphysema   The presence of air or gas in the subcutaneous tissues of the body.

Subdural Hematoma   A hematoma positioned between the dura mater and the arachnoid meningeal layer.

Subluxation   An incomplete or partial dislocation.

Subtractive Pathology   A radiographic term used to describe diseases that are easier than normal to penetrate.

Supernumerary Kidney   A relatively rare anomaly consisting of the presence of a third, small rudimentary kidney.

Surgical Jaundice   Jaundice that occurs as a result of biliary system blockage, which prevents bile from entering the duodenum.

Swan-Ganz Catheter   Specialized, multilumen catheter inserted usually via the subclavian vein for positioning outside the pulmonary artery for purposes of evaluating cardiac function.

Sylvian Triangle   An anatomic landmark in cerebral angiography, created by the middle cerebral artery and its branches.

Symptom   Any subjective evidence of a disease as perceived by a patient.

Syndactyly   A webbing or fusion of digits.

Syndrome   A group of signs and symptoms that occur together and characterize a specific abnormal disturbance.

Systole   The phase of the heart cycle in which the myocardium is contracting.

Tendinitis   Inflammation of a tendon.

Tenosynovitis   Inflammation of a tendon and its sheath.

Tension Pneumothorax   A pneumothorax in which air enters the pleural space but cannot leave because the tissues surrounding the opening into the pleural cavity act as valves; it results in a complete lung collapse and a mediastinal shift to the opposite side of the pneumothorax.

Teratoma   A neoplasm comprised of different types of tissue, none of which is native to the area where it occurs, commonly found in the ovary or testis.

Tetrology of Fallot   A combination of four congenital cardiac defects: pulmonary stenosis, ventricular central defect, overriding aorta, and hypertrophy of the right ventricle.

Thrombocytes   Platelets.

Thrombolysis   An interventional angiography procedure where urokinase, a high-intensity anticoagulant, is dripped over a period of hours directly onto a clot to dissolve it.

Thrombophlebitis   The presence of inflammation and blood clots within a vein.

Thrombus   A blood clot that obstructs a blood vessel.

TNM System   A recognized, standard system for clinical classification of cancer.

Torus Fracture   A fracture in which the cortex folds back upon itself, with little or no displacement of the lower end of the bone.

Toxic Megacolon   An acute dilatation of the colon from paralytic ileus, particularly susceptible to rupture.

Toxoplasma gondii   Intracellular parasites of sporozoa origin that affect tissue and organs of mammals and birds.

Trabecula   The spongy substance found within a bone; it gives a characteristic appearance to bony detail.

Traction Diverticulum   A localized bulging of the full thickness of the esophageal wall, caused by adhesions from an external lesion.

Transesophageal Echocardiography (TEE)   A newer type of echocardiography procedure in which the patient swallows a mobile, flexible probe. The heart's structure can then be readily visualized without having structures such as the skin, rib cage, and chest muscles interfere.

Transjugular Intrahepatic Portosystemic Stent (TIPS)   An interventional angiography procedure in which a catheter is used to connect the jugular vein to the portal vein to reduce the flow of blood through a diseased liver.

Transient Ischemic Attack (TIA)   A temporary episode of neurologic dysfunction that can precede a cerebrovascular accident.

Transitional Vertebra   A vertebra that assumes the characteristics of the vertebrae on each side of a major spine division.

Transposition   Displacement of a viscus to the opposite side.

Transposition of Great Vessels   Congenital malformation of the cardiovascular system in which the aorta arises from the right ventricle and the pulmonary artery from the left ventricle.

Transverse Fracture   A type of complete, noncomminuted fracture that occurs at right angles to the axis of the bone.

Traumatic   Pertaining to the effects of a wound or injury, whether physical or psychic.

Tripod Fracture   A fracture of the zygoma at its three sutures: frontal, temporal, and maxillary.

Tuberculosis   Any of the infectious diseases of man and animals caused by *Mycobacterium tuberculosis*, generally affecting the lungs in the human body.

Ulcerative Colitis   A chronic, recurrent ulceration of the colon mucosa of unknown etiology.

Unicornuate Uterus   A uterus whose uterine cavity is elongated and has a single uterine tube emerging from it.

Uremia   The retention of urea in the blood, as characteristic of renal failure.

Ureteral Stent   A tube used to maintain patency of the ureter with the proximal end placed in the renal pelvis and the distal end placed in the urinary bladder.

Ureterocele   Cystlike dilatation of the terminal portion of the ureter as a result of stenosis of the ureteral meatus.

Urethral Valves   Congenital presence of mucosal folds that protrude into the posterior urethra, which may cause significant obstruction to urine flow.

Urinary Tract Infection (UTI)   The most common of all bacterial infections, a UTI is an infection in the urinary tract usually caused by a gram-negative bacillus that invades by an ascending route through the urethra to the bladder to the kidney.

Uterus Didelphys   Complete duplication of the uterus, cervix, and vagina.

Vena Cava Filter   A specialized basket placed in the inferior vena cava during interventional angiography to catch clots before they enter the heart.

Venous Thrombosis   The formation of blood clots within a vein.

Ventricular Pacing Electrodes   Either temporary or permanent, they provide electrical pacing of the heart in situations in which the normal electrical system of the heart is misfiring.

Vesicoureteral Reflux   The backward flow of urine out of the bladder and into the ureters.

Viral Pneumonia   Pneumonia caused by a virus, spread by an infected person to a nonimmune individual.

Virulence   The ease with which an organism overcomes body defenses.

Volvulus   An intestinal obstruction caused by a twisting of the bowel about its mesenteric base.

Whiplash   Hyperextension-flexion injury of the spine.

Wound   An injury of soft body parts associated with rupture of the skin.

Zenker's Diverticulum   A pulsion diverticulum located at the pharyngoesophageal junction.

Image Credits and Courtesies

American College of Radiology, Reston, Virginia

Figs. 2-9 to 2-13, 2-17, 2-20, 2-21, 2-24A, 2-26, 2-32, 2-34 to 2-38, 2-42, 2-43, 2-46, 2-47, 2-49 to 2-51, 3-5, 3-8, 3-10 to 3-12, 3-27, 3-31, 3-32, 3-34, 3-36A, 3-38, 3-40, 3-42, 3-43, 3-48, 3-50, 4-25, 4-26, 4-28 to 4-40, 4-42, 4-43, 4-46, 4-47, 4-49, 4-51 to 4-54, 4-56 to 4-59, 4-61, 4-63 to 4-65, 4-67, 5-24, 6-11, 6-13, 6-34, 6-36, 6-38, 6-43, 6-48, 6-60, 6-61, 7-14, 8-2, 8-3, 8-6, 8-7, 8-38, 8-41, 9-4, 9-5, 10-7 to 10-11, 10-23, 11-4, 11-5, 11-8, 11-26, 11-32, 11-41, 11-43, 11-44, 11-50, 11-61, 11-62, 11-64 to 11-66, 11-69 to 11-71, 11-75

American College of Surgeons Committee on Trauma, Chicago, Illinois

Fig. 11-1

Bontrager KL: *Textbook of Radiographic Positioning and Related Anatomy,* ed 5, St Louis, 2001, Mosby.

Figs. 2-1 to 2-4, 3-1, 4-1 to 4-8, 5-1, 5-2, 6-1 to 6-4, 6-47, 7-1, 7-3, 7-24, 7-25, 8-1, 8-5, 10-1 to 10-6

Children's Hospital, Columbus, Ohio

Figs. 8-32, 8-34, 8-36, 10-24 to 10-26

Crowley LV: *Introductory Concepts in Pathology,* Chicago, 1972, Mosby.

Fig. 1-2

Damjanov: *Anderson's Pathology,* vol 2, ed 10, St Louis, 1996, Mosby.

Figs. 10-22 and 11-14

The James Cancer Hospital and Solove Research Institute, Columbus, Ohio

Figs. 7-16 and 7-17

McCance, KL, Huether SE: *Pathophysiology: the Biologic Basis for Disease in Adults and Children,* ed 4, St. Louis, 2002, Mosby.

Figs. 4-6, 8-27, 8-29, 8-30, 8-31, 8-33, 8-35, 8-37, 8-42, 8-49, 11-12, 11-25, 11-29

Ohio State University Medical Center, Columbus, Ohio

Figs. 2-7, 2-8, 2-14, 2-22, 2-23, 2-24B, 2-25, 2-27, 2-28, 2-30, 2-31, 2-33, 2-40, 2-41, 2-52, 2-53, 3-2, 3-3, 3-6, 3-9, 3-13, 3-15 to 3-24, 3-26, 3-28 to 3-30, 3-33, 3-35, 3-36B, 3-39B, 3-41, 3-44 to 3-47, 3-49, 3-51 to 3-53, 4-9, 4-10, 4-14, 4-15, 4-18 to 4-20, 4-27B, 4-41, 4-60, 5-4, 5-6 to 5-8, 5-11, 5-15, 5-16, 5-18, 5-19, 5-22, 6-5 to 6-9, 6-12, 6-14 to 6-17, 6-19, 6-21 to 6-23, 6-25, 6-31, 6-32, 6-37, 6-39, 6-40, 6-42, 6-44, 6-46, 6-49, 6-51 to 6-53, 6-63, 6-64, 7-11, 7-18, 8-8, 8-15 to 8-17, 8-39, 8-43, 8-46, 8-52 to 8-55, 9-1, 9-3, 9-6 to 9-9, 10-12, 10-14 to 10-21, 10-27, 10-30, 10-32, 10-34, 10-35, 11-2, 11-3, 11-6, 11-7, 11-18, 11-20 to 11-24, 11-30, 11-31, 11-33 to 11-35, 11-37, 11-38, 11-51, 11-53 to 11-55, 11-57 to 11-60, 11-63, 11-67, 11-74

Riverside Methodist Hospitals, Columbus, Ohio

2-5, 2-6, 2-15, 2-16, 2-18, 2-19, 2-24A, 2-29, 2-39, 2-44, 2-45, 2-48, 3-4, 3-7, 3-14, 3-25, 3-37, 3-39A, 3-54, 4-11 to 4-13, 4-16, 4-17, 4-21 to 4-24, 4-27A, 4-44, 4-45, 4-48, 4-50,

4-55, 4-62, 4-68, 5-3, 5-5, 5-9, 5-10, 5-12 to 5-14, 5-17, 5-20, 5-21, 5-23, 5-25, 5-26, 6-10, 6-18, 6-20, 6-24, 6-26 to 6-30, 6-33, 6-35, 6-41, 6-45, 6-50, 6-54, 6-55 to 6-58, 6-62, 7-2, 7-4 to 7-10, 7-12, 7-13, 7-15, 7-19 to 7-23, 7-26 to 7-35, 8-4, 8-9 to 8-14, 8-18 to 8-26, 8-28, 8-40, 8-44, 8-45, 8-47, 8-48, 8-50, 8-51, 8-56, 8-57, 9-2, 10-13, 10-28, 10-29, 10-31, 10-33, 10-36 to 10-53, 11-9 to 11-11, 11-13, 11-15 to 11-17, 11-19, 11-25, 11-28, 11-36, 11-39, 11-40, 11-42, 11-45 to 11-49, 11-52, 11-56, 11-68, 11-72, 11-73

Rudy EB: Advanced neurological and neurosurgical nursing, St. Louis, 1984, Mosby
Fig. 11-12

Bibliography

American Academy of Pediatrics: Diagnostic imaging of child abuse, *Pediatrics*, 105(6), 2000.

American College of Radiology: *Index for radiological diagnoses*, ed 3, Reston, Virginia, 1986, The American College of Radiology.

American College of Surgeons Trauma Committee: *Injury prevention saves lives*, Chicago, 2000, American College of Surgeons.

American Joint Committee on Cancer: *Manual for staging of cancer*, ed 3, New York, 1988, JB Lippincott.

Atlas SW: *Magnetic resonance imaging of the brain and spine*, New York, 1991, Raven Press.

Benson R, Peronll M: *Handbook of obstetrics and gynecology*, New York, 1994, McGraw-Hill.

Black R: *Rose and Black's clinical problems in nephrology*, Boston, 1996, Little, Brown and Co.

Bontrager KL: *Textbook of radiographic positioning and related anatomy*, ed 3, St Louis, 1993, Mosby.

Bradley W, Brant-Zawadzki M: *The Raven MRI teaching*, Vols. I-III, New York, 1991, Raven Press.

Braunwald E: *Heart disease*, ed 5, Philadelphia, 1997, WB Saunders.

Brenner BM: *Brenner and Rector's the kidney*, ed 5, Vols 1 and 2, Philadelphia, 1996, WB Saunders.

Bullock B: *Pathophysiology: adaptations and alterations in function*, ed 4, Philadelphia, 1996, Lippincott-Raven.

Cawson RA: *Pathology: the mechanisms of disease*, ed 2, St Louis, 1989, Mosby.

Centers for Disease Control and Prevention: *National Hospital Ambulatory Medical Care Survey 2000, Advance Data No. 326.31.* Hyattsville, Maryland, 2001, U.S. Department of Health and Human Services.

Centers for Disease Control and Prevention: *National Vital Statistics Reports*, Vol. 49, No. 3, Hyattsville, Maryland, 2001, U.S. Department of Health and Human Services.

Centers for Disease Control and Prevention: *National Vital Statistics Reports*, Vol. 48, No. 11, Hyattsville, Maryland, 2000, U.S. Department of Health and Human Services.

Centers for Disease Control and Prevention: *Trends in causes of death among the elderly*, Hyattsville, Maryland, 2001, U.S. Department of Health and Human Services.

Chey WY: Functional disorders of the digestive tract, New York, 1983, Raven Press.

Chopra S, May R: *Pathophysiology of gastrointestinal diseases*, Boston, 1989, Little, Brown and Co.

Crowley LV: *Introductory concepts in pathology*, Chicago, 1972, Mosby.

Crowley LV: *Introduction to human disease*, ed 4, Boston, 1997, Bartlett.

Dalen J: The pulmonary artery catheter – friend, foe, or accomplice? *JAMA*, 286(3), 2001.

Gitnick G: *Gastroenterology*, New York, 1983, John Wiley & Sons.

Gore RM, Levine MS: *Textbook of gastrointestinal radiology*, Philadelphia, 1996, WB Saunders.

Greenberger N: *Gastrointestinal disorders: a pathophysiologic approach,* ed 3, Chicago, 1986, Mosby.

Hatfield P, Wise R: Radiology of the gallbladder and bile ducts, In *Golden's diagnostic radiology,* Baltimore, 1976, Williams and Wilkins.

Heptinstall R: *Pathology of the kidney,* ed 3, Volumes I-III, Boston, 1983, Little, Brown and Co.

Hinshaw HC, Murray J: *Diseases of the chest,* ed 4, Philadelphia, 1980, WB Saunders.

Hurst JW: *Current therapy in cardiovascular disease,* Vols 1 and 2, Philadelphia, 1991, BC Decker, Inc.

Jacobson HR, Striker GE, Klahr S: *The principles and practice of nephrology,* St Louis, 1995, Mosby.

Jaffe R, Pierson R, Abramowicz J: *Imaging in infertility and reproductive endocrinology,* Philadelphia, 1994, J.B. Lippincott.

Jariwalla G, Fry J: *Respiratory diseases,* Lancashire, UK, 1985, MTP Press Limited.

Lapides J: *Fundamentals of urology,* Philadelphia, 1976, WB Saunders.

Lieberman J: *Inherited diseases of the lung,* Philadelphia, 1988, WB Saunders.

Latchaw R: *MR and CT imaging of the head, neck, and spine,* vols 1 and 2, St Louis, 1991, Mosby.

Levine D: *Care of the renal patient,* ed 2, Philadelphia, 1991, WB Saunders.

Maier R: Evaluation of abdominal trauma, Chicago, 2000, American College of Surgeons Trauma Committee,

Marcove A, Ralph C, Arlen M: *Atlas of bone pathology with clinical and radiographic correlations (based on Henry L. Jaffe's course),* Philadelphia, 1992, JB Lippincott.

Margulis A, Burhenne I: *Alimentary tract radiology,* ed 4, Vols 1 and 2, Philadelphia, 1994, WB Saunders.

Mellors RC: Congenital and hereditary bone disorders, New York, 1999, Weill Medical College of Cornell University.

Merck manual of diagnosis and therapy, ed 17, Whitehouse Station, New Jersey, 1999, Merck & Co., Inc.

Mulvihill M: *Human diseases: a systemic approach,* ed 3, East Norwalk, Connecticut, 1991, Appleton and Lange.

National Center for Health Statistics, *Health: U.S.,* Hyattsville, Maryland, 2001, Public Health Service.

National data archive on child abuse and neglect: Ithaca, New York, 2003, College of Human Ecology, Cornell University.

Norris H: *Pathology of the colon, small intestine, and anus,* ed 2, New York, 1991, Churchill Livingstone.

Nursing Standard: Central venous lines quick reference guide 6, *Nursing Standard,* 13(42), 1999.

Overwalder PJ: Intra aortic balloon pump counterpulsation, *The Internet Journal of Thoracic and Cardiovascular Surgery,* 2(2), 1999.

Payman S, Cox AJ, Ostendorf R: *Influence of airbags and restraining devices on the pattern of facial fractures in motor vehicle accidents,* Birmingham, Alabama, 2001, University of Alabama.

Pomeranz S: *Craniospinal MRI,* Philadelphia, 1991, WB Saunders.

Purtilo D, Purtilo R: *A survey of human diseases,* ed 2, Boston, 1989, Little, Brown, and Co.

Robbins SL, Cotran RS, Kumar V: *Pathologic basis of disease,* ed 5, Philadelphia, 1994, WB Saunders.

Saul T: *Management of head injury,* Chicago, 1998, American College of Surgeons Trauma Committee in conjunction with the Joint Section on Neurotrauma and Critical Care of the American Association of Neuroligical Surgeons and Congress of Neurological Surgeons.

Scheld WM, Whitley RJ, Durack D: *Infections of the central nervous system,* New York, 1991, Raven Press.

Sheldon H: *Boyd's introduction to the study of disease,* ed 11, Philadelphia, 1992, Lea & Febiger.

Sherlock S: *Diseases of the liver and biliary system,* ed 8, Boston, 1989, Blackwell Scientific Publications.

Silver M: *Cardiovascular pathology,* New York, 1991, Churchill Livingstone.

Sleisenger M, Fordtran J: *Gastrointestinal disease: pathophysiology, diagnosis, management,* ed 3, vols I and II, Philadelphia, 1983, WB Saunders.

Snively WD, Beshear D: *Textbook of pathophysiology,* Philadelphia, 1972, JB Lippincott.

Sutton D: *A textbook of radiology and imaging,* ed 4, London, 1987, Churchill-Livingstone.

Swash M, Kennard C: *Scientific basis of clinical neurology,* New York, 1985, Churchill Livingstone.

Taussig MJ: *Processes in pathology,* Oxford, 1979, Blackwell Scientific Publications.

Tattersfield AE, McNicol M: *Respiratory disease,* New York, 1987, Springer-Verlag.

Wallach E, Zacur H: *Reproductive medicine and surgery,* St Louis, 1995, Mosby.

Walton J: *Brain's diseases of the nervous system,* ed 9, New York, 1985, Oxford University Press.

Wilson R, Alexander J: *Management of trauma-pitfalls and practice,* ed 2, Baltimore, 1996, Williams and Wilkins.

Yochum TR, Rowe LJ: *Essentials of skeletal radiology,* ed 2, Vols. 1 and 2, Baltimore, 1996, Williams and Wilkins.

Zuger J: *Positron emision tomography in lung imaging, PCCU Lesson 15,* Vol. 13, Northbrook, Illinois, 1999, American College of Chest Physicians.

Index